INPATIENT CARE
FOR THE
PSYCHOTIC CHILD

THE LANGLEY PORTER

CHILD PSYCHIATRY SERIES

INPATIENT CARE FOR THE PSYCHOTIC CHILD

Edited by
S. A. Szurek, M.D., I. N. Berlin, M.D.,
and Maleta J. Boatman, M.D.

The Langley Porter Child Psychiatry Series
Clinical Approaches to Problems of Childhood
Volume 5

SCIENCE AND BEHAVIOR BOOKS, INC.
Palo Alto, California

INPATIENT CARE FOR THE PSYCHOTIC CHILD

Library of Congress Card Catalog Number: 78-88175

ISBN: 0-8314-0024-2

PREFACE

This volume, like the ones that preceded it, results from the encouragement we have received from our own students and graduates to make available to them our papers, published and unpublished, past and present, and from the continuing demand from others in the field for reprints no longer available or journals no longer in existence. It is our hope that these materials will be of use to all professional persons concerned with children and their clinical problems.

We should like to take this opportunity to thank Helen L. Casey, Margaret M. Forcade, Carol H. Heald, and Mary J. Polf for their considerable help in the preliminary preparation of the manuscripts. We wish particularly to acknowledge the excellent help and the great effort of Mrs. Linda A. Hinrichs in the final work of preparing the manuscripts.

We also wish to express our appreciation to friends and colleagues who contributed to the Child Psychiatry Fund of the University of California San Francisco Medical Center and thus helped to make publication of this series possible.

FOREWORD

This volume on the development of inpatient care for severely disturbed children presents in logical sequence the evolution of the various aspects of comprehensive child psychiatric residential treatment over a period of more than twenty years at the Langley Porter Children's Services, under the direction of Dr. S. A. Szurek.

Chapter 1, which presents a revision of the Report of the Committee on Treatment to the 1956 Conference on Inpatient Psychiatric Treatment for Children, serves as an excellent background for fully appreciating the value of clearly defining and adhering to a basic philosophy in setting goals and in establishing treatment methods for severely emotionally disabled children. Dr. Szurek and his staff have been eminently successful in developing their program within the conceptual framework that serious emotional disorders in children are rooted predominantly in early parent-child interactions and therefore require the collaborative treatment of the child and his parents as well as well-coordinated, therapeutic daily living experiences for the child in relation to mature adults. This persistent theme is prominent as the program unfolds and is shaped in response to certain realities such as the administrative structure of the ward; the changing psychodynamics and behavior of the patients and the gradual formation of some group interaction; the vicissitudes of staff changes; the development of training programs; the elaboration of treatment methods; and the integration of additional personnel.

In Dr. Szurek's view of the therapeutic process, specifically his fascinating parallel in the process of identification by incorporation and imitation as it occurs in the treatment of the very disturbed child, in the candidate in training analysis, and in normal child development, there are important implications for the further refinement of treatment and educational methods.

An excellent presentation dealing with the intake process and the selection and preparation of patients and their families clearly describes how the parents' active participation is of crucial importance at the very beginning of the diagnostic and therapeutic process. This contribution is equally pertinent to all child psychiatric work, whether on an inpatient, outpatient, or day care basis. In addition, two papers on staff and family interactions, which emphasize family contacts with nurses, point up the specific ways in which ongoing parental involvement throughout child inpatient care enhances the treatment of both the child and his parents.

In this hospital setting, the therapeutic milieu centers around the nursing staff. The key position of the nurse as a member of the therapeutic team is highlighted by the fact that ten of the nineteen papers are concerned with the therapeutic milieu and the specific functions and attitudes of child care personnel, especially the nursing staff. The presentation on education is especially important for its emphasis on the flexibility required of the teacher of emotionally disturbed children, the need for good communication with other staff, and the necessity for teachers and nurses to collaborate closely without losing professional identity.

The development of a truly therapeutic milieu as a major component of child psychiatric inpatient treatment is an intense, challenging process, which is often more frustrating than rewarding; but by sound planning at each step and dedication to a common goal, Dr. Szurek and his staff have had considerable success in realizing this aim.

Throughout the volume and particularly in the section on staff inter-action, the detailed descriptions of the dynamics and problems of staff relationships and of the several methods used in achieving effective collaboration add significantly to an understanding of the complexities of child psychiatric inpatient care.

This volume constitutes a greatly needed and important contribution to the field of inpatient care as well as to all the professional disciplines concerned with the development, education, and treatment of emotionally disturbed children. At the same time it serves as an outstanding example of the skillful integration of programs of treatment, training, and research.

Othilda Krug, M.D.
Professor of Child Psychiatry
Department of Psychiatry
University of Cincinnati

Director, Children's Psychiatric
Center of Cincinnati

INTRODUCTION

Hospital care for psychotic children is a relatively recent development in the young specialty of child psychiatry.

Psychotic children have long been hospitalized in state mental hospitals and hospitals for the mentally deficient. Hospital wards to assess and treat severe childhood disturbances began to open up in the early and mid-1930's, and in 1946 a number of inpatient units were opened to meet the needs of various communities. Many of these inpatient units were considered the most suitable places of treatment for children with severe neurosis, socially troublesome, impulsive behavior, psychosomatic problems, and psychotic disorders.

With the arrival of the present Director, S. A. Szurek, in 1946, the Langley Porter Children's Inpatient Service began its exploration of methods to utilize all elements of the inpatient setting to help the psychotic child as well as the impulsive, neurotic, emotionally disturbed, and organically impaired child. As the staff became more experienced in outpatient treatment of children and their parents, a strong preference developed not to hospitalize neurotic and delinquent children, both because it seemed better for them to remain in their families, and because of the space and grouping problems in the rather small, confined ward setting available. As a result, the focus of the ward program became the care of the most severely disturbed of the psychotic children.

The basic hypothesis that motivated all subsequent efforts in inpatient care was that the severe emotional disturbances of childhood were largely psychogenic in origin. The belief that the disorder had its genesis in the child's relations with the important adults in his life called for simultaneous treatment of the child and his parents. A wide variety of therapeutic and restitutive experiences of the child with the child care personnel, usually nurses and attendants, as well as with teachers, occupational therapists and recreational and other specialists in speech, dance, and music, were found to be essential in the treatment program. The child psychiatrist's direct treatment of the child in play therapy was seen as the integrating and consolidating experience for the child. One of the functions of play therapy was to make more clearly conscious to the child his motivation, which was brought to his awareness not only in the playroom with the psychiatrist but also through the integrating activities and behavior of the psychiatric nurse, teachers, and other specialists.

One feature of the program was the encouragement of parents' visits to the ward and weekend and holiday visits of the child with the family at home. A later development was the mutual exchange of experience and learning between nurses and parents regarding the child's activities and behavior on the ward and at home.

What has been learned in the inpatient setting has been translated to outpatient work. As the continued need for parental involvement with the disturbed child and its therapeutic implications and uses became clear, the trend has been to treat more and more severely disturbed children with outpatient and day care.

CONTRIBUTORS

BERLIN, I. N., M.D., Professor of Psychiatry and Head, Division of Child Psychiatry, University of Washington School of Medicine, Seattle. Formerly Associate Clinical Professor of Psychiatry, University of California School of Medicine and Coordinator of Training, Children's Service, Langley Porter Neuropsychiatric Institute, San Francisco.

BOATMAN, MALETA J., M.D., Assistant Professor of Psychiatry, University of California School of Medicine, and Assistant Director, Children's Service, Langley Porter Neuropsychiatric Institute.

CHRIST, ADOLPH E., M.D., Associate Professor of Psychiatry and Director of Child Psychiatry Inpatient Services, Albert Einstein School of Medicine, Bronx, New York. Formerly Assistant Professor of Psychiatry and Director of Psychiatric Day Care Service for Children, University of Washington School of Medicine, Seattle.

CRITCHLEY, DEANE L., R.N., M.S., Ph.D., Faculty Member, Child Psychiatric Nursing, Graduate Division, New York University; formerly, Psychiatric Nurse on Mental Retardation Training Project, Children's Service, Langley Porter Neuropsychiatric Institute.

DAVIS, MARY B., A.C.S.W., Chief Social Worker, Department of Social Work, Langley Porter Neuropsychiatric Institute.

ENG, MARIETTA C., M.S., O.T.R., formerly Occupational Therapist, Children's Ward, Langley Porter Neuropsychiatric Institute.

FORBING, SHIRLEY E., B.A., M.A., Ed.D., Assistant Professor, San Diego State College. Formerly teacher on Children's Service, Langley Porter Neuropsychiatric Institute.

GIANASCOL, A. J., M.D., most recently Professor of Child Psychiatry, University of Pennsylvania Medical School and University of Pennsylvania Postgraduate School of Education. Formerly Assistant Clinical Professor of Psychiatry, University of California School of Medicine, San Francisco. Now in private practice in Monterey, California.

HARRIS, JOANNA GEWERTZ, B.S., M.A., Ph.D. Candidate, Lecturer in Dance, Stevenson College, University of California at Santa Cruz; formerly, Volunteer Leader of Children's Creative Rhythm Movement Group, Children's Service, Langley Porter Neuropsychiatric Institute.

MEJIA, BERTA, R.N., B.S., Associate Specialist I, Children's Ward, Langley Porter Neuropsychiatric Institute.

MILNES, ESTHER OMACHI, B.A., O.T.R., M.A., formerly elementary teacher from San Francisco Unified School District, assigned to the Children's Ward, Langley Porter Neuropsychiatric Institute. Later Head Teacher, then Director and Training Supervisor, San Francisco Children's Center, Community Effort for Disturbed Children.

PARSONS, CORINNE, R.N., B.A., Superintendent of Nursing Services, Langley Porter Neuropsychiatric Institute.

PAYNTER, JANE, R.N., B.S., Supervising Psychiatric Nurse, Children's Ward, Langley Porter Neuropsychiatric Institute.

PHILIPS, IRVING, M.D., Clinical Professor of Psychiatry, University of California School of Medicine, and Coordinator of Children's Service Mental Retardation Training Program, Langley Porter Neuropsychiatric Institute.

SHEIMO, STANTON L., M.D., Clinical Associate Professor, Department of Psychiatry, University of Washington School of Medicine, Seattle; and Clinical Director, Child Study and Treatment Center, Western State Hospital, Steilacoom, Washington. Now in private practice in Tacoma, Washington.

SZUREK, S. A., M.D., Professor of Psychiatry, University of California School of Medicine, and Director, Children's Service, Langley Porter Neuropsychiatric Institute.

CONTENTS

SECTION ONE

AN OVERVIEW

INTRODUCTION

The development of a hypothesis about inpatient treatment for psychotic children is intimately related to a general view of the psychotherapy of emotional disorders and to a basic hypothesis about the genesis of the severe disorders of childhood, especially childhood psychoses. This development is traced in these papers. A brief review of more recent developments in this general field and some theoretical ideas of other authors are here and there appended, and mention is made of therapeutic results reported at dates later than the papers included here.

CHAPTER 1

SURVEY OF INPATIENT PROGRAMS FOR PSYCHOTIC CHILDREN*

S. A. Szurek, M.D.

EDITORS' NOTE

This chapter is included in order to place the development of the inpatient treatment service for preadolescent and adolescent children at Langley Porter Neuropsychiatric Institute into historical perspective. It is a summary, written in 1956, by the chairman of the commission on treatment for the conference on Psychiatric Inpatient Treatment of Children held in that year [1]. A volume outlining the findings of this conference was published in the following year. Necessarily, the reports of each of a number of commissions was edited and integrated into the book as a whole. In this process several of the separate commissions were left somewhat dissatisfied by what remained in the resulting volume of their own data.

The following summary was itself but the apex of a pyramid, the base of which was composed of individual descriptions, some of them rather detailed and lengthy, of the practices and underlying theories of nineteen treatment centers (two of them for adolescents) considered representative of those then existent in the United States. These nineteen descriptions formed the source for secondary documents on various aspects of treatment in these centers that were written by some of the members of the commission on treatment. The secondary documents in turn were the source for the chairman's summarizing report, delivered at plenary sessions of the conference, which is represented by this chapter.

---

*Unpublished paper, 1956.

This summary of the rather sizable mass of accumulated data of the commission on treatment was duplicated and distributed to all members of the conference along with similar reports of other commissions. Recorded discussions in small groups of conference members during five days of meetings further digested all these reports.

Thus, it is understandable that some discontent followed the publication of a book on the conference. From time to time subsequent to the conference, members of several commissions expressed the wish for the publication of the individual commission reports, hoping to preserve more details of their findings. For a variety of reasons this was not done. Hence, the opportunity offered by the present volume was seized to satisfy a part of the long-standing wish.

The variety of practices, auspices, and theoretical positions among the nineteen centers summarized herein forms a spectrum that is still present in this country.

In the ten or twelve years since this summary was prepared, the use of electroshock therapy with preadolescent children has almost disappeared, though drug therapy continues to be reported. Psychological forms of therapy continue, with a form known as behavioral therapy being introduced in some centers.

The institutions studied are considered to be a representative sample of those operating under psychiatric direction and primarily serving preadolescent children. Only a few institutions that maintain separate units for adolescents were included, although the field of inpatient treatment of this age group was regarded as sufficiently large and discrete to make it suitable for separate study.

GENERAL CONSIDERATIONS

Treatment in any psychiatric facility is rooted in medicine and based on biological data and principles. The fact that modifications of the behavior of the human being occur as a result of processes we call learning, or mislearning (which we term psychological events), and that such learning is profoundly influenced by experience with other persons (which we term variously as group, social, or interpersonal events), does not change the fundamental orientation of the psychiatrist as a physician, namely, that his work is concerned with a living organism. Hence, psychiatric treatment implicitly, if not always explicitly, seeks hypotheses and evidence that will span or include all those intraorganismic events that we narrowly term physiological, as well as those manifested in the behavior of the total organism and expressive of its drives in relation to others of its kind.

Therefore, with children as well as with adults, the psychiatrist studies and uses for treatment any and all influences that offer any hope of modifying disordered biological processes, with a view of promoting health and the fullest development of the genetically given potentialities of the human being. To this end the child psychiatrist always studies his patient carefully, to exclude impersonal disease, and some psychiatrists, in addition to using other methods, experimentally utilize chemical and electrical agents (somatic therapies) to modify processes that are conceived of as expressions of impersonally determined disease. Other methods can be described as falling into two broad general categories: the study or diagnosis and treatment of deficiencies in educational achievement; and, perhaps of greater importance and interest, the efforts at definition and treatment of personality disorder. In children, personality disorder manifests itself not only in signs of somatic and psychological malfunction, but especially in nondevelopment or in maldevelopment of personality—that is, in failure or distortion of that growth as persons living with and among others that somatic maturation makes possible. The child psychiatrist works collaboratively with nonmedical specialists, who integrate all their efforts toward the goal of reducing the child's disease, if any, and his disorder of somatic, psychologic, and social functioning. In terms relevant to the subject of nonsomatic treatment procedures, several different aspects can be discerned, though it may not be possible to isolate them from the operation of any unit studied. None of these aspects is altogether absent in the operations of any institution; however, considerable variation in emphasis upon one or another of them is found.

These nonsomatic treatment procedures are reducible to three basic aspects: direct or individual psychotherapy with children, some kind of work with parents or surrogate parents, and what could be called the milieu therapeutic measures—child care, group work, remedial educational efforts, activity programs, and so on. Differences among the institutions in such matters as intake, duration of inpatient treatment, termination, and what follows thereafter, are the expression of several factors, including size of plant and location. The particular historical origin of the institution for a specifically defined purpose of the community; the legal control of this function and the attendant financial subsidy; any change in the original purpose; the particular staff direction and its continuity, with its individual theoretical orientation; the growth or development in a given period in any or all of these factors, which affect not only staff-patient ratio, but also what the staff does, are all additional recognizable influences upon how a child is admitted, how long he remains, what he experiences, and what happens after he leaves.

The remainder of this report will review briefly these aspects of treatment in the following order:

1. Somatic therapies
2. Participation of parents; intake and duration of inpatient care
3. Therapeutic atmosphere or milieu
4. Direct individual psychotherapy with the child
5. The problem of treatment of adolescents

The effort here is to survey and represent the different ideas and practices in the field as well as space permits.

SOMATIC THERAPIES

Although only a minority of the institutions studied use somatic therapy, a survey of the present treatment would be quite incomplete without a review of this approach, which historically has an important place in inpatient psychiatric practice with children in this country. To quote from a report submitted to this commission:

> The philosophy underlying the use of physiological therapies is basically that behavior is the resultant of the reciprocal inter-action of biological, physiological, and environmental forces, and that improvement in any one area will eventually result in improvement in the other two. These areas imperceptibly merge. The use of physiological therapies such as drug and electroshock treatment attempts to influence directly the biological compo-nent of behavior. In general, the indications for physiological therapy are: to relieve anxiety, to control and pattern impulses, to encourage homeostatic equilibrium and relieve autonomic imbalance, to correct perceptual distortion and, if possible, stimulate maturation.
>
> It is clear that with the above philosophical concept, physio-logical therapy, i.e., the biological approach, is but one aspect of the total treatment situation. The above considerations are valid also in dealing with schizophrenia in childhood, whether the etiological framework of this condition is considered psy-chological or biological. The concept found useful at Bellevue views schizophrenia as a profound disturbance of maturation basically biological, with the retention in the organism of 'embryonic plasticity.' As has been stressed by Lauretta Bender, these patterns include a disturbance in the establishment of homeostatic, autonomic, and respiratory equilibrium, a reten-tion of motility based upon tonic neck and neck-righting

reflexes, and a doughy muscle tonus. With this basic biological concept of schizophrenia, physiologic treatment is clearly indicated.

The details of the manner in which various drugs, electroshock, and (in one surveyed institution) surgery are used and the clinical experience with these agents will not be reviewed in this summary. Only a bare summary of the drugs used for various disorders will be given.

For the diagnostic category known as childhood schizophrenia, barbiturate sedatives are now reported as being used less than the tranquilizing drugs, chlorpromazine, reserpine, azacyclonol, and mephenesin. The last two are reported as less effective than the first two. In addition to these, antihistamines (benadryl particularly), used for their action on synapses, have been reported as effective in curbing motor restlessness and agitation and in improving sleeping and eating patterns. In order to dampen the stimuli from the vestibular apparatus (its overactivity is considered as one of embryonic patterns of functioning in schizophrenia), a group of drugs, exemplified by dramamine, are also administered.

Only four of the nineteen institutions reported the use of electroshock with schizophrenic children or adolescent catatonic patients. The institution with the longest and most extensive experience reports that a series of twenty grand mal convulsions, one treatment a day for six days a week, seems to cause no anxiety in the child, and that it has immediate and long-range results. Panic states, anxiety, and anorexia are often, though not always, quickly reduced, and impulse control and patterning are improved. Anxiety may be increased after several treatments, which is considered to be the result of an organic perceptual depression and the breaking up of neurotic defense patterns, with consequent emergence of the very basic anxiety of schizophrenia itself. Immediately, too (within twenty-four to forty-eight hours), a drop in intellectual functioning (measured by nonlanguage multimental tests) and the dissolution of body image (in the Draw-A-Person test) as organic effects are found. When treatments are continued, these effects are reported to disappear rapidly. On later follow-up study, the IQ following shock is significantly greater than before shock, and the primitive body image gives way to a more integrated one, in which characteristic schizophrenic features (e.g., ego-boundary and motility problems) are less prominent.

Long-term follow-up study of over five hundred schizophrenic children treated with electroshock, compared with those who did not receive this treatment from this hospital, suggests a better prognosis for shock-treated children, although other studies do not confirm this impression.

The amphetamines (benzedrine) produce favorable results in the brain-injured child, in the child with hyperkinetic impulse disorder (considered an organic disease process), and in the preadolescent child who is sexually very active or preoccupied. Finally, anti-convulsants are generally used in the case of children with convulsive disorder, if these children are accepted by the institution for treatment. Of this group of drugs, dilantin sodium is also used by a few institutions for children diagnosed as manifesting the above-mentioned hyperkinetic impulse disorder with either an epileptic or an immature, high voltage slow-wave electroencephalographic pattern. In these instances the drug is reported to cause a decrease in restlessness, better motor patterning, and increased ability to concentrate.

It is noted that in several of the units reporting considerable use of these somatic therapies, there are considerable differences in mode of operation from those who report no use of somatic treatment. This concerns the nature of admission of the patients, the average census, and the average length of the patient's stay in the hospital. In general, in those units that report not using somatic therapies, rate of intake is low (four to six patients per year), census is low (up to fifteen children), and duration of hospitalization is long (up to one year and more). In contrast, in one institution that uses most of the somatic therapies described above, intake is at least 350 patients per year, daily census is generally at a minimum of fifty children under twelve years of age, and the duration of stay averages only one month.

One final fact related to somatic therapy can be mentioned here. As could be expected of any medically directed activity, all the institutions studied make provision in some way, through the services of the staff or visiting pediatricians and other consulting specialists, for somatic medical study on admission, for continual attention to the maintenance of the patient's general bodily and dental health, and for treatment of any intercurrent illness or injury. This is true even of those units in which the theoretical orientation of the staff emphasizes experiential rather than genetic-congenital-constitutional etiological factors of the disorders seen. Alertness to signs of possible organic disease in the former units is stressed as much as attention to experiential psychogenic factors in the latter. Any medical treatment indicated for the severe organic symptoms of psychosomatic illnesses are, of course, used especially in the treatment center that is at present entirely devoted to the study and treatment of these syndromes.

PARTICIPATION OF PARENTS, INTAKE, AND
DURATION OF INPATIENT TREATMENT

The kind and amount of participation of the parents or surrogate parents in the treatment program, and the work done with them by the staff varied among the units studied along a gradient of emphasis that in some measure was inversely related to the contrasting mode of operation of the units mentioned in the previous section. Such work tended to include more parents and to be more intensive in the unit where rate of turnover of patients and census was low and the duration of inpatient stay long. Other factors that influenced the work with parents were the possibility of control of intake and duration of inpatient treatment, the location of the institution in relation to the home of the child, the size of the staff available and trained for such work, and the theoretical orientation of the staff with respect to the importance of the parents, both as regards the etiological contribution their emotional state made to the child's disorder and the possible advantages of their participation in total treatment.

Clearly, if admission of the patient to the inpatient facility is entirely or largely by order of a court or by authority of some other agency or institution, participation of the parental persons in the decision for admission and in the subsequent work is absent or very difficult to obtain. As more and more psychiatrists directing such inpatient facilities become aware of the importance of work with the parents in the total treatment of the child, it may be possible to increase the number of families participating with the staff. Joint studies, discussions, and conferences between staff and others such as juvenile court judges, probation officers, and staffs of other agencies may lead to at least partial resolution of obstacles that now seem insurmountable. In any case, it seems evident that one of the differences in practice as regards treatment has its roots in these factors. It is not implied here that experienced professional opinion is now unanimous, or even growing in the direction that the work with parents constitutes an absolutely essential element in the treatment of the child. It is still quite possible that direct treatment of the child within an inpatient facility may in many instances be quite efficacious even though return of the child to the family after discharge may be either impossible, longer delayed, or fraught with the probability of exacerbation of the disorder. In this respect, further research on these questions seems clearly desirable.

THE THERAPEUTIC ATMOSPHERE OR MILIEU

Under the term "therapeutic atmosphere" in this report are included all those activities and experiences for the child patient within the inpatient facility that were planned or considered as contributory, ameliorative influences upon his disorder—exclusive of somatic therapies and direct psychotherapy. Milieu, management, control, and programming are other terms that were used in the same connection to emphasize various parts of this aspect of inpatient treatment of children. The variety of "nonpsychotherapeutic" professional personnel and the details of their work with the patients were studied. Some effort was made to examine the degree and manner of the integration of their combined activities and the theoretic basis of such work—if any coherent one was expressed or discernible—and of its relation to direct psychotherapy with the child. A partial list of these activities includes the following: the role of the child care workers; educational and remedial work; occupational therapy and other activity programs, including recreation; the routine or schedule of the day and the role of the social worker and psychologist in planning it, the attitudes of the staff toward symptoms, and staff integration. This chapter will be a bare digest of the principles underlying this aspect of treatment.

First, there are a few facilities that place primary reliance on the effect of the orderliness and organization of the child's living experience within the institution upon his behavioral disorder, rather than on direct individual psychotherapeutic work with him. The reasons for this vary from a continuing conviction that this is sufficient with the particular forms of disorder admitted to an inability to provide direct psychotherapy in addition to the general inpatient program. In most of the units studied, however, there is both a recognition of the importance of direct psychotherapy and provision of this modality of therapy for at least some of the children. A good number of the centers expressed a wish to provide more intensive psychotherapy.

Second, several units definitely stated that the primary and only purpose of the child's living in the treatment center was the opportunity for psychotherapeutic work with him in a setting which would not only enhance direct work with him but would also provide a milieu that might make a critical difference in the result. This was contrasted with psychotherapeutic work with the child living at home. In some of the units that provided long-term inpatient care, treatment, research, and teaching were given equal emphasis. In these instances, the institutional aspects of treatment were regarded as opportunities for learning with those methods readily available and for training all types of staff personnel concerned in such work.

Among the facilities surveyed there was a graded discernible variation in the use of the inpatient milieu, from eclecticism to a commitment to test a definitely formulated hypothesis about the genesis and maintenance of a child's disorder, using methods developed from a logical derivation of theorems from basic postulates. In other words, certain aspects of the inpatient milieu, such as the daily routine (the biological functions of feeding, rest, activity, and so forth), educational and remedial work in school, the effects of grouping, and the conscious use of principles of group dynamics in various activities and recreation, were utilized in two ways or in some varying combination of the two ways: either these were primarily opportunities for a prescribed treatment, for correction of deficiencies in the child's experience prior to admission, or they were primarily opportunities to study and to understand the child's behavior as symptomatic of his central disorder and then to use these situations in ways that were consistent with the same psychodynamic theory on which direct psychotherapy was based.

Rather than listing the differences among the centers studied with respect to such matters as types of professional and auxiliary personnel employed, provisions for the patients' schooling, use of recreational or occupational therapy, and flexibility of patient routine, this report will be concerned primarily with the ideas implicit in the differences of practice explicitly described in the basic reports.

The attitudes—about to be described—that the physical plant and the staff personnel concerned in the various milieu activities offered to the child do not exist in pure culture in any unit studied, and bald delineation of opposites is made here only for greater clarity of exposition. Nevertheless, isolation of these attitudes has some basis in that in whatever measure they are combined in practice, they are to that extent discernible.

The Closely Scheduled Milieu

One of these milieu attitudes could be described in the following terms: external control and restraint of any eruptions of hostile, destructive behavior of the child is to be provided, as well as opportunities for more orderly and more satisfying relations with adults and peers. In such a context the daily schedule, from arising, through meals, school, recreation, medical procedures, and free play, to bedtime, is fairly definitely prescribed for each day in the week. Conformity to the schedule by the hour, to rules of behavior, and performance of activities is expected and is generally attained. Visits with parents at or near the center or at home are clearly defined, as is the period of inpatient stay (where this is possible). Classification as to age, sex, intelligence, and already attained individual skills may influence the assigning of a child to a particular group; and continuous membership in a certain group is felt to provide continuity, order, expectation, encouragement, group pressure, and rewards of more or less friendly exchange with coevals and equals. Control or management is imposed upon the child, and he is expected to adapt to the environmental restrictions and opportunities for satisfactions. Occasional individual discussions with the child by some authoritative adult in the institution, either at the time of admission or after troublesome behavior, may be the only individual sessions the child experiences. Direct individual psychotherapy is unavailable for various reasons.

With certain children who show difficulties that can be described in rather objective, impersonal terms, such as impulsive disturbances or behavior disorders, some measure of reduction of the unorganized patterns resulting from deprived and disorganized backgrounds undoubtedly occurs. Perhaps even some learning of academic or nonacademic skills results, and follow-up studies could reveal some improvement in self-direction outside the institution. Whether in these instances closer studies would also reveal an increase in neurotic symptoms poses an interesting theoretical possibility.

The Need-Responsive Milieu

The polar opposite of the described attitude above is more likely to emerge or develop in efforts at therapy with the more inhibited (psychoneurotic) and withdrawn (psychotic, autistic) patients. In some ways, perhaps, this attitude confronts more difficult dilemmas about the hostile, aggressive eruptions and other symptoms of such disorders. For this attitude in the milieu to be positively contributory to the therapeutic goal, these latter dilemmas require careful further study and theoretical and practical reduction. Otherwise, there may be less than the appropriate degree of internal consistency and clarity of application of methods to the realities of the patient's disorder.

In addition, this second attitude also faces the hard realities of shortage of trained and experienced people and the high cost involved in maintaining an adequate staff-patient ratio. The staff provides the personal aspects of the therapeutic atmosphere that respond to whatever the symptomatic activity or bodily function of the child is at the moment in a manner consistent with the psychotherapeutic goal, rather than merely providing control and orderliness of overt behavior. Paradoxically, both the shortage of personnel and the nature of the child's disorder contribute a great deal to the emergence of the "controlling" attitude, even in those units in which psychiatric philosophy is diametrically opposed to it.

A brief delineation of the "noncontrolling" milieu's goal might be formulated somewhat as follows: the aim of every staff person—whether the child-care worker, the schoolteacher, the remedial therapist, the recreational therapist, or the group worker—is to help the child to reduce the internal (conflict) disorder, however it manifests itself in the activity in which the particular staff member is concerned. It is postulated that after the child has taken some steps toward the reduction of his internal disorder the energy freed from symptomatic binding makes it gradually possible for him to learn and to become eager to act with less self-destructiveness.

More and more is being learned about how this goal may be achieved, what period of time is required for the therapeutic process, and what personal attributes of the staff and external nonpersonal circumstances are necessary or desirable for the process even to begin. Such formulations need to be clear, specific, and concrete, or they may give the impression of being platitudes. It should be remembered that conceptual work—desirable as it may be for further development of methods—is never a substitute for the knowledge that comes through actual experience.

In spite of these considerations, it may be added further: 1) that the theory underlying this attitude postulates the disorder as largely or entirely psychogenic, that is, arising out of postnatal experience of the child, primarily with other persons; 2) that the child's destructive or self-destructive activity, although symptomatic, requires firm, nonretaliatory, promptly protective restraint, which is gentle and continuously personal, if at all possible. This restraint needs to be of such a nature that it takes account of: (a) the immediate frustration that precipitates the destructive activity, if known, (b) the total background in the child's past experience with the staff person involved, and with other persons prior to admission, (c) the total duration of the immediate disturbing tension, and (d) the need to differentiate it carefully, sharply, and continuously, from any hint of punitiveness (despite the patient's great tendency to react to any restraint in terms of his own internalized, impatient, derisive self-punitiveness). Further, this restraint needs to be so applied that it leads the child to reduction of his projected fears about his own sensual wishes for contact; in short, that it leads to the child's greater relaxation, trust, and self-confidence, as well as greater confidence in the staff; 3) the sensual (regressive?) self-gratifications of the child that are not destructive, which often appear after the type of restraint described, need to be so understood that they will not be supressed by any action of the staff. In short, that anxious tensions of the staff about both destructive and self-gratificatory activity of the child can be ideally minimal or absent. Such attitudes of the staff will then on every occasion constantly discriminate between (a) protecting the patient against any injurious consequences of his own activity, and (b) accepting the nondestructive, e.g., verbal, expression of even violently destructive or passionately intense sensual desires; 4) that the constant attentiveness to every observable detail of the child's behavior will provide opportunities: (a) to permit any apparently necessary self-absorption and withdrawal; (b) to offer timely help in any of his own efforts to master any and every skill towards self-care and satisfying activity; (c) to redirect any such efforts to reduce his self-frustrations; and (d) to watch, follow, and encourage any of the child's own emerging interest and spontaneity; 5) and that, nevertheless, in all these aspects of the staff's work, each staff member needs to discriminate so clearly his own role in the child's experience that it will in no way interfere with his relation to the child's parents. This means that the satisfactions of the staff are derived from their own technical contribution to the child's achieving a reduction of his inner emotional turmoil, and from their own increasing technical development and proficiency; in short, that any of the patient's "dependency" attitudes appearing in such work are recognized as transient phenomena in his own progress toward more and more complete resolution of his disorder.

Finally, all this requires that kind of technical collaboration with other staff members that could be termed an integration of the entire staff in the work toward the goal defined. It means lack of competitiveness with any other staff member who contributes his share to the "milieu" or "atmosphere" of the treatment center, as well as with the individual psychotherapist of the child or parent. It means clear definition of the particular staff member's part in the whole of the child's experience in the institution. Under such circumstances, problems of "confidentiality" with respect to what each staff member learns from and with the child or parents may either not arise or be more easily solved.

There are variations in the kind and degree of relation that the staff has or wishes to have with parents, referring persons, and agencies. The particular members of the staff having such contact with persons responsible for the child will also vary. Where contact with parents by the staff of the unit is minimal or absent, various difficulties about discharge and follow-up may be greater, and treatment procedures during the child's stay may differ a good deal. Where contact with parents does exist prior to admission, the social worker has the primary responsibility for such casework as is done with them. In a few institutions, the psychiatrists undertake regular therapeutic work with both parents, and an explicit agreement on the part of the parents to do such work is often a condition of inpatient work with the child. In one institution, rather rigid requirements are set that the absence of serious neurotic or psychotic illness of the parents or threatened divorce be established before a child can be admitted to the facility.

Contact of the parents with other members of the staff of the unit may be limited to necessary communication about various arrangements and details of the child's care or visits home, or almost entirely excluded. In those instances where the family home is at a great distance, where the staff considers work with the parents unimportant for its work with the child, or where the parents are already involved with private practitioners of therapy, any work with parents during the child's stay in the institution may be delegated—not always by preference—to professional persons not connected with the staff.

In general, those units with low census, larger staff-patient ratio, low rate of intake, longer periods of inpatient treatment, and commitment to training and research (especially when part of a university-medical school setting) seem to regard regular sessions with one or both parents as an integral part of inpatient treatment of children. In these instances, mutual decisions of parents and staff about admission of the child are sought in contacts with parents, in visits of the family to the facility, and so on. After admission, visits of parents with their child on or off the unit's living quarters for the patients may or may not be rigidly prescribed. The length of visits home of the child may or may not be weekly, becoming longer as the clinical situation indicates. Termination of inpatient work then merges into continued outpatient work, and the hospitalization is then only one phase of the entire therapeutic work with the family.

In the theoretical formulations of some of these last-mentioned units, there is postulation of an etiological connection between the disorder of the child and that of his parents. In one of these the staff has made explicit theoretical formulation of clinical data obtained from concomitant therapeutic work with the child and both his parents and from some results of such work. This formulation includes not only statements about the origin of the disorder, but also a statement of the ongoing nature of the balance of integration and malintegration of all three members of the family. From this point of view, the work with the parents is essential for research, and probably an advantage in therapy with the child; although it is not denied that effective therapeusis of the child's disorder may also result from work with him alone.

The above description of the milieu is not complete. Practice with regard to record-keeping, the essential communication between staff members of different professions and on different shifts, the routine and variety of activities, the manner of physical and medical care, the methods of psychological testing and of educational remedial measures, and collation of all the work with the patient and with the parents differs in detail from one unit to another. It is hoped, however, that the above gives some idea of what therapeutic "atmosphere" means in this context.

DIRECT OR INDIVIDUAL PSYCHOTHERAPY

All the centers reported that there was some type of individual work of a psychotherapeutic nature practiced in their units. In the majority of the units all children were seen from two to three times a week by a variety of professional personnel: general psychiatric residents, full-time fellows in training for child psychiatry; psychiatric social workers; psychologists; and psychiatrists trained and experienced in psychotherapeutic skill. In a few of the centers the psychotherapists were not integral members of the inpatient unit. Many of the last group (a good number of them psychoanalysts) were predominantly occupied with training the other personnel mentioned and supervising their work with individual patients. In those units having a small total census, a good deal of the time of such senior staff psychiatrists (in some, visiting consultants) was devoted to the development of psychotherapeutic skill among the psychiatric trainees by means of individual supervisory sessions of up to two hours per week, seminars, treatment review conferences, and, in one instance, continuous case seminars.

One treatment center specified that its approach to psychotherapy was eclectic. Most of the centers, however—as might be expected from the background of the senior staff and consultants—defined their psychotherapeutic approach as psychoanalytically oriented. In spite of this, it remained difficult to determine the precise nature of the psychotherapeutic work.

The difficulty in defining the nature of psychotherapeutic work was due to several factors. Understandably enough, descriptions of this work in the basic studies was in many instances limited. For more detailed information, a review of published work from these centers would be necessary for which there was no time. The fact that a large proportion of the psychotherapy was performed by personnel in training was another probable reason for the paucity of more detailed descriptions from many of the units. Further, it is clear from what data was obtained that there is a fairly wide range of mental disorders admitted to the various units: from rather severe psychoneurotic and psychosomatic forms of clinical syndromes through the character or impulsive behavior disorders to very severe psychoses such as autism and schizophrenia. The nature and severity of the disorder certainly affects and determines the character of the therapeutic process as much as other factors do. Among these other factors are: the skill and experience of the psychotherapist, the frequency of therapeutic sessions, the duration of therapy, the theoretical orientation of the therapist, and the degree of integration of the rest of the staff with respect to theoretical orientation.

All of these factors vary considerably from one unit to another (and probably from time to time in the same unit coincident with changes in staff personnel and in the skill of such staff as remains) and are the ground for a broad spectrum of patient experience. These experiences range from those termed "ego-building"—efforts to assist the child in acquiring more effective modes of adaptation to the intra- and extra-institutional reality— to those in which more thoroughgoing efforts are made at resolution of conflicts through such processes as establishment of a therapeutic situation for the development of transference, its detailed study and its resolution after appropriately adequate interpretive therapeutic behavior; and the development of insight. How much of the latter processes actually occurs with how many patients, and especially with those manifesting the more severe disorders such as impulsive character problems, psychosomatic illnesses, and psychotic disorders, it is not possible to estimate from the data available. It can be stated, however, that this is the direction of the effort of a number of those training-center facilities with an adequate and appropriately trained and experienced senior staff.

From these considerations, it could be said that such inpatient treatment institutions for children offer clinical opportunities that might make significant contributions to the field of child psychiatry specifically, and to the whole field of psychiatry generally, insofar as the therapeutic study of parents is included (with further development that adequately supported programmatic therapeutic research and research into training methods could make possible).

The previously mentioned factor of the variation in severity and form of the mental disorder of the children admitted to the various units in many respects forms the heart of the problem of treatment in an inpatient setting. It is related to any generalized statement of the criteria for admission, and it is related also to the theories of etiology and psychopathology, that is, to the question of rational therapeutics.

Although space precludes a thorough exposition, it seems nevertheless of some importance to consider in brief outline some general theoretical problems that underlie all aspects of treatment, but particularly this aspect of individual psychotherapy—or at least to touch upon the various theoretical approaches available at present.

These approaches vary from a so-called biological point of view through a frank eclecticism to what could be called a thoroughgoing psychological hypothesis. The proponents of the theory that psychosis in childhood is fundamentally rooted in a somatic maturational lag of genetic-constitutional origin state that psychological aspects—and hence, psychotherapy—are included in their conceptions of the disorder and in their treatment practices. The quoted statement in the chapter on somatic therapies of this report represents this point of view. On the other hand, those holding the more purely psychological theory—that is, that postnatal experiential factors are at the root of the genesis and maintenance of the disorder—also include in their practice study of each patient by every clinical method available for possible genetic-constitutional disease of differences. Naturally, to the extent that the important urges or instinctual drives, as expressions of the biological equipment of man, are considered as the energic basis of the conflicts postulated for the disorder in this psychogenic hypothesis, the differences in opinion are narrowed between these two points of view. However, even those centers that described their theoretical and practical approach as psychoanalytically oriented might differ among themselves as to what factors produce the dynamic conflict associated with severe ego distortion and atypical development.

Finally, those psychiatrists who do not hold any of the theoretical positions described as absolute frankly apply an eclecticism in which somatic therapy, therapeutic milieu, and direct psychotherapy are utilized together or differentially, according to clinical indications. In this instance, learning about clinical problems is in part acquired in ways other than by formulating a hypothesis about the disorder (e.g., the biological lag theory or the psychogenic theory) and testing it by appropriate clinical and therapeutic methods. Research in such eclectic institutions may then have another meaning in which discrete, smaller questions are asked and answered by projects that often are distinguished from therapeutic work. This is in contrast to those institutions in which research is programmatically synonymous with the entire clinical effort with a given patient and his family and with the work with trainees.

It is to be expected that even in more complete reports of psychotherapeutic work in such units there would be differences of practice, differences in statement of results, and differences in expectations from given psychotherapeutic methods in work with different kinds of patients. Psychotherapy and its results with patients whose disorder is psychoneurotic, even though very severely so, would be describably different from that with patients whose disorder is psychotic or patients who are extremely ill with a psychosomatic illness. Whether such differences in clinical data collated from various units will eventually definitely support some current theory is, of course, for future work to decide.

THE PROBLEM OF TREATMENT OF ADOLESCENTS

Although at the outset it was hoped that descriptive studies of five treatment units for adolescents could be obtained, in the end it was only possible to study two such units. One of these included two different wards or treatment units within a state hospital—a treatment ward for those psychotically ill, and one admitting impulsively disturbed children not exclusively in the adolescent age range, largely from courts and other similar agencies. A third indirect description from published literature was a unit under psychiatric direction but not primarily designed for treatment—a diagnostic center for a state youth authority. As previously stated, the subject of inpatient treatment facilities for this age group was considered a subject large enough for a separate conference. In any case, the problem of inpatient treatment of preadolescent children occupied the available energy and time, and hence, the subject of adolescents has been much less well studied.

Most of the present treatment centers exclusively operated for this age group seem to be on state hospital grounds. Those adolescents who are admitted to mental hospitals that are training centers associated with university medical schools are generally placed in wards for adults. Several of the centers for preadolescent children studied admit some patients beyond twelve years of age within a plant facility used for younger patients, but to some degree separate from it. However, no special comments about the problems presented by this placing of age groups were made. One university medical school that contains a teaching, treatment, and research mental hospital (still in the planning stage) will have a unit for adolescents as part of its section for child psychiatry.

The study of the few adolescent units emphasized the unique problems that this period of life presents to the psychiatrist in charge of an inpatient center. The fact that most treatment facilities for adolescents are closed-ward facilities stems from the differences between adolescent and preadolescent patients. The differences mentioned are the adolescents' greater size, strength, and sexual maturity; their propensity both to violence against others and to suicide; the intensity of their conflicts about authority, independence, and dependence; and, especially in the group of impulsive behavior disorders, their greater tendency to make use of group identity and activity. The relative frequency of the impulsive, as compared to the psychoneurotic and psychotic, disorders in this age group would also be of considerable interest to study; certainly the more obvious difficulties posed by the rebelliously impulsive adolescent are more often noticed by the public as well as psychiatrists in institutions for the teenager. The imminence of adulthood and consequent greater need for choice of vocation, for decisions about schooling or training for careers, as well as the problems of sexual activity and the possibility of parenthood in or out of marriage, were also underlined as constituting factors in treatment additional to those encountered in treatment of pre-adolsecent patients. Some attention was given, too, to the relatively lesser knowledge and literature about normal personality dynamics and about psychotherapeutic work with adolescents. An integral aspect of this problem of psychotherapeutics is the possibly greater likelihood of countertransference difficulties of psychotherapists generally, but perhaps more especially of those who are removed from this period of their own lives by less, or little more, than a decade.

Despite the difficulties that this age group presents to the psychiatrist in charge and to the milieu staff, the nonpsychotic adolescent constitutes an interesting therapeutic challenge because of his readiness to respond to adults and to form new identifications, his capacity to achieve re-organization of personality as part of the rapid development of his body, and his consequent rapidly increasing opportunities in social living.

The various aspects of inpatient treatment that the present report has summarized in previous sections for work with preadolescent children are, of course, equally important with adolescents. The influence of the atmosphere or milieu of the institution, of the attitudes of the personnel, their integration as a staff, and their degree of understanding of the particular sensitivities of the adolescent may spell the difference between relative success and relative failure of the inpatient treatment. The rules about behavior within the institution, especially about defiant acts, the number of these rules, the specific satisfactions they deny or prohibit, and the manner in which they are promulgated by the staff and, if possible, accepted and practiced by the patients themselves are a particularly important focus of attention of staff and patients. The relations within the unit between the sexes, both within the patient population itself and between staff and patients, the way in which gang formations occur around a particularly defiant leader, the use of appropriate psychological testing for abilities and aptitudes, adequate schooling, remedial tutoring of special educational and academic deficiencies, the teaching of crafts, vocational training, and recreation to channel energies from destructive to constructive activities, are all obvious and extremely important elements of the treatment program.

Similarly, the role of the somatic therapies, direct psychotherapy with the patients and the work with parents, and collaboration with other agencies in the community are part of the possible armamentarium of the staff of such a treatment center. All of these require closer study as to indications for their use, their effectiveness, and refinement of application.

As regards work with parents, there is evidence of the negative effect of the lack of parental participation in the treatment program of the institution. Especially in the case of the impulsively disturbed adolescent, where commitment by a juvenile court or other authoritative agency, without much or any consultation or continuing participation of the parents, is the predominant or sole mode of admission to the unit, treatment may either not begin or may be prematurely interrupted. Elopement from the facility, aided or abetted by the family in a fair proportion of instances, is reported as the denouement to the efforts of the staff. Other factors, such as insufficient staff, or inadequately trained staff, and great distances between the family home and the facility, also militate against more frequent work with parents, even where the psychiatric director and his staff is convinced of the value of such work.

Direct individual psychotherapy, especially with impulsive character disorders and psychoses among the adolescents, is still relatively undeveloped. Here further theoretical and practical therapeutic research is necessary into such questions as the "normal" adolescent neurosis, if there is one; the need for close collaboration between psychotherapist and milieu staff, and between the inpatient staff and the staffs of other agencies, such as probation officers, school authorities, employers, and so forth; and the particular techniques, if any, that help psychotherapists in training resolve any special countertransference difficulties with patients of this age group.

Considerable difference of opinion exists among clinicians experienced in psychotherapeutic work with adolescents, for example, on the question of whether neurosis is an inevitable development, or only an overwhelmingly frequent occurrence, during the teenage years of life in all cultures. The answer might profoundly affect many other theoretical and practical problems of psychiatric treatment, especially the psychotherapeutic work with the adolescent. Space does not permit an extensive discussion of this problem; however, some of the theoretical questions raised in this connection in the discussion of psychotherapy with preadolescent children would also be relevant here. It may be mentioned that the consequence in practice might be greatly different if healthy emancipation from parents were regarded as occurring either by way of progressive integration of the increased sexuality after puberty through reduction of anxieties about all manner of bodily functions in preadolescence and through more thorough learning of skills relevant to self-care and productive participation in the culture, or by way of a phase of rebellious, self-destructive sexual and nonsexual behavior. In other words, is the solid establishment of inner self-direction possible only through destruction of even unambivalent and effective identifications with parents and other adults with whom experience in the first decade was on the whole integrative? Or are the defiant and usually anxious drives against outer authoritative limits and laws of the adolescent always related proportionately to and are directly the consequences of unresolved conflicts in which anxieties about bodily functions and sensuality constitute the relentless inner self-prohibitions that are never resolved in symptomatic, impulsive activity? Are the *deficiencies* in learning all kinds of skills, or the regressive loss of their availability, always associated with such *conflicts,* or are they part of the intensifications of such conflicts secondary to increased thwarting in current living? And are such deficiencies in skill or regressions in learning capacity the basis for very deep doubts about one's own value, competence, and lovability, the sources of the uneasy and destructive drive for independence, as are social- and self-frustration of the reproductive urges that increase with pubescence?

The answers to these questions might also help in the solution of the other problems of the treatment of adolescents, namely, authoritative intervention against destructive behavior (in contrast to nondestructive expression of feelings) that would not be incompatible with psychotherapeutic work, and the particular kind of countertransference problems that psychotherapists experience with the adolescent.

REFERENCES

1. *Psychiatric inpatient treatment of children.* Washington, D.C.: American Psychiatric Association, 1957.

CHAPTER 2

A NOTE ON RECONSIDERATION OF PSYCHOANALYTIC METAPSYCHOLOGICAL ASSUMPTIONS*

S. A. Szurek, M.D.

For those who undertake psychological therapy with very severely disordered preadolescent children, particularly with psychotics, there are not only the difficulties of technical, practical procedure with the patient and those stemming from the generally discouraging, grave prognosis, but there are also theoretical obstacles.

For the psychoanalytically trained or psychoanalytically oriented child psychiatrists who venture into this thorny field, a number of problems arise concerning metapsychological assumptions. For the present writer these problems take the form of the following questions: whether there are variations in inheritance of strength of instinctual drives; whether there is among these phylogenetically given drives one that is destructive (thanatos, death instinct), or whether the clinical phenomena of destructiveness, hostile-anxious aggression, and sado-masochistic behavior arise as developments secondary to frustration of more primary drives in postnatal experience; and whether the libidinal drives (eros) of infancy and early childhood are relatively immutable and require repression and other transformations (such as sublimation) for any important degree of ego development or integration to occur.

These metapsychological problems are not academic. They are important because each of the basic postulates leads both to basically different interpretations of the results of clinical psychotherapeutic work and to basically different expectations of such work. With different expectations, practice may differ both as to details and as to duration of therapy. These considerations appear important not only for the psychoses

---

*Unpublished paper, 1956.

but also for the psychoneuroses; for the character or impulsive disorders as well as for the severe psychosomatic illnesses.

To illustrate this point, one might say that if it is postulated that an excess of the destructive instinctual drive is inherited (an assumption that poses difficulties in biological thinking), then the drive can never be fully fused with or neutralized by the "normal" quantity of eros or libido. Presumably, then, the only possibility of reduction of the disorder is to supply and perhaps continuously maintain external support to strengthen defenses for the suppression or repression of id drives. Similarly, if it is assumed that infantile erotic drives are wholly or relatively immutable in every human being, and that repression or transformation of them is required for ego development, then one is led into a similar logical dilemma, namely, that the dynamic relations (repression of id impulses and its consequences) are the same for both healthy and pathological personality development.

THE UNITARY POINT OF VIEW AND PSYCHOTHERAPY

On the other hand, if instead of this phylogenetically given internal, irreconcilable opposition between basic instincts only one energy is postulated, and those phenomena in human behavior that are derived from the postulated death instinct in the previous assumption are differently explained, then the logical deductions as a basis of therapy can be quite different. With this latter point of view one could say, for example, that psychopathology results not from defusion of eros and thanatos, or from the latter's inadequate neutralization, but from the *fusion* of libidinous (sensual) impulses with both the rage consequent to their thwarting in experience and the *anxiety* that is partially the consequence of the biologic state of helplessness in early infancy and childhood.

This complex of active, biologically essential id impulses, combined with the rage and anxiety aroused by repeatedly thwarting experience, may be assumed to lead to sado-masochistic transformations of libidinous impulses. How much repression of such fused impulses and inevitable pressure towards return of the repressed into consciousness and into overt action and therefore interference with learning (ego growth or integration), and what other compromise formations result from additional experiential factors then could be seen to determine the particular form and severity of the disorder. The time of the occurrence of the original traumatic thwarting (that is, the developmental phase in which it occurs) and the repetitiousness, frequency, or duration of operation of the pathogenic circumstances and their intensity (severity and duration of parental conflicts) would then be the determinants of: the severity of the child's disorder; and in inverse proportion, the amount of integration or degree of conflict-free ego development.

In this latter theoretical position, the *possibility* of reduction of every mental disorder would be the first logical consequence. How *probable* such a result might be in any given child would then depend upon such factors as: available degree of psychotherapeutic skill; the intensiveness and duration of psychotherapeutic work, which would include the effectiveness of therapeutic influences of the milieu, and the effectiveness of concomitant psychotherapeutic work with those parents who have not yet experienced a complete extinction of their parental impulses toward their emotionally ill child under the pressure and duration of their own internal and external difficulties; and the time at which therapeutic intervention entered the child's life.[1]

Hopefully, this latter theoretical position is clearly enough outlined so that it will be also obvious that even with this hypothesis, problems of great magnitude still remain. Among the problems in inpatient psychiatric units that are also training centers for child psychiatrists are the following:

1. More thorough psychotherapeutic training, at perhaps an earlier age, of psychiatrists and all other professional ("milieu") personnel in the psychiatric inpatient unit; this training needs to be with the severe disorders admitted to such inpatient units. Nevertheless, it is of some importance to emphasize that the aspect of training that includes review of the student therapist's reactions to his work with patients in supervisory sessions is important and requires much further development. As far as this writer knows, only at Langley Porter Children's Service is this use of supervisory sessions with trainees being made. It seems possible that various solutions to the problem would be suggested if an effort were made to collect reports on the practice and thinking of training centers.
2. Adequate time for work with each patient and his family, begun early in the history of the disorder.
3. A suitable plant.
4. Opportunities for frequent sharing and exchange of clinical experience with colleagues who labor in the same field in other institutions.
5. Further development of methods of integration of the entire milieu staff.

---

[1] For further elaboration of these factors and their interrelations, see [1].

Although definitive evidence to support the reformulation of theory is not offered in this chapter, subsequent chapters contain clinical data that are consistent with it. Other more detailed clinical data from work with individual patients and their families over the past decade at Langley Porter have been collected, and a statistical study of a group of psychotic children is planned. Reports of this work still to be completed will be published in due course.

At present one can only report that the theoretical position outlined has thus far proved useful to the writer in understanding the behavior of patients and their families in therapy, and has been a fruitful source for further direction of such work.

* * * * *

ADDENDUM, 1970

For a more recent (1969) effort to reformulate the classical psycho-analytic metapsychology of Freud, the reader is referred to John Bowlby's first volume on *Attachment and Loss* [2]. This has been reviewed by one of the present editors [3].

One of Bowlby's salient modifications of psychoanalytic metapsychology is his elimination of two of the five viewpoints that Rapaport and Gill [4] have identified as essential to classical psychoanalytic theory. These five are the structural, the genetic, the adaptive, the dynamic, and the economic viewpoints. It is the last two, the dynamic and economic, that are eliminated in Bowlby's reformulation. This he does because, he says, they require an assumption of a "psychical" energy. Although these two viewpoints and the psychical energy model form a possible explanatory model for clinical facts, it is, according to Bowlby, one which is not testable by direct, prospective observation or by experimental study of young children. Such studies and observations have been made to test an alternative model: for example, the observation of the phenomena of Protest, Despair, and Detachment as a predictable sequence in children from fifteen to thirty months of age after temporary separation from the mothering adult toward whom they have developed an instinctive behavior that Bowlby designates as "attachment" (the young of higher primates, other mammals, and birds exhibit this sequence also).

For the explanatory hypothesis of this instinctive behavior, Bowlby draws upon more recent data and theory from the "neighboring" biological disciplines such as ethology, comparative psychology, control theory in living systems, and so on. It is of interest to note Bowlby's comment that Freud did not derive his psychical energy model from his clinical data but only from the scientific climate of his time (e.g. the physicalists, Helmholtz, Brücke, Meynert, *et al.*).

In acknowledging that his alternative model is derived from the scientific climate of the present time, Bowlby points out that his model requires only one energy, that of physics, to make it work. It is at this juncture that Bowlby's concepts and those of the foregoing Note tend to agree in basic assumptions. Both Bowlby and the present writer also agree that this assumption of a single energy is more compatible with the natural sciences and modern biological data and theory, even though the Note, written fourteen years ago, makes no effort to specify the biological data and theory at that time.

Although Bowlby does not concern himself much with the problem of a destructive drive, which is one of the central issues in the Note, his emphasis on distinguishing between the *function* of instinctive behavior as a phylogenetic pattern and the *causation* of such behavior in an individual organism—or rather in a pair of organisms (the young and the mothering adult)—is of considerable relevance to the primary theme of the Note. This emphasis of Bowlby's book cannot be elaborated in detail here.

It must suffice to mention only that the distinction between a phylogenetic pattern appearing through evolutionary processes of mutation and established in the progenitors of the two phyla of birds and mammals in the processes of natural selection, and the mechanisms of *causation* in the course of the life cycle of individual organisms, opens the door to a study of the development of normal and pathologically deviant behavior. The mechanisms of causation, that is, of initiation and termination of behavior, such as hormonal levels, the unlearned and learned components, the control systems dependent upon reception of signals from both internal and external sources and of the results of action taken, constitute a broader and more comprehensible basis for further study of clinically important syndromes of disorder. In particular the psychogenic theories of the etiology of the most severe psychotic disorders of early childhood find additional guideposts for closer, more precise exploration for evidence to support them or to define their limits of applicability.

In this distinction teleological assumptions are unnecessary. Furthermore, the concepts of instincts or of instinctual drives and their vicissitudes and transformations are analyzed, simplified, and clarified further into the elements determining the development and maldevelopment of instinctive behaviors. Most important for the thesis of the Note and the theme of this volume is the data in Bowlby that points to the presence or absence or the degree of a "social" (affective?) responsiveness of the mothering adult to the child's initial social gestures (in the first year of life) as the determining factors in whether the child develops attachment toward that adult.

Thus, the theoretical basis for understanding and for study of normal behavior and its myriad paradoxical deviations in pathological syndromes is further delineated. In other words, testable hypotheses can be formulated by deduction from such assumptions to guide therapeutic maneuvers. From this the possible effectiveness of particular therapeutic procedures of psychological approaches, their timing and necessary duration, as well as indicated preventive measures may get more refined definition. In this way, then, there seems to be a basic compatibility between Bowlby's thesis and that of the Note.

Bowlby's contribution is not likely to be any more readily accepted by psychoanalysts generally [5] than the foregoing Note was by the Commission on Treatment (of the Conference on Inpatient Treatment of Children) when offered to it for consideration.

It was perhaps an evidence of this writer's naïveté that he was surprised when this theoretical position was opposed by the Commission on Treatment for inclusion in its summary report to the general Conference. This opposition to its inclusion was the more surprising and incomprehensible inasmuch as examples of the spectrum of the theoretical positions of each of the nineteen centers was not only inquired about of the reporters of each center at the outset, but also examples of these theoretical positions—especially the more "organic" and the eclectic—included in the summary report were acceptable to the Commission on Treatment (see Chapter 1 of the present volume). Hence, the opportunity to publish the Note here, though belated, is welcomed.

Some of the implications of the rather condensed and abbreviated statement in the Note are repeated in more detail in other publications by the writer [1, 6], and in other chapters of this volume.

REFERENCES

1. SZUREK, S. A. *The roots of psychoanalysis and psychotherapy.* Springfield, Illinois: Thomas Publishing Company, 1958.
2. BOWLBY, JOHN. *Attachment and loss.* Vol. 1. *Attachment.* New York: Basic Books, 1969.
3. SZUREK, S. A. Review of John Bowlby's *Attachment and loss.* Vol. 1. *Attachment. Am. J. Orthopsychiat.,* **40**:531-534, 1970.
4. RAPAPORT, D., and GILL, M. M. The points of view and assumptions of metapsychology. *International Journal of Psycho-Analysis,* **40**:153-62, 1959. Cited by John Bowlby [2].
5. KAPLAN, J. LOUISE. Attachment and instinct (Review of John Bowlby's *Attachment and loss.* Vol. 1, *Attachment*) in *Psychiatry and*

Social Science Review, January 27, 1970, 4(1), 19-25.
6. SZUREK, S. A. Playfulness, creativity, and schisis. *Am. J. Ortho-psychiat.,* **39**(4), October 1959.

CHAPTER 3

A CHILD PSYCHIATRIST'S COMMENTS ON THERAPY OF SCHIZOPHRENIA

S. A. Szurek, M.D.

EDITORS' NOTE, 1970

This is a previously unpublished paper, delivered at the October 1953 meeting of the West Coast Psychoanalytic Societies as a part of the discussion of a paper by E. D. Hoedemaker [1]. It is published here as a tribute to Hoedemaker after his recent death.

The patient's incorporation of and identification with the analytic experience and particular attitudes of the analyst, so clearly delineated by Hoedemaker's report, "The therapeutic process in the treatment of schizophrenia," indicates that this process was certainly not limited to analytic work with patients so severely disordered as to be classified as schizophrenic. It is probable that most, if not all, analysts working with patients who are themselves psychiatrists have had the experience that in the course of the work, evidence of such incorporation and identification with the analyst appears. This may be particularly evident in the clinical work of such psychiatrists-analysands with their own patients. Certainly the indiscriminate "swallowing" of a teacher in psychiatry and in psychoanalysis by students of these disciplines, or the reverse—the resistance against either learning anything at all, or against giving any evidence of such learning in analytic sessions—occurs frequently enough and can have unfortunate results both for the student-analysand-psychiatrist and for his patients, often disrupting the analyst's or teacher's relations with his colleagues on the faculty.

On the one hand, such "swallowing" is a first effort at learning to perform a task; on the other hand, it is also defense against uncertainty.

As such it consists of a desperate clinging to a "technique" to relieve one's sense of helplessness and impotence in some moment of panic in reaction to patient attitudes that appear threatening. Parenthetically, one might add here that the triangular situation of two teaching analysts or teachers of psychiatry and their student, who is more or less unconsciously fostering or exploiting for his own reasons any conflict or difference of opinion between them, is reminiscent of the innumerable similar phenomena in families seen in a psychiatric clinic for children. It is also reminiscent of the report by Stanton and Schwartz [26] some years ago of severe, acute excitements in adult psychotic patients who formed a third in a triangular situation between two members of the staff—whether psychiatrists or nurses—of a mental hospital. Some of these excitements, as those I have seen repeatedly on psychiatric wards for children, subsided within a few hours after the triangle was dissolved, whether by one of the two staff members being transferred or resigning from the hospital, or by resolution of the conflict between them.

In the analytic situations with psychiatrist-analysands as well as with nonprofessional patients, one may understand that a peculiarly obscure piece of behavior of the analysand is a reflection, often remarkably caricatured, of the analyst himself. And this sort of thing occurs perhaps universally despite observance by the analyst of all technical measures designed both to reduce such a possibility to the minimum and to await the *development* of the transference phenomena specific and characteristic of the patient's significant past experiences with others.

In this connection some remarks of Anna Freud and Dr. Emmy Sylvester seem relevant. On a visit to America, Anna Freud pointed to some similarities between analytic problems in work with children and in work with candidates in training for psychoanalysis. She referred to the relative inexperience of children with life and the relative inexperience in professional work of candidates in training. She spoke of the continuing importance of parents, other adults, and perhaps of the analyst himself in the further growth and learning of the child in the first instance, and of the training analyst, the supervising analysts, and other faculty and more experienced colleagues in the second instance. The importance of such people in both cases was different and beyond that of an analyst as therapist with other analysands. Dr. Sylvester is inclined to think that for completion of the analysis of the child, the child's experience with the analyst in the earlier phases of the analysis itself requires analysis.

Hoedemaker, with his report of psychotherapy of a schizophrenic, joins a progressively lengthening list of psychoanalysts who have engaged in such therapeutic work—some of whom have reported their experience and have made some effort to place this experience in a theoretical

context. These psychotherapeutic efforts have been made with schizophrenic patients of all age ranges, namely, with preadolescents, adolescents [4], and adults [3, 5].

There are still disagreements among students experienced with the
problem as to whether the psychotic disorders of preadolescents are to
be considered schizophrenic or instances of atypical ego development.
This lack of agreement about the nature of the disorder of preadolescents
perhaps finds its parallel among students of schizophrenia of adolescence
and adult life who still question or doubt the validity of the diagnosis if
improvement occurs with psychotherapy. Nevertheless, in spite of these
continuing disagreements, it is fair to say that there is a gradual change in
the climate of opinion about schizophrenia among students of this disorder.

The fact that undoubted movement towards integration with psychological therapy occurs in schizophrenic patients of all ages—as in the case
reported by Hoedemaker—raises for fundamental reexamination three
inseparably interrelated aspects of theory. Hoedemaker has commented
upon all of them; a very brief comment about each may be of value here.
The first concerns the problem of etiology; the second, that of psychopathology and psychodynamics; and the third, that of therapeutics.
Opinion is still divided between two etiological notions—the constitutional-
hereditary hypothesis and the notion that the disorder is entirely the
result of experiential (psychogenic) processes. There are, of course, many
who would prefer to consider some combination of both of these factors
or, as has been more recently fashionable, to consider every disorder as
multifactorial but with different values placed on some factors due to
the available evidence or data. The psychogenic theory, which for the
present writer is more consistent with major basic psychoanalytic postulates, immediately involves the patient's experience with his parents. This
is an hypothesis that seems susceptible to considerable testing by therapeutic efforts based on analytic principles.

Data is accumulating from various sources to substantiate the idea that
Hoedemaker tentatively raises about the role of the mother in his patient's
case. Time permits one only to mention in passing the nature of this data.
Tietze [27] and others have studied mothers of hospitalized adult schizophrenics both by interview and questionnaires concerning the frequency
of certain basic attitudes among them. Psychoanalytically trained child
psychiatrists have studied parents, especially the mothers of psychotic
children, with the assistance of caseworkers or, as at Langley Porter
Clinic in the past twenty-four years, by concomitant psychotherapeutic
work with both parents and child.

The following statements partly summarize some of this clinical data [2]:

1. The psychotic child often manifests in his disorder the incorporation and identification with the disorders of both parents' personalities.

2. The schizophrenic makes a futile effort from the oral phase of development onward both to live up to, and in a futile way to rebel against, the often incompatible phantastic solutions each of his parents strives for in his own unconscious conflicts, and in the neurotic mal-adaptation between the parents.

3. On first anamnestic review, the disorders of the parents may not be as obvious to some who tend to concentrate attention upon the patient alone as to the trained and experienced clinician, who can fairly promptly detect it. In addition, recent effort to place each disorder in a develop-mental framework gives one increasing data about what critical develop-mental experiences have or have not been mastered, and may also reflect some parental difficulties in these areas.

Some general factors, suggested by the Langley Porter experience with these families, may explain the fact that the child's disorder is more ob-viously severe than that of either parent or of any sibling. The first is that events external to the family intensify the neurotic disorder of each parent (which is usually obsessional or schizoid) during the earliest years of the child's life, when he is most susceptible. The second factor is the con-verging of the influence of the neurotic disorder of each parent upon the child—though it may, so to speak, be funneled to him primarily through the mother.

Concerning therapeutics, one may say that it seems that in the Hoede-maker case, what was of critical moment was the analyst's attitudes to-ward himself and the patient. His realistic, firm, and just consideration for his own time and welfare where this was relevant; his courage to reveal his actual reactions to her behavior, as about her unprepossessing appearance in new clothes; his probably correct evaluation that the con-tinuing burden of care for younger children would make progress in therapy difficult for her; and his clear and firm offering to her of a choice about the conditions under which continuing work with him would be available (as well as his firmness in regard to her impulses to act out with respect to the gifts for the youngest child at the time of the wedding of her older daughter), were all examples of the analyst's integrity and self-consideration, which were the only qualities compatible with unambivalent consideration for the patient's welfare. These attitudes and procedures of the analyst, undistorted by phantastic anxieties of his own, were greatly needed by the patient in order to simplify her own living, and were prob-ably quite different from those that she had experienced with her own mother.

In this context this writer doubts whether these attitudes, particularly the flexible firmness, have anything to do with aggression or aggressivity (words used by both Wexler and Hoedemaker) in any hostile or destructive sense. The essence of firmness is in its realism, in the absence of anxious hostility, in the absence of the brittle rigidity of a reaction formation, and, finally, in the absence of coerciveness as to what another person may feel. However, it contains a clear indication to the patient of what consequences, as far as the therapist is concerned, will follow from one or another action of his together with the readiness to continue contact and work in the event that the action of the patient does not make the work altogether impossible.

The reality base of such firmness may be an important and therapeutic ingredient. It raises the question, too, of whether this patient and other schizophrenics lack the capacity to perceive unconsciously—if such a phrase can be used and understood—the actual and total reality about themselves and others. The reality the patient seemed to be unconsciously testing was whether the analyst would, like her mother and her own superego, underestimate her judgment, underestimate her perception of herself, and underestimate her capacity either to tolerate a kindly but just and correct evaluation of her appearance or to do something about her appearance that was less ludicrous, less self-deprecatory, and less self-derisive.

In these various ways it seems, as Anna Freud might say, that the analyst maintains a psychological position equidistant between all three of the psychic instances of the patient. He is then in a position to lend whatever assistance he can offer to whichever one of them—ego, superego, or id—is at the moment in need of it. All this is in the overriding interest of the whole psychic apparatus to be integrated (instead of divided and split against itself) in its energies toward the task of obtaining vital gratifications of the organism's basic needs in consonance with internalized, realistic ethical principles and in consonance with the available opportunities of cooperative other persons in the real world.

All this reminds one of the quip of the humorist, "No matter what we teach our children, they insist on behaving the way we do"—which may have some relevance for psychoanalytic work.

Some analysts question whether the same analyst can continue with the patient who has achieved sufficient integration in the first phase of therapy to be able to participate in analytic work with the classical method. The present writer is, for one, glad that Hoedemaker is continuing with his patient, and hopes that we will hear of the results in a few years. The fact that he is willing to continue means that he has conducted himself in the first phase of the work with his patient so that he himself feels no contraindication to the trial. It is only in such experimental work that this question can be settled.

This brings one to the final comment about therapeutics. The method of science consists in examining all available data and reflecting upon them with the purpose of seeing whether existing theories of etiology, psychopathology, and therapeutics will explain the reported findings or whether some modifications of theory are necessary. Of course, theoretical conceptions supported by a large mass of experience are not to be lightly modified unless a sufficient amount of new data demands it [2, 24], and even then, any new concept must explain both the old and the new data. However these questions are finally to be settled, it does not at the moment seem necessary either to maintain that the procedures of the analyst in the first phase of therapy with schizophrenics are in the classical form, or that, on the other hand, such procedures must necessarily be incompatible with it.

* * * * *

ADDENDUM, 1970[1]

Many of the foregoing views expressed in the discussion of the paper read by E. D. Hoedemaker in 1952, almost twenty years ago, contain together with Chapter 7 the beginnings of the theoretical framework within which Langley Porter's work with psychotic children developed (see Chapter 7). Other publications of the writer ([2], see also Chapter 2) expanded the theme foreshadowed here. This unitary view of at least some of the psychoses, uncomplicated by any signs of organic disease, of all phases of the life cycle of man had already been suggested by H. D. Sullivan [3] and others [4, 5, 7a].

There was and is considerable opposition to this view, which does not make the effort to test the idea of the psychogenic theory by clinical therapeutic work any easier. Hence the discussion may be of interest as a bit of the history of the climate of local and national professional opinion regarding the psychotic disorders of childhood, within which the therapeutic program described in this volume evolved.

Since those days, work by many others reporting on the psychological and psychogenic aspects of the schizophrenic psychosis has been added to the literature. This literature concerns work with such disorders both in childhood [6] and in later life [7, 7a]. These contributions, many of them

---

[1] The author acknowledges the cooperation of his co-editor, Dr. Berlin, in preparing this Addendum.

later than the date of the discussion, add much to our beginnings in this field. In the volume just referred to [7], published a decade ago and edited by Don D. Jackson, the chapter by Jackson himself and the section on "Family Dynamics" are particularly noteworthy examples of these contributions to the psychological thesis.

Jackson's study, "A Critique of the Literature on the Genetics of Schizophrenia," is of special interest. The data he analyzed were the reported occurrence of schizophrenic disorder in both of several sets of identical twins reared apart. This data had been cited, prior to Jackson's study, as additional evidence for the theory of an hereditary transmission of the psychosis. Among other considerations about the reliability of the statistics resting upon the care and thoroughness of the original observations upon which they are based, Jackson unearthed the fact that the twins were reared in homes of close relatives of their biological parents, and these relatives also appeared to have indications of emotional disorder.

In his conclusion Jackson states in part: "Although the statistics that have been gathered in twin studies are impressive, there are, as we have seen, reasons to suppose that they have been inadequately controlled for *nongenetic* factors. . . . Possible environmental causes and particularly psychic identification have been ignored in favor of possible genetic causes" (italics ours). Also he states that his review had been written "in an attempt to raise questions rather than to answer them, and, in particular, to question the assumption that seems to be widely made that there is overwhelming factual evidence for a strong genetic component in the etiology of schizophrenia. Although it seems likely that hereditary factors do play a part in at least some of the schizophrenias, *it remains to be established* in what forms, how vital is a hereditary 'vulnerability,' and what the phenotypical expression is of the genotypical defect" (italics ours).

Jackson's section on "Family Dynamics" includes summarizing chapters of the clinical work and inferences of Lidz and his co-worker ("Schizophrenia, Human Integration, and the Role of the Family"); Murray Bowen ("A Family Concept of Schizophrenia"); John H. Weakland (who writes for the project group that included Gregory Bateson, Jay Haley, Don D. Jackson, and William F. Fry on "The 'Double-Bind' Hypothesis of Schizophrenia and Three-Party Interaction"); and Maleta J. Boatman and S. A. Szurek ("A Clinical Study of Childhood Schizophrenia"). The last-mentioned chapter is a report on twelve years of work: methods, clinical findings, theoretical influences, and results of therapy in the setting of the Langley Porter Children's Service.

(For a more detailed statement of the results of the psychotherapeutic work of this center, the reader is referred to p. 429 of this report, which is later than most of those included in the present volume.) It may be noted that of the one hundred preadolescent children seen, twenty had shown major improvement. By this was meant that these twenty had been able to function in their homes, in their community, and in public schools for several years with fairly integrated behavior. An additional thirty-four of this hundred, although unable to function without supervision, had manifested considerable improvement in such major symptoms as self-mutilation and mutism; had been able to begin to learn in school and to play; and had become affectively responsive, with occasions of laughter and weeping as appropriate reactions to events in their lives. A still more complete statistical report of results of a study at a still later date, of analysis both of the variety of clinical syndromes and demographic characteristics of 264 patients seen for brief assessment, and the differential results of therapy with 135 of these patients and their parents is in preparation for publication.

All these chapters, together with their bibliographic references, comprise a rich source for study of the problems alluded to in the 1953 discussion. Despite the varying emphases and the somewhat different terminologies used by the authors of these chapters, the congruence of the clinical data and the essential similarity of the theoretical assumptions and inferences is quite clear.

Among recent additions to the literature concerning clinical therapeutic work with psychotic disorders of preadolescent children, the contributions of Goldfarb [8 and 9] and Bettelheim [10] are especially relevant. Goldfarb explores both the psychogenic and "organic" concepts of etiology in his clinical studies and reports differences in patients and in their families between the two groups. For what he terms the "organic" group, he postulates that the child "may be somatically restricted in his intellectual potentiality, his ability to give perceptual form to his environment, to conceptualize, to perform motor acts, and to exercise control." These limitations "in turn evoke reactions in other family members" in a way determined by the motivational psychodynamics of each of the parents. "In the 'non-organic' group, the child begins life with intact physiological equipment; and experiential and interpersonal factors are of greater importance in explaining his ego deficits." The data he presents to support the "organicity" of the first group needs further study and confirmation by others. In the later book [9], Goldfarb describes the therapeutic procedures used in his facility, which he calls "corrective socialization."

Bruno Bettelheim's contribution, reviewed by the present writer [11], is in large part a compilation of clinical data from his experience, which forms the basis for the most uncompromising psychogenic theoretical position in this field. His emphasis on the importance of the child's achieving an autonomous self seems similar to the concept of integration stressed by Lidz and the Langley Porter students of the problem.

Those somewhat contrasting psychological approaches to the psychotic disorders of children that stem from Skinnerian principles (i.e., behavioral modification theory) may be said to be represented by the work of Lovaas [12]. Disregarding any theorizing about etiological factors, Lovaas and other workers of this persuasion record their treatment procedures in a more quantified form than the other clinicians mentioned. Except for this emphasis on quantification, however, there seems considerable basic similarity in therapeutic efforts between Bettelheim, Goldfarb, and the Langley Porter group in persistence in the repetitions of demonstrations (modeling), the use of "prompting" and "reinforcement" (or rewards) for changes in the behavior of the child, and the stress placed on the here and now in the transactions between therapist and child. This similarity is only partly acknowledged by Lovaas. He states, for example, "When the two approaches (the psychodynamic and behavioral modification) are considered on an empirical level, *vis à vis* the therapist's behavior, the differences become more obscure and conceivably diminish [12, p. 155]." At the same time he acknowledges "obvious methodological problems involved" in the extension of his work as regards "phantasy behavior and spontaneity." Other problems, said to be conceptual in nature, are illustrated by the reply of a child who after two years of treatment by Lovaas became facile with language: to a question about his making "crazy faces," he replied that he was trying to "scare away a particular school task which had given him considerable difficulty [12, p. 154]." Lovaas sees this as a conceptual problem for him, since he does not see "how this interaction could be treated within reinforcement theory. It demands empathy [12, p. 155]." With this statement Lovaas appears to move toward the psychodynamic school of therapeutic work, however much he rejects its theory as untestable in practice.

Project Re-Ed, under Dr. Nicholas Hobbs's [13, 14, and 15] direction has sought to deal with the critical manpower problem by training teachers for nine months at Peabody College to work effectively with disturbed school-age children in a residential school setting. The teacher-counselors and the liaison counselor, who works with the regular school and family prior to admission, are key figures. These disturbed children, usually not containable in school or at home, remain five days a week at Project Re-Ed schools for an average length of seven months before returning home permanently. Staff members of local agencies work with the family and community schools prior to the child's admission, and the liaison counselor continues to work with them during the period of readjustment after return of the child to the family and school.

The dedication of the staff, the educational emphasis, and the powerful effect of group interaction combine to enhance the child's competence. Perhaps least successful in altering the child's ecology is the work with parents, since this is done by a variety of local agencies. However, communication between the teacher-counselors and the liaison counselor, who work with a group of eight children for twenty-four hours, is facilitated by informal talks with parents when children are picked up or returned from weekends at home. These are not the most disturbed children; however, they are seriously malfunctioning and Project Re-Ed does enhance the sense of mastery in learning and socialization vital to their continued development.

The common elements of intense therapeutic involvement of concerned adults, the milieu support, the work with parents, and the follow-up work are not very different from the essentials in all good inpatient settings. Further, in Hobbs's latest brief summary [15] he states, "The children are normal to superior in intelligence, but they have all been in serious trouble in school or have been unable to attend school. Labels such as emotionally disturbed, behavior problem, antisocial, withdrawn, schizoid, and schizophrenic appear in the children's records." Also he states, "A careful follow-up of children at discharge and eighteen months after indicates a most satisfactory rate of improvement." A quotation is included from the conclusions of a "panel of visitors," professionals (Eli M. Bower, Reginald S. Lourie, Charles R. Strother, and Robert L. Sutherland), who "followed the project from the beginning, visiting the schools and comparing observations." This reads in part, "That Project Re-Ed represents a conceptually sound, economically feasible, and demonstrably effective approach to helping emotionally disturbed children, including the moderately disturbed *and some seriously disturbed* (italics mine)."

Such statements about the severity of the disorders of the children included in this program raise the issue of the comparability of patients [16] in Project Re-Ed and those described in this volume. Until criteria for diagnostic classification of patients are more clearly defined, not only at each center but also between representatives from the various centers in regional, national, and international conferences, reports of therapeutic results and hence of prognosis for new patients cannot be quantitatively assessed in ways that could be called warranted scientific statements [17].

Explorations in the treatment of childhood psychoses with psycho-pharmacological methods are represented by the work of Barbara Fish [18, 19 and 20].

Dr. Barbara Fish and her co-workers have for more than ten years employed phenothiazines, especially trifluoperazine, with psychotic children. Using the double-blind method, they have found marked improvement in young psychotic children, especially in developmental deficiencies of speech and socialization. These workers emphasize the fact that drugs do not cure the disorder, but do make the child more amenable to therapeutic engagements of various kinds. They feel that outpatient drug therapy is helpful also in permitting more effective psychotherapeutic work.

On the side of biological determinism of the nature versus nurture debate about etiology, Rimland [21] terms "psycho-genesis as an inadequate and pernicious hypothesis [p. 61]." He adds that "the damage and torment . . . wrought upon parents whose lives and hopes have already been shattered by their child's illness is not easy to imagine nor pleasant to contemplate. To add a heavy burden of shame and guilt to the distress of people whose hopes, social life, finances, well-being, and feelings of worth have been all but destroyed seems heartless and inconsiderate in the extreme [p. 65]."

In commenting on Rimland's statements, Bettelheim [10] remarks that since the etiology of autism, psychogenic or any other, has not yet been definitely established, "to make them [parents] guilty will only add to the misery of all and help no one." Further, "[even] if it turned out one day that the parents' contribution is indeed crucial, they did as they did because they could not help themselves to do otherwise [p. 404]."

If Rimland's remark implies that to offer parents an opportunity for psychotherapeutic work is to add to their shame and guilt, then it is difficult for this writer to agree. Many parents coming to this center are not only seriously disturbed but also accept such an offer of help with relief or even eagerness. Quite regularly they present themselves as already burdened with guilt and shame prior to the beginning of any therapeutic work, even though in some it is evidenced by conflictful, defensive attitudes. A trained and experienced therapist accepts their initial unsolicited statements about their conflicting feelings concerning their own parenting attitudes and behavior toward their child as discontent with themselves. Such genuine wishes as they have to resolve these conflicts form the basis for beginning and continuing the arduous effort. Whether such conflicts have indeed contributed to the child's disorder is then a hypothesis to be explored in the therapeutic work. It is frequently clear that with repeated evidence the parents come to see ever more clearly in each episode examined together with the therapist how their guilt and shame may be alleviated if the work continues long enough toward a more thorough resolution. This is especially true if the child is young and, in terms of development, still has opportunities to learn speech. The issue of critical periods in childhood is yet to be clearly delineated, although clinical experiences validate the hypothesis.

Space precludes presenting the detailed clinical data showing how even small steps toward such resolution are frequently accompanied by more integrated behavior, often transient at first, on the part of the child and the parents toward each other, and between the parents themselves (such data is being prepared for future publication). But it would seem that anyone who equates therapy with adding guilt and shame is guilty either of a strange perversion of terms, or of expressing an insufficient degree of training, experience, or comprehension of the psychological therapy described here.

In any event, Rimland makes the effort to separate a syndrome of autism from that of childhood schizophrenia. This he does by analyzing, with the aid of keys and scales, the data he obtains from checklists of the child's symptoms submitted to the parents in questionnaire form. He postulates a lesion in the reticular formation of the brain stem as the source of autism, and suggests that such lesions may either be inherited from highly intelligent parents or be related to "fairly overt postnatal brain damage" such as excessive oxygen in infancy or severe infections early in life.

He asserts that "a careful review of evidence has revealed no support for the psychogenic point of view. The evidence is instead highly consistent with expectation based on organic pathology [p. 61]." However, he "does not presume to have shown that autism is biologically determined, and that the psycho-social environment plays no part in its etiology." More recently it appears he is suggesting efforts at treatment with high doses of vitamins and dietary regimen [21a].

In contrast to Rimland's opinions about results of psychological therapy in the early stages of severe psychotic disorders, the reader is referred to Bettelheim's report of his results [10, pp. 405-416], as well as to the aforementioned 1960 summary of the work at Langley Porter [7] and the initial, preliminary statement included in this volume (Chapter 7). Rimland, of course, might be expected to reply that the patients who have improved were not adequately classified as autistic according to the criteria he defines, which is probably true in large measure. How reliable his classification can be, based as it is on questionnaires from parents and not on direct contact with the child and its parents by trained and experienced clinicians, is left to the reader's judgment.

For further discussion of how etiological problems can be solved and how the overlapping sets of clinical pictures within the spectrum of a syndrome presented by groups of patients thoroughly studied by clinicians can be accurately represented and counted for quantitative assessment of therapy and prognosis with techniques utilizing the "new" mathematics of Boolean algebra and Venn diagrams appropriate to such problems, the reader is referred to Alvan Feinstein [16]. A discussion of Feinstein's conceptual barriers to clinical science as applied to the problem of psychotic disorders of childhood by the present writer is in preparation for publication. This discussion is particularly germane to Rimland's arguments concerning his suggestions [21a, p. 16ff.] about elucidating a syndrome and obtaining clues to etiology. With regard to inquiry concerning etiology of organic diseases, Feinstein points out that clues obtained from clinical work with patients under treatment in hospitals require more accurate testing by epidemiological studies in the populations outside the hospital and the clinic—that is, they require comparisons of the frequency of the occurrence of the disease in groups exposed and not exposed to the suspected etiological factors.

The same kinds of studies of very young children (under two or three years of age) in the general population outside the hospital and clinic, difficult and expensive though they would be in terms of trained manpower, time, and money, are more likely to produce data of crucial importance in answering the etiological questions about the spectrum of psychotic disorders of early childhood. Some research in this direction has already begun to gather data about prevalence [22]. It may be, however, that the problem with respect to the psychogenic aspects of etiology in the psychotic disorders of childhood may be in some respects different from the impersonal causes in the majority of organic diseases.

Several matters become clear to the psychotherapist or clinical team working with the psychotic child and his family. The data of the initial anamnestic review becomes progressively more complete as it emerges during subsequent therapeutic work with richer, more convincing detail, and paradoxical and conflicting historical reports become clarified and resolved. New information comes to light that was earlier unavailable, either because of repressive exclusion from recollection by the parents or because of their intense shame, guilt, and anxiety about being blamed (as they blame themselves) for their past behavior and attitudes toward the child and each other. Moreover, the essential congruence and similarity of past events in the life of the child in his family with the current mode of his living within the home during therapy becomes evident. When an effective working alliance between therapist and parents is progressively established, ongoing episodes, repetitive of the past, are usually the subject of much exhaustive exploration and detailed mutual study. Thus at least some of the original pathogenic influences and the continuing pathologic processes unfold in the course of successful therapy. Even early in therapy, transient resolution of such conflictful trends toward more integrative behavior occurs, or may gradually become more durably established. In short, changes in both the child's and the parents' behavior follows from such resolution. These developments, repeatedly observed, serve as additional supportive data for the etiological hypotheses that are elaborated from the data in therapeutic sessions in the course of such work. The clues about psychogenic etiological factors are thus further clarified, although they require confirmation and quantitative substantiation from the epidemiological type of studies mentioned.

There is a need for considerable clinical acumen among the students performing such studies, if they are to identify and establish the diagnosis of psychotic disorder and to collect the necessary data about the presence or absence of the subtle and not always easily identifiable psychogenic factors. Training in the appropriate methods of obtaining data about possible hereditary or impersonal disease factors is also essential; the possible presence of several of these factors requires careful collation of observations and analysis of effects.

One cannot resist commenting on Rimland's reference to the two papers from Langley Porter previously referred to. He states that "Szurek, who started in 1946 'to test the hypothesis that the etiology of psychotic disorders of childhood are entirely psychogenic' [7, p. 389] *takes a much weaker stand today* (italics ours) in stating that certain 'facts' . . . seem to lend weight to the possibility that psychogenic factors are at least important' (p. 430) [p. 66] ." The reader may wish to see these "facts."

The present writer (author and co-author of the papers Rimland refers to in this quotation) was amazed that a statement of a hypothesis that was as clear and succinct as he could make it should be interpreted by anyone as "stronger" than a later statement of inference from additional data bearing upon the hypothesis. To Rimland, a statement of clinical data (as distinct from a hypothesis) that includes as careful somatic assessments as it is possible to obtain apparently is not factual. One may anticipate here data being prepared for publication that a relatively small minority (17.7 percent) of 135 psychotic children with *identifiable* organic findings did not improve with psychological therapy nearly as frequently as did those in whom there were no such organic findings.

In further comment on the aforementioned remark of Rimland, it is of interest to note here briefly a Langley Porter experience with a child first seen at the age of three and a half years, who improved a great deal in two years with the psychological therapeutic procedures described in the present volume and in the Boatman and Szurek report of 1960 [7]. Briefly, his parents reported him from the earliest months as avoiding eye contact, affectively unresponsive to them and his sibling and peers, and preserving sameness in limiting his eating to certain foods, in ritualistic play with blocks, and in preferring his crib. They also reported that he manifested echolalia, little speech, and pronominal reversal after the first year, as well as other symptoms of autistic disorder. When he was five years of age and had improved much in many of these symptoms, Rimland's questionnaires and scales became available, and they were used with mother, father, and the nursing and psychiatric staff who knew the child when he was first admitted. He was classified, following Rimland's directions, as extremely autistic, with ratings of +44 by mother, +36 by father, and +40 by our staff. This retrospective procedure we assume was essentially like that used with many respondents to Rimland's questionnaires. The rating of +44 by mother placed the boy in the highest range of Rimland's own published data of children classified by him as autistic [21a].

Three months later, when the patient was five years and three months old, another assessment by mother and staff of his behavior at that time resulted in ratings of +5 and +6 on the Rimland scales. These ratings placed the boy below the range of what Rimland defines as autism (+20 to +41), in a range of scores he designates as "non-autism" [21a, p. 6a] or schizophrenia.

Clinically the staff's assessment then and later was that, despite considerable improvement, the boy and his family were not sufficiently improved to allow him to be discharged from inpatient therapy, although he spends weekends at home. He is at the present writing still in the hospital, but he is speaking normally, attending a regular school part-time near the hospital and learning, and going home on weekends; he is generally affectively responsive to the staff, his family, and his peers.

Of course one such clinical instance can only be an indication of possibly unsolved problems of Rimland's methods and theory concerning autism. Much more work on many more patients will be required by many clinicians to test Rimland's thesis. (A number of other psychotic children also in inpatient therapy at the same time as the above-described patient were similarly assessed with Rimland's instruments. These data may form the subject of a later report when time permits its study and collation.)

Also on the hereditary side of the etiological debate, in a much more recent contribution with a review of earlier literature (especially European), Heston [23] begins his article with the categorical statement, "The contribution of genetic factors to the etiology of schizophrenia has been confirmed decisively." His argument for the hereditary transmission of the disorder is based, among other considerations, on regarding "schizoidia as the basic inherited trait [p. 252]." Since data he presents supports "a crude but critical conclusion" that he considers "inescapable," namely that "monozygotic twins of schizophrenics are about as likely to be schizoid as schizophrenic," he considers that "at the very least, a prima facie case has been made for considering the whole group of schizoid and schizophrenic disorders as alternative expressions of a single geno-type. Moreover, because monozygotic twins are identical genetically, there is presumptive evidence that the range of variability within pairs can in principle be accounted for by environmental factors. The genes allow a range of outcomes."

For the details of Heston's data and further details of his argument, the reader is referred to his paper, which is of interest in the context of the perennial nature-versus-nurture debate. The latter Heston acknowl-edges as unreal. In short, he agrees "that phenotypic traits depend on interaction between gene and environment [p. 254]." In his summary, he states among other things that "schizoids and schizophrenics occur with about the same frequency among monozygotic twins of schizo-phrenics. About 45 percent of the sibs, parents, and children of a schizophrenic are schizoid or schizophrenic, as are about 66 percent of the children of two schizophrenics." Also he states, "The proportions of affected first degree relatives and the segregation of affected individuals within families closely approximate theoretical expectations based on the hypothesis of a defect in a single autosomal dominant gene. However, modifying traits play a significant role." His thesis, therefore, is "that the same genotype is compatible with either schizophrenic or schizoid disease." In such wise does the approach to the notion of a "spectrum" of clinical similarities and differences between patients mentioned in a later chapter of this volume (Chapter 7) come from theorists and workers in the field of genetic etiology of psychosis. These clinical similarities and differences of patients are of course based upon degrees of severity of the disorder and of maldevelopment, the age of onset, the duration of the dis-order, and the responsiveness to therapy.

It seems possible at present that the whole question of whether heredity and prenatal and postnatal factors noxious to integrated development are etiological of psychotic disorders both of childhood and of later periods of life may eventually be approached in a more adequately defined and differentiated manner. That is, the etiological question may not lead to such global, dichotomous positions as those of heredity vs. psychogenic origin, nature vs. nurture, and the like. This direction is now already implicit in the many careful efforts to detect organic or somatic factors of disease in addition to studying and treating the psychological disorder.

The whole issue of nosological criteria still concerns workers in the field.

This direction is also implied in Bowlby's theoretical reformulation [24, 25] of basic psychoanalytic postulates in the light of more modern biological data and theory (see "Addendum" to Chapter 2). His redefinition of *instinctive* behavioral systems (some of which are "environmentally labile," i.e., having learned components) as evolved within a species through processes of mutation and subsequently of selection in adaptaing to particular environments lays a more refined groundwork for such inquiry. As Bowlby makes clear, such behavioral systems have a marked potential for maladaptive, psychopathological distortion in particular individuals, as a reaction to special circumstances in early developmental phases. Data from ethological studies of many species of birds and mammals, and especially of the primates, support the clinical data on man. Future advances in genetics, elucidating more precisely the effects mutations of particular chromosomal segments or genes, may make their contribution as well.

REFERENCES

1. HOEDEMAKER, E. D. The therapeutic process in the treatment of schizophrenia. *J. Am. Psychoanal. Assoc.,* **3**:89-109, 1955.
2. SZUREK, S. A. *The roots of psychoanalysis and psychotherapy.* Springfield, Illinois: Thomas, 1958.
3. SULLIVAN, HARRY STACK. Therapeutic investigations in schizophrenia. *Psychiatry,* **10**:231-233, 1947.
4. KNIGHT, ROBERT P. Psychotherapy of an adolescent catatonic schizophrenia with mutism. *Psychiatry,* **9**:323-339, 1946.
5. ROSEN, JOHN N. The treatment of schizophrenic psychosis by direct analytic therapy. *Psychiatric Quarterly,* **21**:3-37, 117-119, 1947.
6. EKSTEIN, R., BRYANT, K., and FRIEDMAN, S. W. Childhood schizophrenia and allied conditions. In *Schizophrenia: a review of the syndrome,* Leopold Bellak (Ed.). New York: Logan Press, 1958, 555-693.
7. JACKSON, D. A critique of the literature on the genetics of schizophrenia. In *The etiology of schizophrenia,* D. Jackson (Ed.). New York: Basic Books, 1960, 37-87, 323-440.
7a. SEMRAD, ELVIN V. *Teaching psychotherapy of psychotic patients.* Supervision of beginning residents in the "clinical approach." David Van Buskirk (Ed.). New York: Grune & Stratton, 1969.
8. GOLDFARB, W. *Childhood schizophrenia.* Cambridge, Mass.: Harvard University Press, 1961.

9. GOLDFARB, WILLIAM, MINTZ, IRVING, and STROOCK, KATHERINE W. *A time to heal: corrective socialization—a treatment approach to childhood schizophrenia.* New York: International Universities Press, Inc., 1969.

10. BETTELHEIM, BRUNO. *The empty fortress: infantile autism and the birth of the self.* New York: The Free Press, 1967.

11. SZUREK, S. A. Review of *The empty fortress: infantile autism and the birth of the self* by Bruno Bettelheim. *Social Service Review,* The School of Social Service Administration, University of Chicago, **42**(2), 241-251, June 1968.

12. LOVAAS, O. IVAR. A behavior therapy approach to the treatment of childhood schizophrenia. In *Minnesota Symposia on Child Psychology,* Vol. 1, John P. Hill (Ed.). Minneapolis, Minnesota: The University of Minnesota Press, 1967, 108-159.

13. HOBBS, NICHOLAS. Mental health's third revolution. *Am. J. Orthopsy.,* **34**:1105-1115, 1964.

14. HOBBS, N. Helping disturbed children: psychological and ecological strategies. *Amer. Psychol.,* **21**(12), 822-833, 1966.

15. _____. Project re-ed: new ways of helping emotionally disturbed children. In *Crisis in child mental health: challenge for the 1970's,* Report of the Joint Commission on Mental Health of Children. New York: Harper and Row, 1969, 310-312.

16. FEINSTEIN, ALVAN R. *Clinical judgment.* Baltimore, Maryland: The Williams and Wilkins Co., 1967.

17. DEWEY, JOHN, and BENTLEY, ARTHUR. *Knowing and the known.* Boston, Mass.: Beacon Press, 1949.

18. FISH, BARBARA. Drug therapy in child psychiatry: psychological aspects. *Comp. Psychiat.,* **1**:55-61, 1960.

19. FISH, B., SHAPIRO, T., and CAMPBELL, M. Long term prognosis and response of schizophrenic children to drug therapy: a controlled study of trifluoperazine. *Am. J. Psychiat.,* **123**:32-39, 1966.

20. FISH, B. Drug use in psychiatric disorders of children: drug therapy supplement. *Am. J. Psychiat.,* **124**:31-36, 1968.

21. RIMLAND, BERNARD. *Infantile autism: the syndrome and its implication for a neural theory of behavior.* New York: Appleton-Century-Crofts, Division of Meredith Publishing Co., 1964.

21a. _____. On objective diagnosis of infantile autism. An unpublished paper sent to author. Intended for prior distribution to a working group in England.

22. TREFERT, DAROLD A. Epidemiology of infantile autism. *Archives of General Psychiatry,* **22**(5), 431-438, May 1970.

23. HESTON, LEONARD L. The genetics of schizophrenic and schizoid disease. *Science,* **167**:249-255, Jan. 16, 1970.

24. BOWLBY, JOHN. *Attachment and loss.* Vol. 1: *Attachment.* New York: Basic Books, Inc., 1969.

25. SZUREK, S. A. Review of John Bowlby's *Attachment and loss,* Vol. 1: *Attachment. Am. J. of Orthopsychiatry,* **40**(3), 531-534, April 1970.

26. STANTON, ALFRED H., and SCHWARTZ, MORRIS S. The management of a type of institutional participation in mental illness. *Psychiatry,* **12**:13-26, 1949.

27. TIETZE, TRUDE. A study of mothers of schizophrenic patients. *Psychiatry,* **12**:55-65, 1949.

SECTION TWO

SETTING, INTAKE, EVALUATION, AND CLINICAL PHENOMENA

INTRODUCTION

The therapeutic process in a particular setting or facility in either inpatient or outpatient child psychiatric care begins with the first contacts with the family and patient, and continues through intake and evaluative phases to the clinical treatment stage. These aspects of the process are described in the following four chapters.

An effort is made to delineate the problems of the child and family in order to understand the meaning of the request for inpatient care in the light of the current degree of family equilibrium and the present crisis and its historical development. The intake procedure is both diagnostic, evaluative, and potentially therapeutic, whether or not the child does become an inpatient. The various aspects of the evaluative procedure itself both expands and defines the clinical problem of the child and his family, carries forward, and in a measure defines the therapeutic potential of the family.

When admission is desired by the family, offered by the staff, and accepted by the family, the therapeutic dynamic of the evaluation merges with the more systematic program of therapy. The latter, of course, continues to deepen the understanding of the psychopathology, its genesis in the past, and its manifestations in the present, and tests the reintegrative potential or prognosis.

The whole process thus provides data not only for or against the original hypothesis, but also for any reformulation or modification of it necessitated by the results of the clinical experiment with the particular family.

CHAPTER 4

A HISTORICAL DESCRIPTION OF THE PROGRAM

Maleta J. Boatman, M.D.

EDITORS' NOTE, 1970

The papers included in this volume were written at various times over a period of more than twenty years. Each refers to some aspect of or to some point in the continuous development of the same in-patient unit for psychotic children. Details have been condensed or omitted wherever the description of such facets as the setting or the patient population were background rather than an integral part of the ideas being presented. The deleted material is combined here. This has reduced, although not eliminated, the inevitable repetitions. It has also given us opportunity to emphasize the unitary and con-stant nature of the principles underlying every segment of the work despite the sequential changes that affected it or were effected by it.

INTRODUCTION

The 20-bed psychiatric ward for children was one of the outstanding features of the Langley Porter Clinic when the Department of Institutions of the State of California dedicated its new 100-bed State Hospital in San Francisco next door to the affiliated University of California Medical Center on February 13, 1943 [1]. The presence of such a ward in this modern training, research, and community service center may have been largely due to the vital role played in its establishment by the respected pediatrician Dr. Langley Porter, Dean Emeritus of the University of California Medical School. The inclusion of a Children's Service was certainly due to the fact that the child guidance movement was at its height throughout the country. The Commonwealth Fund made a generous $15,000 annual grant to the University Department of Psychiatry, which permitted the immediate hiring of a recently standardized [in 1943] child guidance clinic team of psychiatrist director, psychologist and social worker, and a secretary to help them. The rest of the staff and supporting services for children were to be provided through State Civil Service positions in enriched State Hospital patterns similar to those in the clinical areas planned for adult outpatients and inpatients. By law, the Clinic's Medical Superintendent was also Professor and Head of the Department of Psychiatry of the University of California School of Medicine. He alone had actual dual positions and the responsibility for dealing with any conflicting interests between the two sponsoring institutions with the help of a Board of Trustees if he should need them. [1]

It is interesting to note that because of the great personnel shortage produced by World War II, few of the wards were opened immediately. Nonetheless, in the first five months over 12 percent of the 83 patients admitted to the hospital were between ages nine and 20 and 46 of the 225 outpatients were children under age 18.

Such was the beginning of the present 12-bed children's ward of the Children's Service of the Langley Porter Neuropsychiatric Institute of the State of California Department of Mental Hygiene, affiliated with the University of California at San Francisco. The subject of this chapter is what has happened on that Children's Ward in the intervening twenty-seven years during which its auspices were renamed. Perhaps the shift in the value of $15,000 may also reflect the degree of the external changes that have affected the program.

UNDERLYING CONCEPTS

Much of the remainder of this volume is concerned with the elaboration of various of the questions and ideas on which the staff's work has been based. It is difficult, however, to discuss even the more objective elements of the program without some brief mention of certain of the concepts that have been operating since very early. These were concepts about clinical work that the Director of the Children's Service, Dr. S. A. Szurek, brought with him in 1946 from his training and from his experiences in children's work in Chicago before the Second World War [2-4; see Chapter 7].

The basic idea was that perhaps all disordered behavior of childhood not definitively stemming from identifiable somatic disease or defect might have its genesis and its maintenance in the child's early and continuing

---

[1] This responsibility was later shared with the Associate Superintendent.

experience with the conflictful attitudes of the important adults in his life, usually his parents. Such conflicts in the adults would stem from their own childhood experience about the impulses characteristic for the maturational age of the child at the time he developed his difficulties. Should the child have identifiable disease or defect, the degree to which his behavior was also emotionally disturbed might result from the degree of conflict he experienced with meaningful adults about his somatic problems.

If this assumption were true, then other concepts could be formulated. First, even the psychotic degrees of disorder in children might be reduced by psychotherapeutic methods. Second, concomitant psychotherapeutic work with the child's parents might be an additional factor in the outcome. Third, every interpersonal experience that the child and parents had with any staff member had a potential therapeutic value. Fourth, this therapeutic potential of every staff-family contact would require a group of staff persons who were free, or at least becoming free, of similar conflicts from their own childhood [5, 6; see also Chapter 9]. Fifth, some ongoing methods for reducing any developing intrastaff tensions would be essential [7-10; see also Chapters 8 and 18].

The Director also believed that providing the most therapeutically effective service possible to disturbed children and their families that could be achieved at any given time would offer both the method and the milieu for training and clinical research.

The effort over the years to utilize these ideas in the context of whatever physical, financial, and administrative realities were present led to the development of a core staff group of the various disciplines, the members of which saw their shared task as one of constant thoughtful observation and scrutiny of their experience. This was their means of learning together, with their concerns being ever focused or refocused on their mutual clinical endeavor.

It seemed that only to the degree that each member of the staff, through personal emotional maturity, really belonged to himself could he effectively belong to the group. The process of staff integration has therefore been perceived as one that allows each member opportunity for individual growth and for reduction of conflict tensions, so that ever-increasing actual communication can occur.

SETTING

The Institute is a four-and-one-half-story reinforced concrete building facing a very busy street. It is situated at the easternmost end of the ever-increasing row of high buildings that comprise the University Medical

Center. As they rise higher and closer together over the years, they increase the effect described by one architect as a wind-tunnel channeling the usually cold, often foggy or rainy, Pacific Ocean air currents in the Institute's direction. The continuous construction interests some children but also produces a very high noise level. Behind the Institute rises a very steep hill covered with a beautiful eucalyptus forest replete with patches of poison oak.

The ward's small fenced-in playground is separated from the building by a rather hazardous driveway, but has a lovely large pine tree. Some playground equipment was installed about 1952. In 1963 it was possible to reconstruct the playground with more carefully planned storage, equipment, and surfacing, including a raised fire pit for outdoor cooking, a grassy plot, some bushes to hide in and dig under, running water, tanbark under swings and slide, a sand box, and a large cement oval for roller-skating and wheel toys. It has not yet been possible to install an easily accessible toilet, although one trial was made at renting a chemical one of the kind used on construction jobs. Since 1961, there has also been a roofed area surrounded by a high fence, shared by all wards and quite suitable for some ward activities.

The entire medical center is located in a middle-class residential neighborhood with typical San Francisco wall-to-wall homes. It is slowly acquiring more apartment and rooming houses. It is served by a public bus and nearby street car. Parking is crowded and presents a major problem for parents, staff, students, and visitors.

Several blocks down the continuation of the steep hill is Golden Gate Park. Its many green acres include a large children's playground, a shallow lake with boats to rent and half-wild ducks to feed, as well as museums, a planetarium, and an aquarium. The swimming pool at the University Student Union is available to the ward about once a week. In recent years, the Institute station wagon or state cars have been available about once a week when outings at greater distances were deemed important.

Because it was very innovative of the planners of the Institute to include a children's ward at all, they may have had little in the way of others' experience to help them. Perhaps they and the architects had visisted some of the few units for neurologically handicapped children. Whatever the reasons, the physical ward has not been the program's greatest asset. It occupies one wing of approximately 5,000 square feet on the fourth floor of the Institute's roughly L-shaped building [11]. It shares this top clinical floor with an adult ward originally used for neurosurgical patients, and with the X-ray department and operating room. With the addition of a building annex in 1961, the adult ward was placed farther down the hall. Part of the intervening space became available for play therapy rooms more convenient than the outpatient ones in the ground-floor basement area. A small schoolroom off the ward was also obtained at this time. An Institute-wide recreation room with built-in kitchen was developed and became frequently available to the children.

The front door opens into a wide corridor that cuts centrally through most of the ward. Four open dormitory areas widen the immediate access area and have a small storage room and a glassed in "nurses' station" partially separating them from each other. In recent years this has been used as the daytime office of the ward clerk and as the communication center for the children and staff. Schedules and pictures are scotch-taped to the glass for display and easy reference. The originally widely scattered bathing, toileting, and dressing areas were consolidated in 1962 into a bathing-dressing-locker room at the far end of the hall.

Opening off the hall are the various living areas: a large play room with screened porch, currently also used as a nursery school area; a dining-room used also as a schoolroom; a small sitting room; a utility and examining room; several converted toy storage areas; one side room used for obtaining privacy with a disturbed or physically ill child; and a nurses' charting and coffee room, long ago converted from its original use as a "continuous-tub" room. There is a laundry room and a staff psychiatrist's office off the locker room. Three psychiatrists' offices are off the ward's small entry hall. Other staff offices are scattered throughout the building, from the basement to the small fifth-floor "interns' quarters."

Meals arrive from a central kitchen by hot cart. They are currently served family style to small groups of children in whatever has become identified as their area of the ward [12; see also Chapter 17].

A small janitorial closet is used by both ward staff and Institute janitors. Ward housekeeping has been most satisfactory during those periods when one specific janitor was assigned and became familiar with the children and the program's special needs. Some clean-up and furniture rearranging related to activities is always the responsibility of the staff and the children.

Occupational therapy activities may occur in the Institute's Rehabilitation Therapies Department. For the past ten years, it has been considered preferable to provide most of these activities in the children's own areas rather than in facilities intended for adults [14; see also Chapter 15].

Other generally used spaces and services shared by all the Institute include administration areas, record room, library, clinical laboratory, X-ray and electronencephalography rooms, and outpatient reception areas. All the consultative services of the Medical Center are available as needed.

The ward has recently been redecorated with lighter, brighter colors. The corridor floor is vinyl and permits roller-skating, hopscotch, and tricycle riding in the middle of the ward. A molding was installed that permits children and staff to hang bulletin boards or other decorations flexibly. With the reduced census of twelve, there has been room to place a small table, a sturdy comfortable chair, and a chest of drawers in each of the four dormitory areas. On order are trundle beds, which will free more floor space for active daytime play; this will further facilitate helping each child gain a feeling of his own bed and his own drawer for treasures within his own group's space.

Other means to make the space more suitable and inviting to young children have been sought and tried. Murals have been painted on the walls several times. Half-doors have been installed where it seemed helpful for ventilation or for intra-ward communication. Some intercom units have been installed to reduce group disruption when one staff member needs to talk to another. Plexiglas window panels were placed low enough in most doors that children could see through them.

There is usually a pleasant feeling when one enters the ward these days; over the years we have learned a great deal about what not to do in planning such a unit. Most importantly, the staff and children find the separation of the ward and the outdoor play space an insurmountable handicap to many aspects of their work.

WARD CENSUS

The 1943 stated census of twenty children apparently included a nursery of four cribs that was never implemented. The functioning census was sixteen until early in 1955. At that time, the Department of Mental Hygiene reviewed its facilities and decided, using the State Hospital figure of fifty square feet per child, that the ward had usable bed-space for only fifteen. Following the incorporation of one side room in the reconstruction of the ward bathing area in 1961, the Institute's administration agreed to a functioning reduction to fourteen patients. Because of space and numbers of personnel and trainees, the Children's Service had been proposing a reduction to ten children. This was never officially requested, but there was concurrence that up to half the population could be day-patients. When the census was again reviewed on January 31, 1964, it was officially set at the current number of twelve. As part of the State Hospital system, the Service has been expected to keep the ward filled to its stated capacity at all times.

Factors Influencing Admissions

Admissions are limited to residents of California and are voluntary. There are no eligibility requirements or restrictions as to race, religion, or income. The fees are set on a sliding scale based on each family's ability to pay. They range from nothing to whatever is figured as current cost to the state per patient day. This latter figure is usually comparable with current private hospital costs, and has seldom been charged.

Within these broad limits, decisions regarding admissions, length of stay, and discharge have been entirely the responsibility of the Children's Service Staff. Using clinical criteria based on their therapeutic concepts, they have admitted children under twelve whose parents or parent surrogates were willing and able to participate in a collaborative psychotherapeutic program. No child has been refused merely on the basis of severity or troublesomeness of his symptoms, including physical disability, if it was considered that hospitalization in this setting and program was indicated for his emotional disorder.

The interplay of six major factors has determined which kind of child the staff felt the program was suited for at any particular time. These factors are: (a) the kind and amount of space in the facility; (b) the inclusion of parental persons in the therapeutic effort; (c) the needs and available resources of the community; (d) the staff's interest in childhood psychosis; (e) the effects of mixing children of divergent ages or disorders; and (f) the number and skill of the available staff persons.

Over the years there have always been two or three times as many boys as girls in both the outpatient and inpatient parts of the program. This reflects the pattern of referrals from the community. Other programs throughout the country report the same experience.

Admissions prior to and soon after 1946 included more impulsive and neurotic children than withdrawn children [7-8, 11, 13]. Before her resignation early in 1946, the first Director had arranged for the admission of several psychotic children, but urgent referrals for impulsive and neurotic children continued to be the order of the day. It was soon apparent that the amount of space was partly relative to its occupants' need and ability to move. Sixteen fast-moving, impulsive children, often boys ages seven to thirteen, with action as their primary mode of anxiety-reduction or avoidance surely filled the space fuller than another group might have. In addition, the exit to the outdoors was by way of the Institute's then-solitary elevator or by an echoing cement ramp. Any spacious area could be reached only by passing either newly planted shrubs or the University research animal cages, and necessitated a race either up or down a hill too steep for even young nurses to manage with ease.

The new Director gradually succeeded in helping the Service's staff more frequently involve parents and community resources actively in treatment planning and participation; it was possible to achieve this oftener with parents of impulsive children, or to clarify sooner that they preferred an alternate kind of program in which their children remained home and were seen as outpatients.

The Director's experience confirmed that it was effective therapy for both child and parents for the staff sincerely to invite parental participation in decisions regarding the child's therapy. With this approach, the parents of neurotic children often chose to have their child home and frequently became involved in the therapeutic process rapidly. The Director's impression, in that day of very scarce psychiatric service, was that it was frequently feasible and that it often supported the strengths available in a family to utilize their home and their community resources as fully as possible. Consultation with a school or agency frequently increased this probability and added a bit to the development of community skills. The end result was that it was usually contraindicated to hospitalize impulsive or neurotic children. In light of today's trends in psychiatry, it seems hard to believe how severely he was criticized for all this—from how many sources for how many reasons.

Severely neurotic and psychotic children tended to remain on the ward for longer periods of time, and vacancies became infrequent. It was at such a point that the staff discovered with the family of one young autistic boy that unexpectedly impressive improvements could occur with outpatient therapy (such therapy had been started while the child was waiting for a ward vacancy; the vacancy was refused when it became available). In view of the required crowding of the ward with sixteen children who were predominantly of latency or early teen age, it began to seem unwise to admit the younger, less disturbed psychotic children. In addition, children of wide age ranges and very diverse behavior disorders did not seem to do well together. It was also more difficult for one staff to provide the range of activities needed by children of different ages and capabilities.

The exploration of various psychotherapeutic methods of treating psychotic children with family participation interested the staff. It was therefore not as dismaying to them as it might otherwise have been to find that hospitalization in this setting seemed contraindicated for all but difficult diagnostic problems and the most profoundly disturbed of the psychotic children seen. Thus by April 1951, a study of residential treatment of emotionally disturbed children by the Child Welfare League of America reported that as a group the children on this ward appeared more disturbed in social functioning and reality adjustment than at any other center seen [11].

Perhaps the conclusions drawn from the interaction of the aforementioned five factors influencing admissions could or would have been different had there been more sufficient numbers of experienced professional staff persons available to work with the hospitalized children. The Director, however, then as subsequently, placed more emphasis on the purely clinical factors than on the given ones of how much space and how much staff was available. The staff and those responsible for the distribution of personnel throughout the Institute sometimes responded to this with the feeling that he was expecting the impossible. He saw his job as that of helping staff members to do the very best therapeutic work they could at any given time, while learning together how to do it better. The ward personnel began to learn that to postpone trying what was difficult, because they did not yet have answers as to "how," actually interfered with discovering how to do it.

The Director did acknowledge that a staff free or *becoming free* of internalized conflicts was essential to such a difficult endeavor. It was for this reason as well as for meeting the Institute's major task of training that the Director devoted almost all his available time and energies to staff development and practically none to efforts to modify the plant, the financing, or the administrative structure. His only request along the latter line had been insistence that in the Children's Services outpatient and inpatient units function together, rather than separately, as in the adult services. He saw hospitalization as only one facet of a child's and family's therapy, which started before and continued after the hospital experience. Again, with today's ready use of the concepts of primary therapists and vertical staffing in treatment centers, it is hard to believe how idiosyncratic his firm insistence on this principle as necessary to the development of an adequate treatment team seemed to many outside the Service.

STAFF COMPOSITION

After 1948, the Children's Ward staff was more or less the same in its composition for a number of years. The clinical program was under the direction of the child psychiatrists, namely the Director and an Assistant Director, whose positions were financed by the University when the Commonwealth Fund withdrew at the end of five years. One or two full-time two-year child psychiatry trainees were available from University-supported grants or affiliations. The basic ward care staff of ten to fifteen persons from the Institute's nursing service included one senior psychiatric nurse in charge of the ward, nine professionally trained psychiatric nurses, and five non-professional workers. There was also one elementary school teacher from the special education department of the city school system. One occupational therapist contributed some time. The clinical psychologist and several psychiatric social workers participated in both in- and outpatient work, as did the child psychiatrists. Social work students, psychology fellows, psychiatric residents, and pediatric residents were involved in the inpatient work less often than in the outpatient work.

By 1950 the Children's Service had a small core of staff persons of the various disciplines (including nursing) who saw treatment, research, and training as interrelated and inseparable aspects of their mutual clinical endeavor. Their work had begun to find focus in the development and study of psychotherapeutic methods with children and families. A major emphasis of the work was, and would continue to be for the next decade, the development of a program in which every aspect of the inpatient care of psychotic children would be a precise and integral part of the total psychotherapeutic work.

PATIENT POPULATION

During these middle years (1950-1964) the population of the ward was made up almost entirely of the most severely disturbed of the many psychotic preadolescents seen by the staff. These children showed serious and persistent psychotic behavior at all levels of functioning. They were extremely sensitive even to apparently minor disappointments and frustrations. Their reaction was often profound withdrawal or destructive rage toward themselves and others—head-banging, kicking, biting, scratching, and tearing clothing. Their manneristic behavior included such isolated activities as rocking, twiddling objects, masturbating, aimless pacing and running, flapping arms and hands, and standing in one particular area in a fixed position. They often repeated certain acts over and over, such as retracing steps or touching, licking, or smelling certain objects. They had many difficulties in eating, sleeping, and elimination. These included near-starvation, day-and-nighttime wetting and soiling, smearing, and retention of feces for days. Their communication was usually nonverbal, distorted, and difficult to comprehend. Even their noises were often loud, monotonous, and inappropriate in affect. Although sometimes disconcertingly sporadic and shifting in its manifestation, such symptomatic behavior persisted almost continuously in one form or another throughout each child's day.

Although children were still always admitted under the age of twelve, they were allowed to remain on the ward into adolescence when progress, however slow, was promising. Where the therapists stayed on the psychiatric staff after their training periods, patients were seen into adulthood.

Two very small and very immature young women, treated since childhood, stayed on or returned to the ward program as their families and the staff worked hard together to consolidate and increase the improvements that had occurred.

CHANGES IN STAFF AND PATIENT POPULATION

During these years the author, as Assistant Director of the Service, was delegated primary responsibility for the day-to-day clinical operation of the Service. Another staff psychiatrist, I. N. Berlin, assisted greatly with the development of training and research and of consultation methods [15-17]. It then seemed feasible to devote some of the staff resources to improving the patient census, the size of staff, the financing of the work, and the availability of research help. With the preparation in 1955 of a request for a grant from the Ford Foundation to expand the research on childhood schizophrenia, the senior psychiatric staff joined in the so-called era of "grantsmanship." This grant was not obtained, but the writing of the request further clarified and consolidated their ideas.

In 1956 additional child psychiatry faculty and full-time trainees, four each year, were regularly assigned from the Institute's Graduate Training Grant from the National Institute of Mental Health (NIMH). The Rehabilitation Therapies Department was also able to assign one occupational therapist one-third time to the Service. In that same year the Nursing Service was able to reassign positions so that fifteen-and-one-half instead of ten to fourteen nursing personnel were available to the ward most weeks. The Children's Ward began making annual budget requests for at least three additional nurses. It was never possible for these to be granted.

It was at this point that it became more truly possible for the ward staff members to work so closely together in their planning and function that their activities with the children often dovetailed or overlapped. Psychotherapist, nurse, occupational therapist, and elementary teacher all collaborated closely. One or several psychotherapists continued to see each family. The parents were seen at least twice a week, sometimes in two individual sessions and sometimes in one individual and one conjoint session with the spouse. Each child was seen at least twice a week in play therapy. Nurses continued to find much of their role with the child centering around self-care activities. They also were in frequent contact with the parents. The occupational therapist offered various craft and recreational activities to groups of children. The teacher saw each child for some period most days and assisted him in readiness or academic work at his level. All of them sometimes worked together around one or more of these activities. Each saw as his goal the need to behave at all times in the precise manner that might help the child to reduce his disorder, i.e., his internalized conflict, however it manifested itself at a given moment or in a given activity, and provide opportunities for the child's development of more integrated behavior at whatever level was timely for his own particular maturational and emotional capacities. Each attempted, in all aspects of his work, to discriminate his own role in the child's experience so clearly that this in no way interfered with the child's relationship to his own parental persons, with the work of the individual psychotherapist of the child or parent, or with any other staff person's contribution to the therapeutic environment [18; see also Chapter 11].

In 1956 the Director and Assistant Director participated in a conference on inpatient psychiatric treatment for children and its year-long preparatory commission on treatment [19]. This and the Assistant Director's earlier work with a committee of the San Francisco Community Chest about residential treatment [20] led directly into careful concentration on further development of the ward nursing staff. The author and the Superintendent of Nursing Services prepared and submitted to NIMH, with the help of all the senior staff of psychiatry and nursing, an application for a Mental Health Project Grant entitled "Nursing in Hospital Psychiatric Therapy for Children" [18]. It resulted in four years (1960-1963) of support for a study of definition and attainment of skill by psychiatric nurses.[2] During this time it also provided opportunities to explore the results of more intensive nursing care and more nurse participation in the total ward program. From 1959 to 1962 the ward staff also participated in the initial establishment of and training in a Masters and Post-Masters Specialty Program in Child Psychiatry in the University of California School of Nursing. Some ward time was available after 1958 from the nurse included in the NIMH grant-supported Training Project in Mental Retardation obtained by the Children's Service.

Following the reorganization of the Institute's administrative staff, the first Department of Mental Hygiene position for a staff psychiatrist was granted the Children's Service in July 1958. This freed the Assistant Director to devote more time to the inpatient work for a few years. It then seemed possible to devote some staff resources to trying to improve the plant. Minor reconstruction plans were submitted that culminated in the 1961 improvements already mentioned. At this point the staff applied to NIMH for inclusion in the new Research Center Program in order to follow up on reconstruction plans and program ideas evolving from the above experiences. This ward was not one of those chosen. A speech

---

[2]NIMH grants OM-234 and No. 5-R11-MH234.

therapist was added to the ward staff, and the occupational therapist became a full-time staff member. Full-time psychiatric trainees increased to three each year, for a total of six.

In 1963 it was apparent to the staff that it was unlikely that they could go much further in the needed steps toward more available staff, fewer children, and an improved plant. Under these circumstances they had tested their work as far as it seemed practical to go with very disturbed children. They also wanted to take the next step of trying what they had learned about a therapeutic activity program with younger, less disturbed psychotic children. They began to work with families then in treatment toward the discharge of all children over twelve. More young day-care patients were admitted, and almost all children went home every weekend. This allowed the more nearly desired concentration of ward staff for the treatment program during the week.

In 1967 the Institute's Evening Nursing Supervisors' positions were reassigned to specific ward programs. This addition of an experienced full-time nurse supervisor to the Children's Ward staff was helpful; although it did necessitate more rotation of nurses rather than non-professional workers through the evening and night shifts to provide professional care to patients at all hours. In February 1968 a second teacher was assigned from the public schools under California's educational program for Educationally Handicapped pupils.

The last shifts in patient population occurred about two years ago. Some children were recommended for discharge before age twelve if therapeutic progress was minimal and sporadic, particularly as regards emergence of speech or effective parent involvement. The staff's experience was extensive enough for them to feel relatively sure that work carried out in this setting with trainees would probably not help a child and family with this magnitude of difficulty by age twelve. Newly admitted children were accepted at as early an age as possible—usually close to age three.

CURRENT PROGRAM

At present the staff is obtaining considerable satisfaction from their work. They are continuing to test and to teach what they think they have learned, but in situations that permit readier feedback than previously. The work is still strenuous, but it is possible to put more emphasis on statistical review of past data, improved documentation of new data, and experimentation with the incorporation of new methods into the same rigorously followed application of psychotherapeutic concepts.

In very recent years the degree of integration in the total ward staff has been stable enough to permit increasing the use of ward volunteers without too much program disruption. One has been as young as eight years old; others have been high school or college students.

It has been possible to include overnight camping trips in the children's spring program for several years.

In 1965 the Mental Retardation Training Program's staff acquired a clinical psychologist experienced in both psychotherapeutic and operant conditioning methods. Subsequently it was possible for him, with other staff members, to test the staff's assumption that these operant techniques were not necessarily alien to the previously-sought precisely therapeutic behavioral responses on the part of the staff members to specific behavior of the children. They were also able to demonstrate statistically that some of the children's aversive behavior was motivational in origin [21].

Recently it has been recommended to parents that children who had been in the day-program several years without being ready for outpatient work become twenty-four hour patients during the week. In the spring of 1970 it was possible to free staff time to offer the long-desired ward parents' therapy group for the first time. It was offered on an entirely voluntary basis.

It has sometimes appeared to new staff members, trainees, or outsiders that the Children's Ward staff sets certain policies and applies them arbitrarily. It has been interesting in working with them to have the opportunity to help them understand that this has not been the case. Precisely applied principles may frequently result in similar decisions under similar conditions. Applied in changed conditions, different decisions may occur: for example, it was not thought that day-care was better than twenty-four hour care, but it had frequently been thought to be the best possible program for some children at a given time.

This period may be the lull before the storm. Already the winds of change are blowing from State Department of Mental Hygiene reorganization plans and from knowledge of impending NIMH grant reductions. No one knows what the child advocacy system may bring. But the present is the current "particular time," and the staff is trying to use it precisely.

REFERENCES

1. THE LANGLEY PORTER CLINIC. *Statistical report of the department of institutions of the State of California for the year ending June 30, 1943.* Sacramento: California State Printing Office, 1944, pp. 91-94.

2. SZUREK, S. A., Critique of *Residential treatment of emotionally disturbed children* by Joseph H. Reid and Helen R. Hagan. New York: The Child Welfare League of America, Inc., 1952, 19-24.

3. BOATMAN, MALETA J., and SZUREK, S. A. A clinical study of childhood schizophrenia. In Don D. Jackson (Ed.), *The etiology of schizophrenia.* New York: Basic Books, Inc., 1960.

4. SZUREK, S. A. Childhood schizophrenia: psychotic episodes and psychotic maldevelopment. *Am. J. Orthopsychiat.,* **26**:519-543, 1956.

5. _____ . Some observations on the dynamics of staff interaction in hospital psychiatric treatment of children. *Am. J. Orthopsychiat.,* **17**:652-664, 1947.

6. _____ . Remarks on training for psychotherapy. *Am. J. Orthopsychiat.,* **19**:36-51, 1949. Reprinted in S. A. Szurek & I. N. Berlin (Eds.), *Training in therapeutic work with children.* Vol. 2, the Langley Porter Child Psychiatry Series. Palo Alto, Calif.: Science and Behavior Books, 1967.

7. SZUREK, S. A., SHEIMO, S. L., and PAYNTER, JANE. Problems encountered in dealing with handicapped and emotionally disturbed children. *Am. J. Occup. Ther.,* **3**:303-307, 1949.

8. SHEIMO, S. L., PAYNTER, JANE, and SZUREK, S. A. Problems of staff interaction with spontaneous group formations on a children's psychiatric ward. *Am. J. Orthopsychiat.,* **19**:599-611, 1949.

9. SZUREK, S. A. The family and the staff in hospital psychiatric therapy of children. *Am. J. Orthopsychiat.,* **21**:597-611, 1951.

10. _____ . Some lessons from efforts at psychotherapy with parents. *Am. J. Psychiat.,* **109**:296-302, 1952.

11. REID, JOSEPH H., and HAGAN, HELEN R. A descriptive study of the program of the Langley Porter Clinic, Children's Inpatient Service, in *Residential treatment of emotionally disturbed children.* New York: The Child Welfare League of America, Inc., 1952.

12. MEJIA, BERTA, and PATTERSON, RELLA B. Lunchtime routine designed to help psychotic children. *Food talks: bulletin of nutrition services,* Department of Mental Hygiene, State of California, April 1962.

13. BERLIN, I. N., BOATMAN, MALETA J., SHEIMO, S. L., and SZUREK, S. A.. Adolescent alternation of anorexia and obesity. *Am. J. Orthopsychiat.,* **21**:387-419, 1951. Reprinted in Geo. Gardner (Ed.), *Case studies in childhood emotional disabilities.* Vol. I. New York: American Orthopsychiatric Assn., Inc., 1953 and in S. A. Szurek & I. N. Berlin (Eds.), *Psychosomatic disorders and mental retardation in children.* Vol. 3, the Langley Porter Child Psychiatry Series. Palo Alto, Calif.: Science and Behavior Books, 1968.

14. ENG, MARIETTA C., O.T.R., and BOATMAN, MALETA J. The occupational therapy program on a ward for psychotic children. *Proceedings of the American Occupational Therapy Association 1960 annual conference.* New York: The American Occupational Therapy Association, pp. 33-36.

15. SZUREK, S. A., and BERLIN, I. N. Elements of psychotherapeutics with the schizophrenic child and his parents. *Psychiat.,* **19**:1-9, 1956.

16. BERLIN, I. N. Some learning experiences as psychiatric consultant in the schools. *Mental Hygiene,* **40**:215-236, 1956. Reprinted in S. A. Szurek & I. N. Berlin (Eds.), *Learning and its disorders.* Vol. 1, the Langley Porter Child Psychiatry Series. Palo Alto, Calif.: Science and Behavior Books, 1965.

17. _____. Some implications of ego psychology for the supervisory process. *Am. J. Psychotherapy,* **14**:536-544, 1960.

18. BOATMAN, MALETA J., PAYNTER, JANE, and PARSONS, CORINNE. Nursing in hospital psychiatric therapy for psychotic children. *Am. J. Orthopsychiat.,* **32**:808-817, 1962.

19. ROBINSON, J. F. et al. *Psychiatric inpatient treatment of children.* Washington: Am. Psychiatric Assoc., 1957.

20. BOATMAN, MALETA J., BYRON, HELEN V., DE VRIES, ROBERT G., and GALLAGHER, URSULA. Some basic characteristics of à residential center. Section II. *Residential treatment for emotionally disturbed children.* Community Chest of San Francisco, 1954, 6-27.

21. MORRISON, DELMONT, MILLER, DALE, and MEJIA, BERTA. Comprehension and negation of verbal communication in autistic children. (In press.)

CHAPTER 5

INTAKE FOR INPATIENT CARE*

Irving Philips, M.D., Mary B. Davis, P.S.W.,
Maleta J. Boatman, M.D.

In our work with the child and his family, we consider that inpatient
psychiatric treatment is always an incident in the total therapeutic work
with the family, which begins before and continues throughout and often
after hospitalization. This paper describes how children are admitted for
inpatient psychiatric treatment to the Children's Service of the Langley
Porter Neuropsychiatric Institute. "Selection" in the ordinary sense of
the word, in that the staff chooses its patients by definite criteria or
policy, does not apply to what we try to accomplish with the child and
his family. No preadolescent child is excluded from inpatient psychiatric
treatment because of the nature or severity of his disorder if staff time
for treatment is available and a vacancy exists.

The Children's Service consists of both inpatient and outpatient facilities. The inpatient psychiatric treatment unit is a fifteen-bed ward for
children—both boys and girls—usually under twelve years of age. Ordinarily, one child is on the ward for a brief diagnostic study and the remaining
fourteen are there for long-term psychotherapy and often stay from three
to six years, the average being three and one-half years. The major part of
the inpatient psychotherapeutic work as well as the diagnostic studies is
done by advanced child psychiatry trainees who remain for a two-year
period of supervised career training in child psychiatry.

Our approach to the treatment of emotional problems of childhood is
through concomitant psychotherapeutic work with the child and his parents. The psychotherapeutic goal is the resolution of internalized conflicts
in each family member.

---

*Unpublished, 1960.

Selection and preparation of patients are aspects of the same process, which begins with the initial contact, whether it be by letter, telephone call, or personal inquiry. Referrals come largely from other medical and social welfare facilities. Since the severity of the disorder in the child or in his family is no bar to admission, the requests for service for psychotic children have increased.

In earlier years we considered hospitalization essential in the treatment of severely disturbed children. At a time when there was lack of space on our inpatient service, we hesitantly tried outpatient therapy for some children. After a period of outpatient therapy some patients had so improved that neither the staff nor the family desired hospitalization for the child when a vacancy became available. We thus found that outpatient therapy for the severely disturbed child is possible and therapeutic movement occurs. As a result of such experiences, we cannot with any surety predict which children might benefit most from hospitalization. Therefore, decision for inpatient therapy is made only after a trial of outpatient study and evaluation and if inpatient space and staff time are available. In only one instance do we recommend inpatient psychiatric study: for those children in whom a diagnostic problem may involve impersonal or purely somatic factors that complicate the behavioral manifestations, and then only to expedite the physiologic studies and to better observe the child's behavior.

Most of our admissions are children whose disorder may be classified among the psychotic reactions of childhood. We have, however, admitted children with phenylpyruvic oligophrenia, postencephalitic and post-meningitic disorders, epilepsy, and other forms of neurologic disease if there are diagnostic problems or if an emotional disorder was the paramount problem disrupting the child's development. We rarely admit children with primary neurotic or conduct difficulties. Although discouraged parents of children with the latter disorders sometimes seek placement of the child, they seldom actively request hospitalization except in a desperate effort to solve a crisis. They may, for example, fear their child's continued destructive and disruptive behavior and the resultant criticism from the community. Usually we explain that it is more helpful to see what we can do if the family works with us as outpatients, with the child living at home. Those parents who are ready, however skeptically, to participate in the work often feel relieved to learn that we do not feel it essential or even desirable to the child's welfare for him to be separated from them. Nevertheless, in rare instances, during an acute family crisis, we may hospitalize such a disturbed child, usually for an explicitly stated brief period of study, until the parents in their work with us are able to deal more effectively with themselves and their child.

THE INTAKE PROCESS

The intake process is hard to describe as a separate process. The first contacts with the family may initiate and become an integral part of the psychotherapeutic work. These contacts may have potentially therapeutic influences, although this potential is not always realized.

The process begins with the social worker, who works with the family in several ways: by answering initial inquiries; by interviewing parents at the time of application and again at the time of admission of the child; and by keeping in contact with a family in those instances where there is an interval between the decision for hospitalization and the occurrence of the anticipated vacancy on which the decision was based. All applications are reviewed by a multidiscipline intake staff.

Certain factors of selection operate from the beginning, in the manner and attitude of persons who answer telephones and letters, since it has become obvious that some social workers succeed more consistently than others in making satisfactory plans with parents of very disturbed children. Some parents can decide from telephone conversations about the problems and our available services whether to make an application or to try other resources. In our experience, however, many parents of severely disturbed children ask for help in such negative and distorted ways as to half-invite rejection. Requests may be phrased: "I am calling just to find out how long the waiting list is." Or, "My little boy is three and a half and doesn't talk. I have taken him to a lot of doctors but nobody will help him. Perhaps he needs his tongue clipped." Or, "My doctor told me to call. I don't want any psychiatric treatment, as my husband and I are very happy. Can you tell me the name of a good school?" Thus, the first problem in the process of selection often is to help such parents formulate their requests. By telephone or letter we plan appointments with attention to such details as time, place, and route, taking care to explain why both parents are to come, and whom they will see, and how the fees are set. Regard for these small details often reduces the parents' anxiety about the next steps and conveys an attitude of interest in the family members.

Another aspect of beginning work that may influence the eventual decision about using hospital care or other resources is the hospital's relationship and activity with community agencies and professional persons who know the child and family and have recommended psychiatric help. We inform them about our available services and ask them to discuss this with the parents, but we also ask the parents to apply directly for the appointments, for reasons of convenience in planning time and in recognition of parental responsibility. In these early contacts with referring agencies we tentatively plan to continue to exchange pertinent information, with the parents' consent, and to share responsibility about further work, so that these persons, without waiting for a clinic recommendation, will continue their help to the family.

Now for an illustration of some early work with one family that resulted in relatively successful treatment:

Mrs. A. telephoned, first asking if we had received her physician's letter. When we said no, she reacted with immediate anger, saying she would not tolerate getting the "run-around" from us. She wanted inpatient care for her six-year-old son, who seemed deaf although she had been told by a school that he was not. We suggested an appointment and asked that the father come too. She agreed, except to say that he would have to decide.

Later the father called to complain about the inconvenience of coming to the hospital. The social worker checked her calendar with his until they could agree on a time. Because of the fear and anxiety suggested by the parents' loud, angry voices, a special effort was made to offer an appointment within a few days.

At the appointed time the father came alone, explaining, "I want to investigate the place first." He appeared tense and frightened. After some talk about the boy's symptoms, he asked to see the ward. He glanced into the playroom, where a few children were quietly occupied, and said his son was not like these children. He left quickly, saying he would look for assistance nearer home, and the social worker told him he could reapply later if he wanted to talk further about the hospital. The referring doctor, who had called in the meantime, was informed of the father's decision.

Two weeks later the father called, asking for consideration of inpatient care, but said that he could not come in because of his work, and that the hospital knew enough about the case by this time to see that the mother was the important parent involved.

The social worker explained the need to plan with both parents and again offered them an appointment. The parents came and were interviewed together. They asked for treatment only for the child. They said various people had told them that something wrong in the home or in the past lives of the parents "causes disturbed children." They felt that this was not their situation because their marriage was happy and gave them the greatest security they had ever known. They saw their only problem as the difficult behavior of the child, who was disrupting the lives of the whole family and causing the younger brother to become disturbed, too.

The social worker asked the parents to describe the difficulties in more detail, saying that although we had reports from school and doctor, parents know their child best. She also explained that the Children's Service offers help directly to parents in understanding the problems and their meaning to the family members.

No specific questions were asked or suggestions made, but the social worker continued to search for what the parents wanted. They now began to describe in a limited way some things they wished they understood better. They referred to the child's ability to do a few tasks well at times, and their own feelings of frustration and despair at having failed to encourage growth of these abilities. They gave examples of their helpless anger and guilt about being unable to deal with the child's tantrums, cruelty, and negativism. Their talk uncovered, fleetingly, some disagreements between them. They agreed that they had reason to examine the situation further, provided they need make no promises.

The social worker then proceeded with such details as filling out the face sheet: the identifying information about the family make-up and social setting, the financial inquiry regarding a fee for the outpatient interviews, and the approximate charges for hospitalization. The discussion was directed to helping the parents think about themselves and the child and how the placement of one family member away from home would affect everyday details of life for all the family, including the child himself. The interview ended with the parents' plans to return with the child for study. The parents doubted that the child could understand why he was being brought to a hospital. The social worker said that the psychiatrists would talk openly with the child about why his parents were bringing him, with the belief that he could understand at least part of the explanation.

This example shows a common situation wherein parents who blame themselves and each other have become so hopeless, after many fruitless attempts to solve their problems, that they talk very little even to each other about getting help. We believe that interviewing the parents together in the early planning stages may enable them to see that their doubts and fears are mutual. As they then share the experience of the initial inquiry and discussion, they begin to lose their fears about fixing of blame and being judged good or bad, and to see that their participation helps in the analysis of the total and complex situation. They may feel some relief from self-blame from this experience and thus become less hopeless.

Indeed, as parents begin to work together, they may regain some self-respect because of their own efforts to help themselves, to pay what they can, and to retain parental responsibility for decisions. When they feel they have some choice and control over their application, their tensions about the child lessen somewhat, so that they can then attend to his preparation for clinic study.

THE DIAGNOSTIC AND EVALUATIVE STUDY

After the application interview, the family is seen for a psychiatric diagnostic and evaluative study on an outpatient basis, however brief that part of the work may be. This procedure evolved from our early experiences in admitting children directly to the ward because of an urgent request. Sometimes the family withdrew the child from the ward within a day or two and terminated contact with us. We believe that this occurred because of inadequate preparation of the family for hospitalization of the child without examination of their fears and expectations prior to admission. Then, too, a brief period of outpatient work with the family often changed the nature of the application. The exploration of the desire and need for hospitalization, as well as a statement about our inpatient and outpatient services and our willingness to try either one, often result in a reduction of the family's fears and apprehensions. They are then able to arrive at a clearer decision for continued work.

The outpatient study usually consists of three to four weekly visits of the child and his parents. The weekly spacing of interviews allows time for the correlation of findings by various staff members and for each parent to begin to regard his own feelings and behavior in the family situation.

At the start, the psychiatrist sees the parents and the child together to outline in a general way what will occur during the ensuing weeks. The procedures are explained in the presence of the child, regardless of his stage of withdrawal or retardation. The psychiatrist thus sees a clear picture of the family as a whole and how they interact; and the family may feel that they are all working together with the staff to achieve the best solution to their problems.

After this introduction, the interview continues with both parents together. The psychiatrist helps them to give as complete a history of the child's life and illness as is then possible. As the parents come to feel that they are not being criticized or judged, they often begin to speak more freely about their own troubles, including their feelings of guilt, shame, and responsibility. As they are given the opportunity to talk about all aspects of their family, they usually begin to explore some of their feelings about the child and themselves. The psychiatrist tries to explain precisely what services, if any, are available, or the approximate interval before either inpatient or outpatient services will be available.

The psychiatrist also sees the child during this first visit, usually in the playroom. He describes to the child his picture of the child's troubles as recounted by the parents, and obtains the child's reaction to this account. He tries to formulate some impressions about the child's disorder. Later, the psychiatrist makes a complete physical and neurologic examination,

72

and laboratory tests are done. The psychologist evaluates the child as completely as is possible within the limits of the child's testability.

If the question of inpatient psychiatric treatment is raised, the parents and the child are invited to see the ward. The psychiatrist goes to the ward with the parents and their child and introduces them to the charge nurse. The ward program is discussed with them. Parents at this point are frequently apprehensive and often perceive that their expectations of the ward and the program may have been unrealistic. Some become more doubtful about hospitalizing their child. Paradoxically, those parents whose children are most disturbed have few doubts and questions. It is with these families that the engagement in therapy may be most difficult.

In the following interviews each parent is seen individually. The psychiatrist listens to the reactions of each to the tour of the ward. He discusses with them as fully as possible the advantages and disadvantages of inpatient treatment. The advantages are: (a) The child will have frequent psychotherapeutic sessions as well as a therapeutic living experience. (b) The welfare of the family is considered when the disturbed child is an extremely disruptive factor in the home or when the parents seem unable to offer enough and consistent control in the case of the child's progressive, self-destructive, and aggressive behavior. (c) The distance of the home from the clinic may make weekly visits for the child impractical. (d) Inpatient therapy time, but not outpatient therapy, may be available.

Some of the disadvantages of hospital treatment involve the parents' fears and anxieties about separation from the child, their guilty feelings about "abandoning" him, their self-condemnation and fears of possible injury to him during his hospitalization. The psychiatrist may state his impression of how the child may or may not fit into the group of children already on the ward. He questions the admission of a child who has had serious difficulties in previous separations from his parents, with increased symptomatology in either the child or the parents. He also questions the advisability of admitting a child who is improving during the outpatient study. He does not stress in any coercive way the advantages of either outpatient or inpatient therapy, and while he does give his professional opinion, he leaves the final decision to the parents.

One additional factor is considered. In a few instances, after psychiatric study and evaluation that may include a brief period of hospitalization, the history and clinical picture indicate that the parents have for the most part already given up all hope of resolving the problem. We do not at that point offer the parents a choice, but recommend a trial of outpatient therapy first. In our experience with such families, hospitalization increases the parental hopelessness, and real therapeutic engagement of the parents is seldom achieved—or is long delayed—unless it begins before the child is admitted.

In the individual interviews the psychiatrist inquires about each parent's biography. Each is encouraged to speak of his own problems, in order to help him take a more realistic view of himself and to give him some experience in the method and meaning of therapy. As the parent gains confidence that he is a person and that his problems can be understood, he then seems to make a more rational and valid decision than before about what is likely to be useful. In each interview, the psychiatrist reviews his impressions, however tentative, of the prior discussions and examinations, discussing in a noncritical way the possible family difficulties, external and internal, that play a part in the child's behavior. He explains how such difficulties might be wholly or partially reversible if the child were seen for psychotherapeutic interviews and if each parent would try in psychotherapy to see what he might gain for himself. Some families raise questions about working in this way. The psychiatrist then frankly acknowledges that other people in other clinics work differently, but that nevertheless, in his experience this method affords the best results. He asks not that the parent be convinced of the value of this method, but rather that he try it.

A few parents prefer not to work in a therapeutic program that requires their participation. If they do not consent to this way of working, we do not undertake treatment. Thus, the parents may or may not select themselves for continued work. With cumulative experience we find that more parents, both fathers and mothers, begin work with us. If the family desires to seek help elsewhere, the psychiatrist accepts their decision and attempts to be as helpful as he can in facilitating other plans. He informs the family that if they desire further service from us, they are free to reapply at any time.

If the family's problems of living together still seem to them to be intolerable, even after several outpatient interviews, the psychiatrist may agree that inpatient therapy be tried. The child may then be admitted for brief observation, usually for three to six weeks. The psychiatrist explains beforehand what further treatment will be available after the brief hospitalization. If inpatient treatment is desirable, but no bed is available for continued treatment after inpatient evaluation, he usually does not suggest admission of the child, but helps the family explore the possibility of more immediate help in the community. However, when a developing crisis in the family threatens to erupt with increasing destructiveness to the child and family, he may admit the child for study even without the prospect for continued treatment. Such brief studies aid the family in stabilizing their situation and allow them time for considering alternative plans. Often, after a period of hospitalization the family may sense that they can care for their child at home and begin to consider the possibility of outpatient treatment or other plans.

The preparation of the child for admission to the ward takes place during the course of the study, as the family moves toward their decision. The child has seen the ward and met the charge nurse prior to his hospitalization, and the psychiatrist has discussed hospitalization with the child; he will therefore see some familiar faces when he arrives.

We consider the work with the parents to be of equal importance, to help them prepare the child in their own way for living away from home. Parents almost without exception react to hospitalization as if it were condemnation of their ability to care for their child, even though they request hospitalization and the advantages are clearly stated. During the course of the study their ambivalence concerning hospitalization may be somewhat reduced; if, however, the family remains indecisive even at the proposed time for admission, the psychiatrist will offer them further outpatient interviews to reconsider their decision. But, if they feel secure in the step they are taking and feel that they have made a good decision, there is usually a reduction of their guilt and anxiety, and they can give the child some assurance. He in turn senses their attitudes and feels less deserted. At the time the child is admitted to the ward, the same social worker who saw the parents for application will see them again and discuss the final arrangements.

After admission, the study continues in much the same way as described for the outpatient study. By the end of the period of brief hospitalization, all findings have been clearly discussed with the family. Each parent in his own experience with the psychiatrist and hospital staff is more able to formulate for himself what he desires in the way of continued treatment, and what may be most helpful to him and the child.

In conclusion: selection and preparation of children for inpatient psychiatric treatment is part of the total psychotherapeutic work with each family, and is a dynamic process to be understood in relation to the psychotherapeutic goal—the resolution of conflict in each of the parents and the child. All the work is directed toward this end.

CHAPTER 6

PSYCHIATRIC EVALUATION OF THE CHILD*

A. J. Gianascol, M.D.

The psychiatric evaluation of a child includes a psychiatric history, a physical examination, pertinent consultation and psychological testing when indicated, laboratory studies, diagnostic play therapy sessions or interviews with the child, and interviews with the parents.

"Child" as here used includes adolescents. Whereas playroom sessions are used with preadolescents, the interview may be used with older adolescents. In the age group from ten to fourteen, transitional techniques involving both play therapeutic techniques and interviewing may be used, with the interview predominating as the child's age increases.

The evaluation process might better be termed brief service or brief therapy, since it usually is an integrative experience for the family and may occasion symptomatic improvement in the child.

Because of the importance ascribed to the history, the reliability of children's histories as obtained from their parents is first discussed. A suggested summary form for recording the evaluation is then presented and briefly discussed.

THE RELIABILITY OF PARENTS' HISTORIES

The inaccuracy and unreliability of histories obtained from mothers has been demonstrated, beginning with the report of Pyles, Stolz, and Macfarlane [1] on mothers of 252 children who participated in a longitudinal study of development. The mothers' answers to a physician's interview were compared to observations made by a nurse who had visited the home every three months during the first year of the child's

---

*Unpublished.

life. The interview included five questions concerning prenatal and birth history, and five related to the child's development.

There was low agreement between mothers' health during pregnancy and their recall of their health. Only two-thirds of mothers whose deliveries required instruments, and about one-fifth with a record of birth injury, recalled these data. (It was not clear, however, that all mothers had known of these complications.) Recall of birth weight tended to be accurate, with exact agreement in 59 percent; age of the first tooth was accurate in over one-third, whereas recall of the weight at one year was accurate in only 9 percent.

About 50 percent were in exact agreement concerning the age of walking alone. Errors in this and in recalling the eruption of the first tooth were in the direction of precocity.

Two mothers failed to recall illnesses in the child, whereas the records revealed respectively "whooping cough and eczema" and "asthma and several colds." Twenty-eight mothers, whose children's illnesses or physical handicaps were considered as "probably slightly modifying development," failed to mention any illness during the first year.

Haggard, Brekstad, and Skard [2] compared independent observations and mothers' reports with mothers' recollections as much as eight years later, and found that items dealing with attitudinal questions, i.e., anxiety concerning childbirth and preference for a boy or girl, showed less reliability than those involving more factual questions such as birth weight and length of breast feeding.

Goddard, Broder, and Wenar [3] interviewed mothers of twenty-five children born at the Hospital of the University of Pennsylvania, whose records permitted a reasonably complete description of early development. Their questions covered pregnancy and delivery, the neonatal period and developmental highlights, the child's weight at the end of each year, and the occurrence of illnesses. Their findings agreed with those of Pyle, except that they found no evidence that mothers tended to report developmental precocity. Gestation time was not reported reliably. Many mothers did not remember the use of forceps (only four of the seven in which it was used reported it), and few accurately reported neonatal difficulties of the infant such as respiratory difficulty (they may not have been informed, however). There were many discrepancies in feeding histories, particularly duration of nursing and formula composition; and many forgot or overlooked a number of illnesses. The mothers' reports were more accurate and in agreement with those of the physician concerning difficulty of labor and delivery, birth weight and subsequent yearly weight, as well as details of motor development.

Robbins [4, 5] compared parents' retrospective accounts of child rearing with behavioral history protocols obtained in the course of the longitudinal study of Thomas and Chess [6] begun in 1956—a study in which interviews were held every three months during the first year and every six months thereafter. The sample consisted of forty-four mothers and thirty-nine fathers. The children's ages at the time of the interview ranged from twenty-nine to forty-five months, with a median of thirty-seven months. Each parent was interviewed individually.

Robbins concluded that parents were inaccurate in many details of child-rearing practices and early development *despite the frequent rehearsal of data in the longitudinal study.* In discussing the findings, Robbins noted a parallelism between the advice of authorities and parental distortion, i.e., parents tended to report demand feeding, late weaning and toilet training, and a permissive attitude toward sucking. On items where expert advice was less specific or irrelevant, errors were more random.

Each parent was inaccurate on items dealing with age of weaning, beginning of bowel and bladder training, stopping of the 2 A.M. feeding, whether feeding was by schedule or demand, and whether or not thumb sucking occurred. Fathers were inaccurate in their recollection of the age of introduction of cereal and the cup, and when the child first stood alone.

The parents' memory of the onset of bowel and bladder training erred from three to six months in being later than that initially recorded. A tendency to shorten the learning process was noted with walking, the age of introducing the cup was placed later, and the completion of weaning was reported earlier than it had actually occurred.

Recall of the presence or absence of a particular practice was more reliable than the estimate of when it was begun or discontinued. Yet no fact was recalled accurately by all parents, and there were two with significant discrepancies: both parents reported a greater incidence of demand feeding than had been recorded, and several stated there had been no thumb sucking, although the records indicated its presence.

These reports reaffirm that historical data from the parents of normal children concerning significant maturational and developmental highlights during infancy may be unreliable. Several of the factors that may contribute to the unreliability have been alluded to, i.e., the influence of child rearing and the interference of parental conflicts and anxiety.

These findings have disquieting implications for theories of personality development and descriptions of child rearing, as well as for the validity of data used in clinical research and case studies where parental histories comprise part of the basis on which formulations are made.

It would be useful, however, to temper the pessimism of these studies by reiterating the role of the history in clinical medicine, particularly since this was not mentioned in the reports cited.

As the physician elicits a history, he concurrently assesses *what other corroborative sources of information might be helpful.* For example, he may contact other physicians who have cared for the patient to obtain an objective account of their history, physical examination, laboratory studies, diagnosis and treatment, as well as records of previous hospitalization, military records, school records, and vocational adjustment. He may also see other family members, or another person whose observations of the patient both prior to the illness and during the illness might be helpful in documenting the history. *These multiple sources of information have traditionally been part of the medical history, and they tend to compensate for the unreliability of the patient.*

The reliability of the informant is (or ought to be) assessed in any medical history, particularly in a psychiatric history, since the anamnestic data more frequently evokes affect and the various defense mechanisms.

An example of the importance of assessing the reliability of the informant, as well as obtaining independent supplemental historical data from other sources, follows:

A four-and-one-half-year-old girl raised by her maternal aunt was referred from a pediatric hospital for evaluation of increasingly bizarre and disturbed behavior. Past history from the aunt, as given in the pediatric records (where the girl had been treated for three years) and the records of the welfare agency, revealed that her mother, a narcotics addict, had died during the patient's birth, and that the father was admitted shortly after the girl's birth to a federal psychiatric hospital, where he had died after several months, for reasons not clear. The girl was adopted by the maternal aunt when she was released from the hospital.

This history had been consistently obtained by several different pediatricians, the welfare agency, prior consultants, a psychiatrist during the intake evaluation, as well as by another psychiatrist during an outpatient study.

With the aunt's permission, information was requested from the hospital where she had been born, as well as from the psychiatric hospital where her father was said to have died. Replies revealed that the girl's mother had not been a narcotics addict, did not die during the patient's birth, and in fact had been recently admitted to the same hospital for the birth of her thirteenth child shortly before the child's referral. Similarly, the child's father, whose name was obtained from the birth record, had never been admitted to the psychiatric hospital and, according to the last information available, was still alive.

An example of the distortion that may occur by informants follows:

A seven-year-old severely disturbed boy was referred for evaluation of the role in his disorder of encephalitis at age three and one half. The referring neurologist discounted its importance, whereas it had received more emphasis in the summary of the family physician. Neither physician, however, had contacted the pediatrician who had cared for the boy during his hospitalization for encephalitis, nor were the hospital records obtained. When this was done, neither the doctor nor the hospital record alluded to encephalitis. The boy had been hospitalized briefly for treatment of a febrile illness. During the early stages, the pediatrician had mentioned to the parents that he was considering endocarditis in the differential diagnosis, but at no time did he consider or mention encephalitis (to the best of his memory), and this was corroborated by his records and those of the hospital.

The parents' misinterpretation occurred perhaps because of their tendency to ascribe the child's behavioral difficulties to heredity or brain damage despite an absence of any evidence either from repeated histories or physical examinations to support their notion. However, from the time of the febrile illness on, they had included encephalitis in the medical history, and this remained unquestioned without further investigation.

In passing, it is worth mentioning that occasionally a head injury or encephalitis becomes the etiologic scapegoat in the history of a behavioral or emotional disturbance, whereas more careful inquiry reveals that the head injury or encephalitis followed by several months or even years the emergence of the symptoms of the mental disorder.

At times the existence of organic brain disease might have been suspected early in the course of a psychotic disorder if a careful history had been elicited, as in the following example:

The onset of progressive psychotic behavior in a three-year-old was preceded by definite gait difficulty, although no definite physical or neurological signs could be elicited at the time of the initial history and physical examination. Subsequently in the course of the illness, definite neurological findings emerged, and following the death of the child, a post-mortem diagnosis of cerebromacular degeneration was made.

When the onset of this disorder is during the third year of life or later, the first signs often are those of cerebellar dysfunction, and fundoscopic findings are often negative. It may be difficult in a severely disturbed child to do a satisfactory physical and neurological examination that might demonstrate the cerebellar nature of the reported gait disturbance.

THE HISTORY AS PART OF THE PSYCHIATRIC EVALUATION

The history needs to be integrated with the other information gained from the physical examination, laboratory studies, psychological testing, the mental status of the child, and observations in play therapy. From these data, a diagnosis will evolve as a help to planning an appropriate treatment regimen. The importance of these various aspects of the evaluation will be discussed.

The outline provided in Figure 1 for summarizing the psychiatric evaluation of the child provides merely the loom on which the evaluation can be woven. The warp and woof, as well as much of the design, rest with the skill and experience of the interviewer and the reliability of his sources of information. The summary form adaptable for clinic or hospital use includes data readily recoverable for statistical recording or reporting. It is based on that developed for the Children's Service at Langley Porter Institute.

DISCUSSION OF EVALUATION OUTLINE

It is seldom a child's concern about himself that leads to his coming to the clinic, and unless he is a ward of the court, his parents share the responsibility for his care. Because of this, the history usually involves both parents, and there are several ways in which this may be done.

Initially, a conjoint meeting with the parents may be held to understand their concerns, and to see if psychiatric evaluation of the child is needed and if they wish to proceed. If they do, a conjoint meeting at which mother, father, and child are present may follow. At this meeting one can further review their concerns about the child, as well as the child's concerns, and then one can outline the nature of the service to be offered and how it will be carried out. Through hearing the history from the parents together, and then individually from each parent, as well as seeing the interaction of the parents with each other and the child, a more objective and less biased understanding may be obtained than through working solely with one parent.

The familial homeostasis involving the parents and the child may be likened to the equation describing the plasma bicarbonate buffer system to maintain acid-base balance, namely,

$$pH = pK + \log \frac{[HCO_3]}{[CO_2]}$$

This equation includes three variables: the pH, the bicarbonate ion concentration, and the concentration of CO_2 dissolved in the plasma. To define any disturbance of the acid-base balance, one needs to know at least two of these variables, i.e., the pH and the carbon dioxide content of the plasma. If only one is known, it does not suffice—i.e., a low pH may be due to a metabolic or respiratory acidosis, and low CO_2 content may indicate a respiratory alkalosis or metabolic acidosis.

In the family, there are also at least three variables—the father, mother, and child existing in a psychosocial homeostasis where any change in one is reflected by compensatory shifts in the others. To accurately assess the nature of these relationships, it is inadequate to study only one family member, i.e., the child or the mother; whereas, if at least two family members are seen, the degree of integration of the third may be surmised. Indeed, there is increasing evidence that if the two parents are seen without the child, one can predict the degree of psychopathology in the child [7, 8].

Although parents may be divorced, one may invite the other parent, with the custodian's consent, to participate in the evaluation. If the child is a ward of the court, and if the court is willing, one might also involve the parents, if available, in the evaluation. There may be times when the unavailability of one parent precludes his or her participation, but this seldom occurs if a therapeutic effort is made to offer the parents the opportunity to participate in the evaluation and study of their child, and to share in its conclusions.

At the conjoint meeting, one might begin with the identifying data. The information about socioeconomic factors implicit in this data may be important, as is the presence of other persons in the household and the actual living conditions (referring physicians or facilities may not mention, for example, that an eight-member family is living in a one-bedroom apartment with a television set).

The source and the conditions under which the referral was made provide valuable information as to the parents' appraisal of their child's difficulties and their feelings about coming. If, for example, it is a school referral, the parents may feel anger and embarrassment at "being forced to see a psychiatrist when the problem is entirely the fault of the school," or if a court referral, the parents' willingness to participate may be at the request of the judge, and their motivation may be more difficult to sustain than that of parents who come voluntarily because of their own concern about the child's adjustment.

It is useful to ascertain what the parents' expectations are concerning the consultation or evaluation—that is, whether their motivational momentum is merely to fulfill a school or court requirement for one visit, or whether they feel they are coming without extrafamilial coercion.

If the referral is other than a self-referral, it is appropriate to obtain the family's consent to let the referring source know that they have followed through with the recommendation, and also to furnish whatever information may be useful to the referring source at the conclusion of the evaluation.

Traditionally, after the identifying data has been obtained and exploration has been made as to how the patient sought medical attention, the physician begins by eliciting what it is that troubles the parents most— their chief complaint.

In enumerating the chief complaints, it is well to elicit that of each parent and that of the child separately. An effort should be made to document the date of onset, duration, frequency, and intensity of the symptoms or behavior the parent is concerned about, and also its relation to stress, i.e., is it related to a change of father's job, a move, death or illness of a significant family member, the birth of a sibling, or what?

The way in which a complaint is presented may also provide insight into some of the family psychodynamics, as in the following example:

In describing the illness of his son, referred for serious fire setting, the father added with a wink and smile, "There's nothing wrong with that—I used to do it myself as a kid." The mother, however, who tended to project and externalize, attributed the boy's difficulties to his teachers at school, who "don't understand him and aggravate him."

The parents may then be encouraged to describe the child's present illness, interrupted perhaps only by questions relevant to the presence or absence of other information whose significance they may not be aware of. The doctor, from the time of the initial complaint, has begun both a psychodynamic appraisal and a differential diagnostic formulation. Although certain principles can be outlined for the history, the significant data elicited are determined in large part by the acumen of the physician. Any attempt to outline the details of this interaction between family and physician would entail a summary of the basic and clinical medical sciences, and much of the outline would have little application for a given patient, since the interview depends on the experience and wisdom of the physician. The attitudes of the parents toward one another and toward the child are often very revealing in terms of the family dynamics and interaction. Significant areas of parental disagreement as to their expectations of the child and their attitude toward child rearing may clearly emerge.

No attempt will be made here to review in any detail the importance of a thorough past history on each parent, including grandparents and collateral lines—but the material should amount to a careful psychiatric history for each parent. It should include a careful assessment of genetic factors, the parents own birth and early development, medical, school, vocational and avocational background, and their premarital histories.

Remembering that parents have come not primarily because of their own symptoms or difficulties, one might preface the eliciting of their histories with a statement that the difficulties a child develops *may be* related to those the parents have had. This may provide an easy transition into the exploration of their own backgrounds, particularly if the physician says he is not sure of the relevance of the material but feels that only through reviewing it can he assess its possible significance. At times when one attempts to focus on the parent, one may find the parent persists in talking about the child. It may be helpful to temper one's impatience with the recognition that anything an individual describes is psychodynamically autobiographical and meaningful, whether it concerns an ink blot, office decoration, or the behavior of a child. With patience and skill one can return to the parent's background information.

Rather than developing two separate histories, one can merge the narrative accounts of both parents at the point where the parents became acquainted with each other into a chronological account of courtship and marriage, and follow with the circumstances around prior and subsequent pregnancies as well as that of the patient, paying careful attention to all prenatal factors thought to be implicated in the etiology of mental disorders. Records of prenatal care, as well as those from the obstetrician who delivered the patient, should be obtained, if possible, to enhance the reliability of the account.

From the point of the marriage, or at least the pregnancy, it may be most useful to develop the history of the child as the main theme concurrently with the history of both parents, so that the chronology of the parents' histories and that of the child remains the same. This contextual development of the child's history makes it easier to correlate the events in the parents' lives with those of the child. If the child's history is developed without these concurrent data, very often significant stresses and psychodynamic interactions may be missed.

Concerning each event in the child's history, including birth, early development, preschool and school adjustment, the parents' attitudes and interpretations may give clues to significant intrafamilial psychopathology. For example, the effects of gross environmental stress—such as father's loss of a job or job change, transient separation of the parents, significant medical or psychiatric illness of either parent, signs of adjustment reaction in the parents, and the like—may be overlooked, or their correlation with significant deviations in the psychological development of the child may be missed. Too often the history of a child may be presented with an excellent chronology of the development of the early symptoms but with no effort to ascertain whether or not these correlate with parental stress or other disturbances of the familial homeostasis.

Significant features of prenatal, natal, and postnatal development should be established from multiple sources, including prenatal records, hospital records, and the records of the pediatrician who cared for the child, as well as from the parent. Rather than merely determining the date of a developmental landmark, an effort should be made to elicit the parents' recollection of the event *in their own words,* because their memories may reveal significant attitudes toward the child. The correlation or lack of correlation between developmental deviations and intrafamilial stress and psychopathology may have differential diagnostic import.

One example of the value of a contextual history was illustrated in that of a seven-year-old school girl referred because of severe emotional disturbance and uncontrollable seizures despite various anti-convulsive regimens. After a careful history, it became clear that her seizures accompanied significant tension and open conflict between her parents, periods in which she served as a scapegoat. This was further corroborated by her being seizure-free without medication throughout visits to a grandmother. Upon return to home, her seizures frequently recurred and were uncontrollable with varied anti-convulsives.

In the histories of emotionally disturbed children, the frank onset of symptoms often may be correlated with intrafamilial psychopathology. Indeed, if one were unable to demonstrate such a correlation, one's suspicion of an organic brain syndrome might be heightened. A carefully woven assessment of the family's psychodynamics is an important part of one's attempt to formulate and understand the genesis of a child's disorder.

Abridged examples of the value of the contextually developed history have been published and may be reviewed [9].

The description of the mental status of the child depends on the age and level of functioning of the child, as well as the background and approach of the examiner. It may be categorized under headings similar to those used for adults, i.e., attitude, appearance, and general behavior; affect and emotional expression; intellectual functions, including orientation, general intelligence and fund of information, vocabulary, recall, memory (recent and remote), ability to abstract, insight, and judgment.

Further evaluations that overlap with the neurological examination also might be included, i.e., a survey of apraxia, agnosia, and aphasia, as well as evaluation of parietal lobe functions including right-left discrimination and orientation, assessment of body image, constructional apraxias, acalculia, alexia, spatial neglect, and the like. Here also might be included examples of the child's spontaneous drawings.

Of importance in the mental status of preadolescent children is the description of playroom activity, the selection and use of play materials and their projective value as interpreted by the examiner, and the patterns of the child's play. Of particular interest are the shifts from one play activity to another and the apparent reason or lack of reason for this shift, as well as evidence of anxiety accompanying the termination of a play activity. The use of specific play situations, such as reenactment of significant life experiences, family dolls, puppets, finger paints, story-telling, "three wishes," and so on depends on the preference and experience of the examiner.

Specific changes in playroom behavior may be highly significant, as illustrated by the evaluation of a seven-year-old school girl referred by a neurologist, who found no neurological abnormalities, because of headaches and vague gastrointestinal complaints including nausea and vomiting. Past history revealed that she had been sexually molested by a relative prior to the onset of her symptoms. Further historical data revealed that her mother had had a similar experience at nearly the same age with the same relative and had reacted with the same symptoms.

In the first play session, the child spontaneously reenacted what might have been considered the precipitating traumatic event of her symptomatology through the use of a doll house and a family set of dolls playing out the relative's sexual advances, followed by her development of headaches and gastrointestinal symptoms, just as her mother had.

The second week of the evaluation, however, she behaved much differently in the playroom, with little interest in the toys and no spontaneity. Her mood shifted from apathy to apprehension, without evident reason. Her response to comments about this change was merely to verbalize her symptoms of headache and vague gastrointestinal distress. Because of this marked shift in her playroom behavior, the examiner did an ophthalmoscopic examination, and found definite papilledema. Prompt reevaluation by the referring neurologist was done, and the diagnosis of a progressive brain tumor was confirmed at surgery the following week.

Another example of how significant a small detail of playroom behavior might be was that of a pre-school, severely disturbed child who hesitantly entered the playroom and stood there rocking to and fro saying, "Goodbye" repeatedly to the examiner. It was a clear expression of the child's ambivalence, reflecting both hesitant warm impulses toward the examiner and distrust and withdrawal from interpersonal contact—an interaction which caricatured his father's paranoid orientation.

Positive physical and neurological findings should be recorded carefully, including data such as the height and weight of the child, deviation from normal growth curve, and the degree of cooperation with the examiner, since often with severely emotionally disturbed children a thorough neurological examination is difficult to carry out and ophthalmoscopic examination, if indicated, may require sedation or general anesthesia.

If abnormalities are present and consultation indicated, a record of the consultant's findings and recommendation should be included along with the date of examination and the reason for pursuing or not pursuing the recommendations further. Psychological testing, if done, should be summarized. If discrepancies between the psychologist's findings and other data exist, they should be commented on and included in the diagnostic formulation. Laboratory findings should be included and assessed, if abnormal.

In describing the course of the brief service or treatment, one can record one's experience with the child and each parent, noting particularly shifts in symptoms, adjustment, school performance, or other indications of improvement or regression. Often these shifts in symptomatology may be important clues as to the role of emotional disturbance producing the disorder of the child even when known central nervous disease exists. In difficult borderline cases of mental retardation, where there is no unequivocal evidence of organic brain disease and where the degree of emotional disturbance precludes adequate assessment of the child's intellectual potential, the remission or improvement of the behavior of disturbance after several play therapy sessions or a course of psychotherapy may give valuable information as to how much of the disturbance in the child may be due to emotional factors. If the behavioral disturbance improves, the child may be amenable to a more accurate definition of intellectual potential.

Often when a family decides to seek psychiatric or other help for their child, significant improvement may occur even before they initiate contact with a clinic or physician. Similarly, even though there may be a waiting period between their telephone call and first visit, improvement may continue in the child, reflecting perhaps the integrative effect on the family of their having recognized the problem and proceeded with its evaluation. The degree of improvement that occurs even after one interview or during a diagnostic evaluation may be a valuable prognostic indicator of the family's potential for response to further treatment. Similarly, during a brief service, one may become more aware of the depth and chronicity of parental disturbance and its relative immutability, as evidenced by the use of denial by the parents or their continued efforts to seek a somatic or genetic origin for their child's difficulty despite repeated demonstration that there is no evidence for these factors.

The diagnostic formulation represents the fruition of the evaluation and includes an integration of all data into a meaningful psychodynamic formulation of the child's strengths and weaknesses—as well as the relative roles of genetic, prenatal, and organic factors, including any central nervous system or other body defect or disorder that may play a contributory role to the mental disturbance. It attempts to assess all factors, including the experiential and socioeconomic, into a summary of one's understanding of the child's disorder. It does not discount potentially relevant genetic factors, the role of prenatal disturbances in the mother that might have affected the developing central nervous system, birth trauma, or postnatal disease, but it does not develop any one of these factors at the expense of others. It includes as comprehensive an attempt as possible to integrate these into a psychodynamic appraisal of the child, along with the role of the child's experience with its parents or their surrogates, in an effort to understand the child's disorder.

In medicine it is seldom that one hears any organ system referred to as normal unless a careful history, physical, and laboratory assessment has been carried out. Yet in psychiatry, too frequently perhaps, one hears statements such as "These were relatively normal, well-adjusted parents doing the best they could with a difficult child"—statements based on impressions gained during an interview but made without a careful historical inventory of each parent and his own psychological development.

Finally, the diagnostic formulation attempts to make up for some of the unreliability of parental histories as reviewed in the initial parts of this paper. For example, not only the parents are used as informants, but other sources of information are used to corroborate the history in as detailed a way as feasible, i.e., other physicians' evaluations, medical and hospital records, school reports, and so on. In addition, this historical information is integrated with data obtained from the child's assessment in diagnostic or therapeutic play sessions (or interviews, if an adolescent), along with the results of the physical and neurological examinations, laboratory findings, and psychological examinations, if needed. Thus, the formulation and diagnosis here as elsewhere in medicine depends on multiple sources of data, not only from the history but from varying levels of direct observation of the child and the family.

In addition, the diagnostic formulation often is tentative and may be modified according to the response of the child and family to whatever course of treatment is recommended. Sometimes the therapeutic process itself comprises part of the diagnostic evaluation, particularly in those children who manifest both central nervous system disease and mental disorder, where the role of each is clouded primarily because of the severity of the child's emotional disorder. Through therapeutic efforts to reduce the child's behavioral and emotional disturbance, one hopes to achieve a more precise definition of the organic factors at a time when the child can more cooperatively participate in their assessment.

FIGURE 1

OUTLINE FOR PSYCHIATRIC EVALUATION OF A CHILD

PATIENT'S NAME _____
CASE NUMBER _____
THERAPIST'S NAME _____

SUMMARY AT TIME OF_____
(End of Brief Service and/or Case Closing. Transfer to New Therapist, etc.)

(Note: All headings should be covered adequately. The material will be more useful if written contextually and succinctly. Headings may be combined and previous summaries may be referred to, if you wish.)

DATE OF THIS SUMMARY:

IDENTIFYING DATA: (Child's age, color, sex, education, religion, and living arrangements; as well as family constellation, including ages of parents and sibs, vocation, educational level, and income with sources.)

DATE OF ADMISSION: (Date last opened.)

DATE OF CLOSING: (If not yet closed, leave blank.)

DATES OF BRIEF SERVICE VISITS: (If during this admission.)

REFERRED BY: (Name and address. Include brief statement of circumstances under which family applied and what they were seeking.)

CHIEF COMPLAINTS: (Enumerate those of child and parents briefly, giving onset, duration, severity, and apparent relationships to stress.)

PAST HISTORY: (Grandparents, parents, collaterals, marital, pre-natal, birth and early development, medical, nursery school, kindergarten, school, vocational, and avocational.)

PRESENT ILLNESS:

MENTAL STATUS OF CHILD: (Description of observation of child at the time first seen by you and at time of writing, if different.)

POSITIVE PHYSICAL AND NEUROLOGICAL FINDINGS: (Date of last examination. Include summary of consultant's examinations, with name and date.)

LABORATORY FINDINGS: (Include EEG and dates.)

PSYCHOLOGICAL EXAMINATIONS: (Dates, briefly summarize conclusions.)

COURSE OF TREATMENT—OR BRIEF SERVICE: (Include a summary of the child's therapy and that of the parents. If day or residential treatment was involved, include brief summaries from all involved, i.e., child care, nursing, special education, etc.)

AGENCY CONFERENCES HELD, IF ANY: (Date, who attended, brief summary.)

TREATMENT REVIEWS HELD: (Dates and recommendations.)

LETTER: (To referring sources and/or other indicated persons, name and address. If none, state why or indicate if phone call(s) made instead.)

DIAGNOSTIC FORMULATION: Briefly integrate the data into a psycho-dynamic summary of the patient's history and illness.

Include family history, genetic, pre-natal and somatic factors, as well as socioeconomic and experiential factors. The account should include contextual family material, i.e., if developmental disturbances or symptoms are noted include parental data that may be related either as cause *or* effect. Summarize the integrative as well as disintegrative aspects of the history, as well as the family and child's current assets and liabilities.

If differential diagnostic considerations are involved, briefly discuss why you chose your diagnosis.

DIAGNOSIS AND NUMBER: Enter the diagnosis and code number from the *Diagnostic and Statistical Manual (DSM II)* of the American Psychiatric Association [10], in conformance with instructions in Section III, Pages 14-52, and *include the complementary evaluation therein described, i.e.,*

Stress:

Predisposition:

Impairment:

CONDITION: (Improved, unimproved, unknown, not treated.)

DISPOSITION AT THIS TIME: (If closing, reason. Plans made with family and recommendations made, if any.)

TOTAL NUMBER OF VISITS: (Count from date opened, including all therapists. Include application, fee setting, testing, and all other visits.)

	BRIEF SERVICE				**TREATMENT**			
	Patient	Mother	Father	Other	Patient	Mother	Father	Other
				(Specify)				(Specify)
Social Service								
Psychiatrist								
Psychologist								
Laboratory								
EEG								
Clinical								
X-Ray								
Total								

_____

(Therapist's Signature and Title)

REFERENCES

1. PYLES, M. K., STOLZ, H. R., and MACFARLANE, J. W. The accuracy of mothers' reports on birth and developmental data. *Child Development,* **6**:165-176, 1935.

2. HAGGARD, ERNEST A., BREKSTAD, ARNE, and SKARD, ASE GANDA. Reliability of anamnestic interviews. *J. Abnorm. Soc. Psychol.,* **61**:311-318, 1960.

3. GODDARD, K. E., BRODER, G., and WENAR, C. Reliability of pediatric histories—a preliminary study. *Pediatrics,* **28**:1011-1018, 1961.

4. ROBBINS, L. C. Parent recall of aspects of child development and of child-rearing practices. Unpublished doctoral dissertation. New York University, 1961.

5. ROBBINS, L. C. The accuracy of parental recall of aspects of child development and of child-rearing practices. *J. Abnorm. Soc. Psychol.,* **66**:261-270, 1963.

6. THOMAS, A., and CHESS, S. An approach to the study of sources of individual differences in child behavior. *J. Clin. Exper. Psycho-Path. and Quart. Rev. Psychiat. and Neurol.,* **18**:347-357, 1957.

7. GIANASCOL, A. J. Psychodynamic approaches to childhood schizophrenia: a review. *J. Nerv. Ment. Disease,* **137**:336-348, 1963.

8. SINGER, M. T., and WYNNE, L. C. Thought disorder and family relations of schizophrenics. IV. Results and Implications. *Arch Gen. Psychiat.,* **12**:201-212, 1965.

9. BOATMAN, M. J., and SZUREK, S. A. A clinical study of childhood schizophrenia. In Don D. Jackson (Ed.), *The etiology of schizophrenia.* New York: Basic Books, 1960, pp. 389-440.

10. American Psychiatric Association. *Diagnostic and statistical manual.* 2nd ed. Washington, D.C.: American Psychiatric Association, 1968, pp. 14-52.

CHAPTER 7

CHILDHOOD SCHIZOPHRENIA:
A PSYCHOGENIC HYPOTHESIS*

S. A. Szurek, M.D.

BASIC PHILOSOPHY OF TREATMENT

For about nine years the staff of the Children's Service of the Langley
Porter Clinic has been testing the hypothesis that the etiology of very
severe mental disorders, particularly those of preadolescent children, is
entirely psychogenic, that is, that the psychotic disorder is due to postnatal experiences that have led to intense, generalized motivational conflict.

The reasons why this etiological hypothesis for these disorders has been
and is still being tested extend back before World War II, to clinical experiences and the conclusions reached from them at the Institute for Juvenile
Research in Chicago. These conclusions were obtained in collaboration
with a number of colleagues, in particular with Dr. Adelaide Johnson [8,
22, 25-27, 49-53, 57]. Briefly, this experience was collaborative psychotherapeutic work with neurotic preadolescent and adolescent children,
some of whom were impulsively aggressive, and with their parents. In this
work we encountered no child whose parents were not also in severe conflict. The particular conflicts of the child, the form and severity of his
symptoms (which expressed futile solutions to these conflicts), and his
degree of emotional integration were all primarily due to the timing, intensity, and duration of his experience with similar aspects of the personalities of his parents.

*Reprinted by permission from *The American Journal of Orthopsy-
chiatry,* **26**(3), July 1956, 519-543. (Copyright, The American Orthopsychiatric Association, Inc.)

Toward the end of the Chicago experience there was an opportunity to begin clinical therapeutic studies with a few psychotic children and some of their parents. This study, though brief and incomplete, suggested that similar but much more intense factors were possibly at the root of the more severe disorders.

And so the question remained. For if the schizophrenic disorder should prove to be as understandable as the neurotic and the impulsive disorder in terms of early continuous distortion of biological tendencies of the human organism after birth by anxieties induced by anxious parents, then perhaps all mental disorder not traceable to impersonally caused disease of the soma would be in the same continuum.

DEVELOPMENT OF NEW PROGRAM

An opportunity for more thorough testing of this hypothesis came at the end of the war, when it became possible to work with a combined facility in San Francisco consisting of both an inpatient and outpatient service for children. I say "more thorough" even though the staff and I cannot say that we are wholly satisfied with all the conditions of our testing. A staff requires training in psychotherapeutics with both children and their parents [55, 56, 58-60]. This training and mutual learning still continues as a progressive refinement of technical therapeutic procedures, which are made necessary by the severity and form of the disorder and the complexity of the family problem. In addition to the problem of therapeutic skill, we are also not satisfied that the factor of frequency of therapeutic sessions for the child, and especially for the parents, has been sufficient or optimal.

I have hesitated to report any of our experience up to this time because the details of our clinical data are still not as accurately and thoroughly collated as we wish. My remarks here, then, are preliminary, impressionistic, and largely unstatistical.

Fifteen staff psychiatrists, five staff psychiatric social workers, and two staff psychologists have participated in the past nine years in this work. Most of the psychiatrists have spent at least two years of full-time training on the service; a few have spent only one year; and three have continued for over seven years, including the time of their formal training periods. Among the social workers, one has been continuously on the Children's Service staff for over six years, two have been here for one year each, and the remaining two have been here three and four years, respectively. One of the psychiatrists returned a little over a year ago after some years of absence from the staff, following his formal training period, to undertake further therapeutic research with a family.

In nine years this staff has seen more than 100 children with a disorder classifiable as schizophrenic or very severely schizoid, along with their parents. The ages of the children on initial clinical contact have ranged from eighteen months to fourteen years; most of them have been under twelve years of age, but in recent years more of them have been six years or younger. The duration of clinical contact with these families has varied from a brief period of study of four to five weeks in the outpatient or inpatient service up to almost nine years. (Incidentally, in recent years our work with most patients begins with such studies before we make definite decisions with the family about longer and more systematic therapeutic work.) Most of the families who have been seen therapeutically have worked with us for periods under three or four years; a smaller number, for five, six, and seven years. In a few instances our work with these families has been entirely in the outpatient service; with some, entirely in the inpatient service; while with the majority, it has been on the inpatient service followed by a period of outpatient work. Sometimes our work has not gone beyond the four weeks' study period, either because of a lack of staff time or because of various reasons originating with the family. I would like to mention here that in a very rough preliminary survey of the total number of children we have seen in this series, there is a preponderance of boys over girls—about three to two. Although we have speculated about the factors underlying this interesting sex differential, shortage of time has precluded closer study and analysis of them.

Complete physical, neurological, and laboratory examinations, and as thorough psychological studies as the condition of the child permitted were carried out at the outset in all of these instances, and in many were repeated during our period of work. During the past few years electroencephalographic examinations have been made routinely. We have had the benefit of expert consultants from the University departments of pediatrics, neurology, neurosurgery, and others. The medical histories of the children have in each instance been closely scrutinized, and reports have been obtained whenever possible from physicians attending any serious past somatic illness. Any uncertain signs or indications of somatic disease, anomaly, or identifiable congenital defect were pursued by every means available. Chemical or other nonpsychological therapy was administered only for a diagnosed intercurrent somatic illness or injury.

As the psychiatric staff gradually increased in the last three or four years, more of these children were seen in individual sessions during their hospitalization—usually in playrooms—as many as three times per week. In those few instances in which the family was seen throughout the course of our clinical contact in the outpatient service, the child was generally seen once a week. With most of these families, both parents were seen weekly in individual interviews throughout our work with the child. In two or three instances, one or both parents have had two or three interviews per week for several years. To the full extent of the skill of the particular therapist, the therapeutic work with the parents has aimed at the resolution of conflicts that each parent has explicitly agreed upon with them.

I shall not speak of the work contributed to the total effort by nurses, attendants, schoolteachers, occupational therapists, and others, which in many instances was considerable [45, 54, 59; see also Chapters 8, 9, and 18]. Their observations and work with the child and such contact with parents as they necessarily had were always correlated in numerous conferences with that of the therapists of the child and of the parents. I shall mention the fact that in the past few years we have decided that it is a useful experience for the same psychiatrist to work with all three members of a family [60].

DIAGNOSTIC DILEMMAS

We can agree with those experienced students of diagnosis who feel that clear-cut criteria for a nosological entity are not easily defined. Differentiation of the disorder from mental deficiency, from disease of the central nervous system (especially in the case of children under five or six years, when speech is minimal or absent), and from severe chronic, psychoneurotic (obsessional or phobic) disorders is in some instances difficult without prolonged therapeutic study. We are coming more and more to the opinion that mild, moderate, or even severe mental deficiency and organic brain disease can be complicated by severe mental disorder or personality maldevelopment [1, 4, 17, 65]; and we are beginning to consider it clinically (that is, prognostically) fruitless and even unnecessary to draw any sharp dividing line between a condition that one could call psychoneurotic and one that could be called psychosis, autism, atypical development, or schizophrenia. For many reasons, the concept of a gradient of severity of disorder, a psychopathological spectrum, is one that fits our experience most closely. The reasons for this stem not only from the "natural history" of the disorder in the various children we have known but also from our experience during therapeutic work with their families.

As far as the "natural history" is concerned, it is as follows: in a few instances the disorder of the child was episodic, with a rather abrupt onset and a variable duration ranging from a few weeks to several years. Here is a brief example of episodic disorder:

A girl almost five years of age within one week became mute, enuretic, and inactive to the point of maintaining the same position for long periods of time. She lost weight, suffered from severe night terrors, and was very destructive toward her dolls. She once threw a kitten into a fire burning in the fireplace, and frequently attacked her mother physically. These symptoms, with only short recessions while she was briefly hospitalized for somatic illnesses, persisted for over a year. She had become gradually less active and less spontaneous during the sixteen months prior to these more severe symptoms. All this occurred in the context of the following events: her father's sudden surgery for a strangulated hernia; her beloved paternal grandmother's becoming ill and leaving the home for good; and the increasing sexual conflicts, homicidal impulses toward the child, and suicidal preoccupations of the mother, who was sixteen years her husband's junior. The father's very anxious and prolonged convalescence from his surgery seemed related to his childhood experience of being hospitalized in a cast for four years for tuberculosis of the hip. Incidentally, the girl's symptoms progressively began to subside even before direct therapy of the child and both parents began, after her mother began to discuss her own difficulties with a minister, a pediatrician, and finally, in correspondence with a psychiatrist.

Generally, in such instances there was fairly clear evidence of a preexisting neurotic personality development. Following a gradual recession of the psychotic symptoms, the disorder then merged into that of a moderate to severe degree of psychoneurosis. The psychotic period in these patients was clinically and psychodynamically indistinguishable from the disorder of those children whose development from the first or second year of life was what we tend to call autistic, except for larger "islands" of greater ego integration. Further, we have seen among several of those whose disorder was more insidious, chronic, and continuous a considerable variation in degree of severity of the disorder, so that either term—psychosis or neurosis—was difficult or impossible to apply for any length of time.

Finally, although we have not worked out any satisfactory "objective" scale as yet, nor applied any measure other than the usual clinical criteria of capacity to work, to play, to learn, and to develop some durable give-and-take relationships with coevals and with adults, we have had varying therapeutic results. In a recent review by those staff psychiatrists with most experience on the service, we agreed that fourteen of the younger children with both insidious and abrupt onset of the disorder can be counted as well or as very markedly improved. They are now in school and have been living at home for several years and progressing rather well. Five of these are without any directed therapeutic program anywhere. Some of these children have never been hospitalized subsequently: in one instance, the second of two therapists treating a child found it difficult to believe that the child had ever had any schizophrenic symptoms. We hear from their parents periodically. One of the children who recovered was a Negro girl whose illness was of abrupt onset at eleven years of age, within a year or so after her parents finally began living together with her in the home. Her illness was marked by rapid grave regression, hebephrenic symptomatology, withdrawal, periods of destructive violence, and bizarre sexual exhibitionism and excitement. Within a year and a half after her illness began, the parents were separated and ultimately divorced, and only the mother remained in therapy. This patient remained in the hospital for four years and four months, continued in outpatient therapy for about a year, and was married two years after all therapy had stopped.

At the other end of the scale, we know of several who are now in state hospitals, usually for reasons other than the staff's conscious unwillingness to continue, and are no better than when therapeutic work with our staff stopped. Some of these are somewhat better than when we first saw them—usually late in preadolescence or early adolescence. Between these extremes is a larger number with varying degrees of improvement from moderate to little, but with some reduction of the most severe symptoms.

Because our experience as to the form of the disorder is so similar to that of other students [2, 3, 5, 7, 9, 10, 12, 14, 18, 21, 24, 28-32, 35, 38, 39, 42, 66], I hesitate to consider symptomatology. Nevertheless, the clinical syndrome that more and more of us tend to call childhood schizophrenia, autism, atypical ego development, or just psychosis is full of paradoxes. One could say it is as full of paradoxes as all human life. The child whose disorder is extreme can be recognized by his marked or extreme unresponsiveness, even negativism, to the approach of others—adults or coevals. Yet at certain times and with certain people, particularly adults, and in reaction to certain attitudes he responds with an intense vigor and speed so disproportionate to the immediate precipitating event that the cause is sometimes difficult to notice or to reconstruct later. He is quite indifferent to others, sometimes particularly so to his mother. Yet on closer observation he is, as we say, particularly "dependent" upon her as well as in an intense struggle with himself and with her, and in tremendous panic on separation from her—panic that is expressed in very devious ways, sometimes through somatic malfunction.

He gives the impression of stupidity at one moment and of Machiavellian precision in his cunning at another. He is phobic about some things and situations and foolhardy in his apparently fearless and heedless activity about others. He appears altogether absorbed in his own inner processes, yet gives evidence of being acutely sensitive to all that goes on around him. He seems at times almost self-destructively content to do nothing for himself, yet suddenly on a few occasions he shows unusual skill and expertness in some activity of his own choice, pace, and timing.

We have seen among these children many gradation of affective expressiveness and responsiveness: from those who evince general apathy, dulling, flattening, frozenness, or apparent absence of all kinds of feeling, through queerly distorted, incongruous feelings with which it is difficult to feel any empathy or understanding, to those children who seem much less disordered much of the time but who manifest periods during which there is obviously considerable suppression, distortion, and explosiveness of emotional expression. In the extreme form or instance of the disorder one rarely if ever sees a simple smile of pleasure, joy, or any eagerness and interest. Nor does one see a simple prompt outburst of tearful hurt, disappointment, discouragement, or sadness, nor an expression of easily understandable anger, obvious revengefulness, or jealousy. Instead, there is often a "dead-pan" indifference, for example, in reaction to the parents' departure from the ward when the child is first admitted. When he is hurt in an accidental fall, he may turn away with anxiously impotent fury from any offer of sympathy from an adult; or a considerable time after he might have been expected to feel disappointed, hurt, angry, or envious, he may suddenly explode into prolonged periods of hollow laughter, queer, gleefully malicious grinning, tearless wailing, or endless rages with murderous destructiveness toward objects, other persons, or himself—sometimes in quick alternation. Yet, when on some occasions during such vengefully sadistic attacks he is quietly but firmly restrained, he may, after a short struggle, suddenly melt into a heap on the floor, against the body of the adult, or into his lap—only to pinch, bite, or smear saliva suddenly later.

During such periods of self-directed savagery a child may slap his own face vigorously, flick his finger against his cheek till it is severely inflamed, or bang his head viciously against walls to the point of severe bruising or laceration. He may bite his tongue or lips until severe bleeding occurs or chronic ulceration results; or he may punch his face and eyes with fists or knees until they are blackened or cut. In one boy a traumatic cataract of one eye developed during a prolonged period of such self-punching. Another boy broke his femur when trying to strike his head with his knee; this occurred while he was begging to be restrained. Another child suddenly slammed a door on her own finger and, without much sign of pain, came to a nurse to show her the terminal phalanx almost severed. Still another child cut the prepuce of his penis.

Similar intensity is directed against others. One patient sat on the back of another, smaller, child, pounding her head violently against a concrete floor; on another occasion, she smashed a kitten against the wall, killing it; and on a third, she threw a skate at another child in a murderous fury.

In some of our patients we have observed that such destructive violence alternates with attitudes of withdrawal, isolation, indifference, or unresponsiveness; or that the destructiveness has replaced the isolation either after longer acquaintance with members of the staff, in response to their continued approaches, or after prolonged efforts at therapy. I have likened it to the thawing and melting of a completely frozen surface of a body of water and its breaking up into dangerously loosened floes of ice. In short, it is as if the frozen state reduces the danger.

In addition to the affective freezing and the affective explosiveness, we have observed in some patients characteristically, and in others episodically, a great deal of very obvious anxiety, occasionally of panic proportions. Such anxiety may be concentrated about specific identifiable, even though not easily comprehensible, situations that persist for long periods, or that appear fleetingly, to recur elsewhere and at other times. Such anxiety may be in a few instances rather diffusely and generally evident in all sorts of endless vacillations about many activities that merge into a variety of what appear to be ritualistic propitiatory acts of undoing or magically protective and avoiding manneristic stereotypies.

We have observed among these patients similar gradations and variations of learned executive functions or of overt behavioral capacity for self-care and for pursuit of self-satisfying activity and freedom to learn. These gradations extend from extreme, generalized nondevelopment to very uneven development. In what appears to be an inverse relation to such skills, capacity, and freedom, we have observed among the patients a preference for extremely isolated activities and interest in their own bodily movements, processes, and sensations. In the most extreme instances of the disorder we have seen queer flailing movements of arms, unusual gaits, self-rocking, and prominent uncertainty in all motor skills. Some of these children may be persistently and monotonously active, while others are quiet, listless, daintily aloof, and difficult to interest in any play, game, or movement. These patients may show an extremely persistent and generally lonely interest: in a piece of string; a self-made twiddler of some sort; a particular kind of toy; a fetishistic object such as a piece of hose, a purse, or a piece of blanket; or in the movement of their own hands or fingers; the touching and smelling of sheets, blankets, or other textile objects; or the manipulation of their own hair.

If certain patients are started on an activity, they proceed without verve, interest, or any obvious pleasure. Yet some of them may suddenly be embarrassingly direct in touching, fondling, or attacking various parts of another person such as the breasts or the genitals, or they may insistently lift the skirts of women. The interest in their own bodies in some takes the form of open genital or anal masturbation, which appears less pleasurable than anxiously and defiantly gleeful [61]. In other children, on the other hand, we have seen excellent coordination, great skill in climbing or jumping, and marked alertness and readiness to engage in all sorts of activity, alone or parallel with others, occurring together with mutism and other signs of marked affective disturbance and great difficulty in durable relations with others.

When still fairly young, say, three to four years of age, or even at a later age, some of these children may still make little or no effort to dress, feed, bathe themselves, or to keep clean—or do so slowly and very reluctantly. At the table they are sloppy and careless, preferring to use their hands and fingers rather than utensils and to snatch food from the plates of others, even though they are offered all the food that they might wish. Some eat anything they can put into their mouths—clay, paint, dirt, or garbage. Others show intense and very persistent particular food preferences or aversions. Their clothes or shoes may be worn in a slovenly fashion, and they may soil or urinate in their clothes, in the bath, or in bed; or, on the other hand, they may retain stools for days until defecation is enormous, inspissated, and painful. We have known a boy of three, for example, with normal dentition, but such inhibition of chewing that his parents still fed him all solid foods in puréed form from a bottle through a nipple. He was not only severely withdrawn and unresponsive to others, mute, and still in diapers for both bowel and bladder functions, but he also collapsed to the ground whenever taken out of his home. He spent long periods lying in bed looking at his own slowly moving fingers held close in front of his eyes. He rarely if ever smiled, and ran off to bed and fell asleep after the slightest disappointment with adults. I might add that during the course of therapeutic work with this family, his mother developed a severe anxious depression demanding hospital care and electroshock therapy, while his father was anxiously helpless about many problems of his life.

The nondevelopment or inhibition of mouth and hand-mouth executive functions as examples of this general phenomenon of the disorder has been strikingly illustrated for us by several patients. We have seen peculiar tremulous or spasmodic jerking of the hands brought to, but not in contact with, the mouth in a young child whose parents were glad that at least he did not put things into his mouth. A frankly unwanted five-year-old boy, who had been weaned abruptly at six weeks, when his mother's breasts dried up suddenly after the illness of an aunt who cared for him, did not use his hands for any activity whatever during the first three and a half years of his life. His hands had been restrained almost continuously from the time he was two months until he was eighteen months of age because of such persistent finger sucking that the skin of his fingers was bleeding and raw.

We have, of course, in common with all other students of the disorder, observed nondevelopment, maldevelopment, and uneven development of the most characteristically human activity, namely, speech and interest in communicative expression and exchange with others. Thus, such a child's speech, if any, may be fragmented, parrotlike, echolalic, devoid of feeling, full of reversals, and often devoid of the personal pronoun "I," or with self-referrals in the third person, and with many self-scolding, self-shaming phrases, warnings, and threats. If largely mute, he may have begun to speak a little at an early age and then gradually or suddenly ceased to do so. If he is then more or less completely mute, his rare vocalizations on tense, strained occasions may be reminiscent of a wild animal in terror or rage, or expressive of inconsolable yearning. Many chronically mute children are so blank in facial expression or other motor signs of responsiveness to the verbal approaches of others that they give an impression of deafness or of severe mental deficiency convincing to many adults, including their parents. Some patients who are not wholly mute may have long periods in which they use a completely incomprehensible jargon without any communicative intent toward another person. Those children who are not mute may be fairly clear in verbal expression of most of their interests, wishes, and observations, although the speech of some of them may at times be not to the apparent point or be wearyingly persistent about some wish or question that seems never to get settled.

A great many of these children apparently learn little or nothing from the usual and persistent efforts at teaching academic skills—skills which are not beyond their intellectual endowment—for discouragingly long periods of time. Yet some show a capacity to learn many things they themselves become interested in knowing and doing. In this case, the child may be extremely, although narrowly, persistent in the pursuit of his own interest, skill, or knowledge, though utterly indifferent to letting any adult know, or particularly insistent about not revealing what he has learned to an eagerly interested teacher or parent. In this respect, as in many other respects, the wishes of others are most persistently denied and frustrated—as are many of his own wishes. One boy who had been on our ward for seven years, for example, and who was characteristically entirely mute during his first two or three years with us, was clearly able to read to himself, to do some arithmetic, and to write. He showed for many months an avid, consecutive interest in several subjects, including geography, interstellar space, factories, and rocket ships. With each of these he was quite single-mindedly and almost exclusively absorbed, but manifested no urge of his own to communicate to the teacher or other adults his reactions to the subjects he pursued.

MALINTEGRATIVE EXPERIENCES AND ETIOLOGY

When we have learned enough about it, we have found each symptom and each special interest in a fetishistic object or skill to be a derivative and an elaboration of particular experiences of the child with some adult, parent or other, that was malintegrative in the first case and in some measure satisfying and integrative in the second.

None of these general remarks and illustrative vignettes of characteristics of individual children are adequate substitutes for the more vivid and perhaps more convincing clinical biographies of particular patients. Nevertheless, for reasons of space, they must suffice here to indicate the nature of the clinical experience that forms the basis of our present attitudes and ideas concerning this problem. We cannot, however, present these ideas and attitudes without indicating in a similar general manner the remainder of our total clinical experience, namely, our experience with the parents of these children.

First of all, as our experience increases, we find that more and more parents are willing and sometimes even eager to begin therapeutic work with us. This willingness is not wholly unambivalent, and resistances and anxieties make their appearance eventually, even with those willing to begin work. Nevertheless, in reaction to our increasing conviction—based on increasing experience—that in the case of every child with mental disorder there is some disorder of both parents, we are finding it possible to begin work not only with the mothers but also with the fathers. This has been progressively truer even with families living a hundred or more miles away from the clinic, and in a very few instances with parents who were divorced.

Secondly, we have known a number of families who had already placed their children out of the home for some years prior to their contact with our staff. In several of these cases it has become apparent after some work that the parents have little further interest in trying to solve their problems, problems which preclude for them considering at least eventually having the child at home. Nevertheless, I have the impression that early in the problem the majority of the parents do not show what could be called simple rejection of their child. Instead we find both parents in conflict— conflict that involves the child, and conflict between themselves, leading in some cases to disruption of the marriage. In those families that have worked with us longest and most intensively, we have what we consider definite evidence that these conflicts are but the overt signs of internal problems. Such intrapsychic conflicts are easily seen in therapy as stemming from the earliest life experiences. These conflicts are usually intensified by various events and experiences seriously frustrating to, or constituting a critical strain for, them both during their marital history prior to—or even after—the birth of the child who is brought for therapy. The intensification of such conflicts of each parent is chronologically related to certain events in the marital history on the one hand, and to the appearance of the child's symptoms or their exacerbation on the other.

Events frustrating to the parents may be of two distinguishable categories. One category would be called external frustration or threat. I mean by this external in origin as far as the parental neurosis is concerned—war, general economic conditions, serious somatic illness of either parent or close relative, and the like. The second category could be called internal in that it is primarily an outgrowth of the parental neurosis that cumulatively has given rise to a more and more difficult situation for each parent, and particularly to repressed but dangerously explosive tensions between the parents that generally involve the child. Obviously, both the externally and internally determined factors are frequently intertwined in the time of their occurrence and duration of their operation.

As bits of illustrative data of such factors, I mention in very brief outline historical data from a few families' experience.

A highly intelligent, very anxiously rebellious young woman with a deep sense of inferiority, queerness, and difference, and doubts of her own value—the result in part of a highly ambivalent identification with her own mother, who felt inferior to the father and who died suddenly of heart disease when the young woman was in her early teens—proposed marriage to an unstable, rather confused fellow student in college after a tense, desperate premarital affair, because she had a considerable inheritance. The husband was said to be reluctant to have children, but twins resulted from the first pregnancy. For many years thereafter the mother felt that she was disfigured physically and sexually unattractive to her husband, who also complained of this. Tension between the young parents was high, and serious differences about the care of the infants appeared. Three months after the birth of the twins, one of them was found dead as a result of what was diagnosed as an enlarged thymus. Both parents had heard some crying earlier in the evening in the children's room while entertaining a guest. Father wished to investigate, but mother irritably stopped him. Afterwards, she had a very severe emotional disorder that necessitated the parents' placing the surviving twin in other people's care and leaving the area for some months. Father was also seriously disturbed, did poorly in his schoolwork, and repeatedly stayed away from home. Both suffered from many neurotic somatic symptoms, felt very isolated and estranged from each other, often did not speak to each other for days, complained of not knowing what the other thought about many of their common problems, and repeatedly considered divorce. In this climate of parental tension, the surviving twin developed autistically. He was almost entirely mute and unresponsive, but had frequent, furious, noisy tantrums. Professional opinions about his condition and development ranged from mental deficiency, deafness, and speech block to endocrine disease, and he was placed in various schools and hospitals from the age of four and a half years.

From work with another young couple, married during the early part of World War II, it was learned that they were both very ambivalently and helplessly dependent on their own parents for many years after their marriage. Father, in an effort to remain out of the service, decided to have children early, and then remained emotionally aloof from the first-born son in order that the child would not be hurt emotionally if he should be drafted. He gave up his remunerative occupation for one more arduous, less remunerative, but more essential to the war effort. Sexual incompatibility between the parents was severe. The mother and son were in a serious neurotic entanglement by the time a daughter was born, when the boy was about four and a half. Within a few weeks the boy developed garbled speech, began tearing at his penis, made efforts to take the baby's place in the crib, and was otherwise so difficult for the parents that within a year he was admitted to a state hospital with a diagnosis of schizophrenia.

In a third family the father, after a great number of combat missions during the war, in which he carried a heavy responsibility and made an excellent record, decided to give up an assignment that would have meant continued promotion and to take instead another job in a climate more beneficial to the health of one of his two children. His dissatisfaction with this position aggravated the preexisting neurotic difficulties of his wife, who bore another son during this period. This child developed autistically amid continuing tensions between the parents that culminated in the father's developing a peptic ulcer, the mother's developing increasing phobias, and both parents' entertaining impulses toward marital infidelity.

In other families, we have seen the absence of a father from home due to military service, prolonged hours at work and study, or considerable pressure to do well in a position that was a marked advance in his career, or a father's illness at a period critical in the family's financial situation— all factors that could be classified as external, i.e., nonneurotic, sources of strain. The mother's reaction to these stresses, of course, exemplifies the internal neurotic component in her personality—frequently resulting in her sexual unresponsiveness—and the father's reaction in turn to both the mother's emotional state and his own situation in and outside of the family has been an intensification of his neuroticisms. In any case, such brief excerpts from the history of events in these families surrounding the birth or early childhood of the patient cannot do justice to the complexity of events we have known in any one family, not even of those in the families from which these excerpts are abstracted. This is particularly true as the multiplicity of factors unfolds itself during therapy with both parents.

The relation of each parent's conflicts to his earliest experience with his own parents is most evident in those families in which the grandparents are either still living, or living close to the child's own family or in the same home. When some resolution of the parents' conflicts occurs in therapy, we then see not only changes in the parents' attitudes toward the child and in the child's attitude toward them and toward himself, but often simultaneous changes in attitude toward the grandparents and, of course, toward the spouse.

I recall here the early paper of Erik Erikson [13] on the subject of the childhood experiences of the Sioux Indians. I was particularly impressed by the manner in which the young Sioux acquired identification with the members of his tribe and especially the trait of generosity toward them. This generosity was important in the days when survival on the Great Plains was so largely dependent upon successful hunting of buffalo. Those familiar with the facts reported by Erikson will recall how the Sioux young were in many instances still being reared, even after being penned up in reservations for a few generations. These rearing experiences had to do with nursing, with bowel and bladder training, with masturbation or other bodily self-stimulation, and with impulses toward possession of toys and the like. The child was on what is now called a self-demand schedule of nursing. He was rarely if ever beaten, and he was not trained for bowel or bladder control by the parents until old enough to be led by older siblings to appropriate places for such functions. He experienced no interference with any bodily self-stimulation, and learned from the behavior of the adults that his toys and other possessions were sacredly his own. Erikson also mentioned instances of some Indian parents who, upon receiving a long-awaited government check, unhesitatingly bought a toy or trinket asked for by the child, at times going without much-needed supplies as a result. Such parents bought the desired toy even though the child threw away the gift shortly after leaving the store. Erikson also observed that when a child was asked to close a heavy door, for example, no adult helped him, because it was considered possible for him or he would not have been asked to do it. The child learned, in short, that his needs, impulses, his bodily sensations and functions, would be gratified as promptly and as often as possible, and that his possessions were his own. He also had the opportunity to learn not only that no one had any wish to estrange him from any of them, but also

106

that no one had much anxiety either about his enjoying them or about his ability to do or learn to do things by himself. All this, of course, was heaven on earth for the Sioux until he was about six years old, after which the world changed a good deal for him. But this first period of his life tended to solidify his own integration (and/or incorporation of his experience) as well as his identification with parents and tribe.

All this is very different from the experience of many children in our culture, but it is particularly different from that of the children who are brought to the child psychiatrist with a psychotic illness or psychotic maldevelopment of personality.

PARENTAL DILEMMAS

Parents of schizoid or schizophrenic children may be in varying degrees, and for good reasons, helplessly guilty about their rearing methods, or for a long time completely unable to see or feel any relation at all between their own attitudes and the child's disorder. Those parents who bring in the most isolated, withdrawn, and silent children with the most bizarre self-preoccupations, the least spontaneity, and the greatest apparent indifference toward their own comforts and toward their parents, especially the mother, are also frequently the parents who show similar traits themselves. They are the parents who have the greatest difficulty in keeping their own daily lives, finances, libidinal economy, and thinking in some semblance of order. The mother has intensified unconscious needs for omnipotent, all-loving care and tenderness from her husband without any demands upon her. These unconscious needs turn into desperately necessary demands because of her own earlier frustrations and inadequate (ego) mastery of her own housewifely or other skills. Such frustrations and inadequacies constantly justify her own buried self-contempt and often make an external scapegoat necessary. She finds all these desperately necessary demands rudely frustrated. They are frustrated by exactly similar difficulties and demands of her mate upon her for comparable reasons of his own. Sapped by her own conflict and her husband's reaction, she may then turn toward the child, in regressive identification with her helpless infant, for all sorts of compensatory (libidinous, narcissistic) satisfactions in her experience with him. But she finds the child reacting with paradoxical negativistic tension to her anxiously rigid and unstable care of him. The child's protectively apathetic withdrawal and reactive nonlearning of basic skills stir further guilt and a sense of failure as a mother. She cannot help her child to experience the passive gratifications his helplessness makes necessary without experiencing a paralyzing fear of herself being destroyed in the process. Neither can she help the child through his regressive reactions of panicky hostility when she herself is in a similar state, alternately overinvolved or frozenly withdrawn. Thus, the child's reaction is a tremendously magnified mirror opposite of the mother's attitudes.

Such parents are also those who have the greatest difficulty in considering, accepting, or finally participating in psychotherapeutic work themselves because of fantastic degrees of anxiety about discovery and about destruction of precarious and inadequate sources of security. They are often not only the most convinced of organic disease etiology of their child's condition and most hopeless about him, as they are about themselves, but they are also the most certain for the longest time that there is not a shred of difference of opinion or attitude between them about the child, let alone any resentment or hostility. These are also the parents who are apt to manifest either overt psychotic symptoms during therapy, or an enormous drive toward divorce with one of them taking the child, or who are able to continue to live together only if the child is more or less permanently extruded from their home. Those parents who, during therapeutic work, are gradually enabled to feel resentment and eventually express it verbally and nondestructively toward each other or their child, are then also more likely to feel some affection, although both kinds of feelings are first experienced with great anxiety. It is interesting to see the child at times begin to cling tenaciously to the parent even before the parent himself is aware clearly of any change in himself. There are, of course, innumerable oscillations even in the relatively more successful cases, with explosive, murderous rages on the part of parents toward each other, toward the child, and vice versa, especially when the parent becomes tremendously anxious and guilty about some act of unconscious disregard or exploitation of his own and of the child's needs. We thus see both exacerbation and lessening of symptoms in the child and in the other parent whenever one parent or the child manifests either increasing tension of conflict or movement toward its resolution in his own therapeutic situation.

Another frequent result of working out conflicts in the therapeutic situation is a convincingly reported change toward integration of the other children of the parents—siblings of the patient not seen in therapy at the clinic. In several instances we have continued therapeutic work with the mother of such a disordered child through a subsequent pregnancy, and afterwards such mothers have reported a marked difference—a greater capacity for satisfactory mothering—in their experience with the new infant, in contrast to their experience with the child in therapy.

DISCUSSION

In spite of continuing disagreements, I think it is fair to say that there is a gradual change in the climate of opinion about schizophrenia among us. The fact that undoubted movement toward integration with psychological therapy occurs in schizophrenic patients of all ages [16, 44, 47, 48] raises for fundamental reexamination three inseparably interrelated aspects of theory. I refer first to etiology, second, to psychopathology and psychodynamics, and third, to therapeutics, before discussing prognosis.

Although opinion as to etiology is still divided between the constitutional-hereditary hypothesis [20, 21, 36, 46, 66] and the psychogenic hypothesis (which is more consistent with basic psychoanalytic postulates), the latter theory immediately involves the patient's experience with his parents. This is a hypothesis that is susceptible of considerable testing by therapeutic efforts based on psychoanalytic principles. Data are accumulating from various sources to substantiate the idea about the role of the mother in the disorder of the child. Space does not permit review of the nature of these data [15, 24, 33, 34, 41, 43, 62]; but data of other students and the Langley Porter Clinic experience suggest a basis for a few formulations.

One formulation would take the following form: the executive (or, as it has been called, conflict-free) ego organization is inversely proportional to the superego-repressed id conflict or conflicts. In other words, the greater the repression of the earliest libidinal impulses, the greater the sadomasochistic distortion of these impulses, with inescapably lessened control and greater likelihood and frequency of breakthrough of such distorted impulses into consciousness and especially into overt behavior that is at once revengeful and self-destructive. This result is self-destructive for at least two reasons. The anxiously defiant behavior (the return of the repressed) is still self-condemned by guilt, shame, and retaliatory anxiety, and therefore does not itself lead to full sensual (libidinal) satisfaction; secondly, it generally provokes further anxiously retaliatory—in effect, repressive—response from others, thus increasing the viciousness of the vicious circle

The more the organism's available energy is bound up in such futile, circular, self-defeating conflicts with itself and with others, the less it is available for learning really effective ways of obtaining biologically essential satisfactions through efforts in collaboration with others. One net result is that even "toward," "affectionate," and "independent" impulses come to be part of a frightening nexus that arouses so great a sense of danger that hostile activity alternates with frozen inability to feel an impulse to any but the most isolated activity.

From the point of view here advanced, repression is always a pathologic process and leads to a dynamic state of affairs that is the antithesis
of satisfactory living through learning, mastery of age-appropriate skills,
and full use of genetic endowment and environmental opportunities.
The schisis that comes about from repeated and intense experiences of
anxiety about many kinds of impulses involving bodily contact with
others and with oneself is, in this conception, one of degree. The amount
or intensity of anxiety experienced is a function of one's actual helplessness with respect to satisfying internal needs. Hence the earlier the developmental phase in which such experiences occur, and the more intense
and continuous or repetitive they are, the more enduringly damaging they
are to further learning and emotional growth, and the more perpetuating
they are of helplessness, despite apparent bodily growth.

Another aspect of the formulation has to do with the source of such
"intrapsychic," "intrapersonal," or internalized psychodynamics. Briefly
stated, the process is one of literal incorporation (in the sense of making
the response of another person a part of one's own corporal or bodily
reaction), the introjection of, and the identification with, both the disorder and the integrated personality of both of the parents, and the futile
rebellion against both. Although this statement depends for its substantiation on more detailed clinical therapeutic evidence from work with
parents and the child, many are aware of its basis, either from their own
experience or from the reports of students of this problem. Without
detailed, prolonged therapeutic experience, one may not be fully persuaded of its validity, since on the face of it the statement appears as a
condemnation of parents rather than as a dispassionate report of their
hidden, internal troubles. Those, on the other hand, with such experience
know how even the smallest detail of a particular child's inner history is
the result of his genetic endowment and his actual experience, intensified
by internalization. Especially important here is the revengeful and frightening caricaturing of the internalized parental image in the sadistic and
inconsistent prohibitions of the superego, particularly with regard to
impulses of the pregenital period. We have, for example, observed mothers
speaking to nurses about their own child who is present as if he were absent, or as if he could not understand. These are the children who speak
of themselves in the third person and behave as if they did not hear or
could not understand what was being said to them. We have also observed
many parents who, during visits on the ward, show much more interest
in other children than in their own child, who in turn reacts by showing
little or no interest in his own parents.

To summarize these remarks, one could say: that the psychotic child
manifests in his disorder the incorporation of and identification with the

disorder of both of his parents' personalities; that the schizophrenic makes a futile effort from the oral phase of development onward both to live up to and in a futile way to rebel against the often incompatible, fantastic solutions that each of his parents strives for with regard to his own unconscious conflicts, and the neurotic adaptation between them; that this disorder of the parents may not be as obvious on first anamnestic review to some who tend to concentrate attention upon the patient alone as to the trained and experienced clinician who can fairly promptly detect it as it manifests itself toward the child and in the child's reaction.

All this, of course, in no way excludes determinants of the character of the child's symptoms which express his genetic endowment as to sex, intelligence, and general vigor, or which express his reaction to such experiences as he may have had with siblings, playmates, or adults other than his parents.

It is possible to restate the results of all this largely in terms of individual or intrapsychic "structural" psychodynamics. Such dynamic, progressively internalized pathologic and pathogenically circular processes clearly interfere greatly with the ego development of the patient. The "weakness" of the ego has been confirmed by many psychoanalysts since Freud. More recently, Pious [37], Wexler [63, 64], and Hoedemaker [23] focus attention upon the extremely pathological characteristics of the superego functions and processes—and Hoedemaker particularly points to the incorporations and identifications giving rise to them—as the important source of the weakness of ego functions in the schizophrenic. Pious speaks of the superego as defective as a container of mortido; Wexler emphasizes its archaic and savage qualities; while Hoedemaker speaks of the ego as imbedded in such pathological tissue that the object of the first phase of therapy is to strengthen it by fostering the incorporation by the patient of a new, more stable, essentially less destructive, "superegolike" image of the therapist.

Such analytic experience as I have had with adult, borderline, or ambulatory schizophrenics—with one of them intermittently over a period of eighteen years—and the previously mentioned experience with families with a schizophrenic child, on the whole tends to confirm this general idea—namely, that the superego is both savage and defective (defective, however, in a sense different from that of Pious), and that the ego functions are either more or less generally smothered or underdeveloped irregularly (i.e., with islets of acquired skills), depending upon the particular experience of the child with the parents.

We need, however, to remember that, in addition to this superego-ego focus of pathology, there is a corresponding qualitative and quantitative difference in the repressed id portion of the schizophrenic personality.

Since the psychoanalytic theory of the personality is a field theory—a theory of a unit system—a shift in the intensity of forces in any one "part" is necessarily associated with an equilibrating or dynamic shift in all other "parts." Given the savage qualities of superego functions, the impulses of the repressed id are correspondingly violent, raw, and intense, with extremely tenacious libidinous fixations, especially at the oral and other pregenital levels. I would describe, all too briefly and inadequately, the defectiveness of the superego in its inconsistency (a kind of corruptibility) and lack of firmness against the violent eruptions of id forces which, upon thwarting or with tempting opportunities, possess the ego functions of motility, and its savagery, in its furious and vengeful punitive possession of the same ego apparatus a moment later. We frequently see in our preadolescent patients a quick alternation between revengefully sadistic attacks upon others and equally severe self-punishment. Excitements of older schizophrenics seem incomprehensible because of the swift alternation and mixture of the two processes. The sudden stillness, interpreted by Pious as an increased rate of dying, is for me more simply understood as a deadlock between the two processes: a squeezing of ego functions by equal intensities of pressures from both sides, the id and the superego, whether into total, catatonic immobility or into a sudden paralysis of particular ego activities. Parenthetically it might be said that the world destruction experience one hears about from recovered or partially recovered schizophrenics is the result of such a dynamic deadlock.

If all this is so, the question of appropriate therapeutics will depend upon all the factors in the clinical problem of the family as well as upon available therapeutic skill and time. Whether therapeutic work with parents will be done, or is even necessary, will depend upon all these factors, including the willingness, the readiness, or the sense of need for it that the parents show. Although such work is not uniformly successful, the matter of entering into therapeutic work with the parents is becoming a technical problem worthy of still greater attention and research.

The dictum that strength of ego means its capacity to serve its three taskmasters—the biologically essential id impulse, the superego discriminations as to cruelty, fraud or deceit, etc., and the actual opportunities and real attitudes of other persons—is fulfilled when one therapist is able to maintain his position of flexible but firm support of whatever component of the personality needs his help at a given time. In this sense Wexler's [63, 64] procedure, first, of actually physically restraining the patient in her revengeful or sadistic sexual assaults upon him, and later, of agreeing with the justified self-criticism of his patient, would promote repair of the defectiveness of the superego. In the same way, actual, gentle, firm, but not punitive (i.e., not anxiously revengeful) physical restraint of the child's destructive assaults upon objects, the person of the therapist, or his own person is essential at first, until verbal intercession becomes sufficient. This attitude simultaneously reduces the superego's savagery, since an actual damage or assault upon another is not committed or consummated, and therefore self-punishment is unnecessary or less necessary. The therapist's continued contact and interest in the patient after such events encourages the ego in the hope that a less sadomasochistic and therefore less dangerous gratification of the id impulse might eventually be possible. In this sense Hoedemaker's idea of the therapist's not only "talking to the ego" of the patient, but himself behaving realistically about himself and his patient regarding every important real issue of the patient's behavior in or toward the therapeutic sessions, offers the patient a "palatable and digestible" object "to eat" and identify with as an example of executive possibility. And whenever the executive ego functions are increased or enlarged, and defensive functions made less necessary, narcissism—that is, a really tolerant attitude toward the self—is increased, and more energy is made available for the ego's task, just as the spontaneous delight of parents upon the appearance of a new skill of their child increases the child's own pleasure at his own achievement.

I once heard Bertram Lewin say that mothering consists of "eating" the child and of "being eaten by" the child.[1] I would modify this a little and add that "good" mothering and "good" babyhood consist of both of them doing this with each other tenderly, and therefore without any retaliatory anxiety about the possible destructiveness implied in this mutual cannibalism for either of them. When the infant develops teeth, the ability to walk, and ability to learn all sorts of other skills necessary to his survival as an individual organism living among and with others more or less cooperatively, the mutually satisfactory previous experience during the infant's helpless state is internalized and solidly assimilated by the child as the anticipation that most of his real needs probably will be gratified by his own activities together with whatever real assistance he actually requires from firm, just, and realistic other persons. When this last does happen sufficiently often in childhood and adolescence, the integration of the personality is further consolidated and fortified. This last experience is in a sense as equivalent to the later phase of the more classical form of psychoanalytic therapy with a schizophrenic—the kind of therapy that Hoedemaker, Wexler, and others have described as equivalent to the fortunate experience of the infant with a "good" (integrated) mother.

---

[1] Lecture on "The Dream Screen Reconsidered" at the meeting of the San Francisco Psychoanalytic Society, August 22, 1952.

It does not at the moment seem to me necessary either to maintain that the procedures of a therapist in the first phase of therapy with schizophrenics are in the classical psychoanalytic form or that, on the other hand, such procedures need to be or must be eventually incompatible with it.

At present this is a frontier for further therapeutic work, sympathetic exchange of experience, and deep mutual thoughtful effort to arrive at a common understanding of terms, and, eventually, at a more precise theoretical formulation.

Finally, prognosis, for us, is beginning to fade as a very essential bit of prophecy when only willingness to begin work on the part of the family and the time available on the part of the staff decides whether the first regular appointment will be made. We are finding predictions about degree of success or duration of the work less and less important for the more experienced clinician, who presents his uncertainty about these questions to the parents, clearly but with calm conviction, and with no eager urging states that nothing less than actual collaborative trial can clarify such questions.

Factors in the prognosis that are probably of equal importance to the various factors in the child's disorder are the skill and experience of the therapist or therapists, and the length of time he or they are available. Somewhat unexpectedly, we have learned that a change of therapists, although generally a negative influence, is not always deleterious to the outcome.

It is perhaps not necessary to emphasize that among the many elements contributing to the skill of the therapist, his having resolved more or less thoroughly the remnants of pregenital conflicts from his own childhood experience is of considerable importance. Such resolution is important for him in order that he may be able to understand and behave therapeutically toward the intensely sadomasochistic distortion of the sensual, libidinal impulses not only of the child but also of the parents, whose guilty projections of their own deeply regressive conflicts onto the child, the other parent, and eventually onto the therapist, are a therapeutic problem of great complexity and magnitude. The training of therapists for this kind of work has been a problem second only to our own learning of the depth and varieties of psychopathology in these families.

We are relearning a truism: the obstacle to progress in therapy that may be contributed by the therapist is the countertransference [19] —in the original sense of the term, inadequately resolved conflicts of his own. And empathy with schizophrenic children and their parents—as with all patients— is inversely proportional to countertransference. In short, other factors being equal, the more thorough the resolution of the therapist's personal problems, the greater the chance that therapy will progress.

114

It may not be obvious from this very brief résumé of our experience of the past nine years what, if any, conclusions are possible. In this effort at testing the psychogenic hypothesis we have learned a great deal; but we do not think that we have "proved" the psychogenic hypothesis to anyone's total satisfaction. We think we have data in the few successful instances that would make the hypothesis more than a mere possibility; and we have continued—with whatever self-criticism we are capable of exercising—to look for the factors in the disorder of the child, in the family situation, and in our methods of work that resulted in the failures and in the instances of only slight or moderate improvement.

Thus far we have failed particularly with those families in which the child's disorder was extremely severe and practically coterminous with his life span, and in which such a child was seen initially late in preadolescence or early adolescence. The advanced age of the parents, or their experience of having the child out of the home for some years prior to our first contact with the family, has also seemed of some importance in these failures. We have failed relatively often with those families who were seen early in our own staff development. We have had less success when the family had a greater number of changes of therapists who were beginning their training in psychotherapeutics.

In contrast, several of us on the staff have had some exhilarating moments when those changes occurred that we hope for in the child and in the family. There have been enough such moments of satisfaction that the hypothesis will continue to be tested.

REFERENCES

1. ANGUS, L. R. Schizophrenia and schizoid conditions in a special school. *Am. J. Ment. Defic.,* **53**:227-238, 1948.
2. BENDER, LAURETTA. Childhood Schizophrenia. *Nerv. Child,* **1**:138-140, 1942.
3. _____. Childhood schizophrenia. *Am. J. Orthopsychiat.,* **17**:40-56, 1947.
4. BERGMAN, M., WALLER, H., and MARCHAND, J. Schizophrenic reactions during childhood in mental defectives. *Psychiatric Quart.,* **25**:294-333, 1951.
5. BRADLEY, C. *Schizophrenia in children.* New York: Macmillan, 1941.
6. BRILL, A. A. Psychotic children: treatment and prophylaxis. *Am. J. Psychiat.,* **82**:357-364, 1926.
7. CLARDY, E. R. A study of the development and course of schizophrenia in children. *Psychiat. Quart.,* **25**:81-90, 1951.

8. DAVIS, ANNE, and SZUREK, S. A. Some observations on the management of hostilities of children. *A.A.P.S.W. Newsletter,* **12**:96-98, 1943.

9. DESPERT, J. LOUISE. Schizophrenia in children. *Psychiat. Quart.,* **12**:366-371, 1938.

10. _____. Thinking and motility disorder in a schizophrenic child. *Psychiat. Quart.,* **15**:522-536, 1941.

11. _____. Prophylactic aspect of schizophrenia in childhood. *Nerv. Child,* **1**:199-231, 1942.

12. _____. Early recognition of childhood schizophrenia. *Med. Clin. Nor. America,* 680-687, 1947.

13. ERIKSON, E. Observations on Sioux Education. *J. Psychol.,* **7**:101-156, 1939.

14. ESCALONA, SIBYLLE. Some considerations regarding psychotherapy with psychotic children. *Bull. Menninger Clin.,* **12**:126-134, 1948.

15. FABIAN, A. Some familial considerations in childhood schizophrenia. Round Table on Childhood Schizophrenia. *Am. J. Orthopsychiat.,* **24**:484-528, 1954.

16. FROMM-REICHMANN, FRIEDA. Notes on the development of treatment of schizophrenics by psychoanalytic therapy. *Psychiat.,* **11**: 263-273, 1948 (and other writings).

17. FULLER, DOROTHY S. A schizophrenic pattern of behavior in a child with brain injury. *Bull. Menninger Clin.,* **18**:52-58, 1954.

18. GELEERD, ELISABETH R. "A contribution to the problem of psychoses in childhood," in *The psychoanalytic study of the child.* Vol. 2. New York: International Universities Press, 1946.

19. GREENSON, R. On Countertransference. Paper delivered at Annual Meeting of West Coast Psychoanalytic Societies at Coronado, California, October 1954.

20. HAJDU-GIMES, L. Contributions to the etiology of schizophrenia. *Psychoanal. Rev.,* **27**:421-438, 1940.

21. HENDRICKSON, W. J. Etiology in childhood schizophrenia: an evaluation of current views. (See especially "References.") *Nerv. Child,* **10**:9-18, 1952.

22. HILGARD, JOSEPHINE, and SZUREK, S. A. Successful psychotherapy of a choreic syndrome. *Psychosom. Med.,* **5**:293-300, 1943. Reprinted in S. A. Szurek & I. N. Berlin (Eds.), *Psychosomatic disorders and mental retardation in children.* Vol. 3, the Langley Porter Child Psychiatry Series. Palo Alto, Calif.: Science and Behavior Books, 1968.

23. HOEDEMAKER, E. D. The therapeutic process in the treatment of schizophrenia. *J. Am. Psychoanalyt. Assoc.,* **3**:89-109, 1955.

24. JENKINS, R. L. The schizophrenic sequence: withdrawal, disorganization, psychotic reorganization. *Am. J. Orthopsychiat.*, **22**:738-748, 1952.

25. JOHNSON, ADELAIDE M., FALSTEIN, E. I., SZUREK, S. A., and SVENDSEN, MARGARET. School phobia. *Am. J. Orthopsychiat.*, **11**: 702-711, 1941.

26. JOHNSON, ADELAIDE M., and SZUREK, S. A. The genesis of antisocial acting out in children and adults. *Psychoanal. Quart.*, **21**:323-343, 1952. Reprinted in S. A. Szurek & I. N. Berlin (Eds.), *Learning and its disorders.* Vol. 1, and *The antisocial child: his family and his community,* 1965. Vol. 4, the Langley Porter Child Psychiatry Series. Palo Alto, Calif.: Science and Behavior Books, 1969.

27. _____. Etiology of antisocial behavior in delinquents and psychopaths. *J. A. M. A.*, **154**:814-817, March 6, 1954. Reprinted in S. A. Szurek & I. N. Berlin (Eds.), *Training in therapeutic work with children.* Vol. 2, the Langley Porter Child Psychiatry Series. Palo Alto, Calif.: Science and Behavior Books, 1967.

28. KANNER, L. Autistic disturbances of affective contact. *Nerv. Child,* **2**:217-250, 1943.

29. _____. Early infantile autism. *J. Pediat.*, **25**:211-217, 1944.

30. _____. Feeblemindedness: absolute, relative and apparent. *Nerv. Child,* **7**:365-397, 1948.

31. _____. Problems of nosology and psychodynamics in early infantile autism. *Am. J. Orthopsychiat.*, **19**:416-476, 1949.

32. _____. Early infantile autism. *Am. J. Psychiat.*, **108**:23-26, 1951.

33. KASANIN, J., KNIGHT, ELIZABETH, and SAGE, PRISCILLA. The parent-child relationship in schizophrenia. *J. Nerv. Ment. Dis.*, **79**:249-263, 1934.

34. LIDZ, R. W., and LIDZ, T. The family environment of schizophrenic patients. *Am. J. Psychiat.*, **106**:332-345, 1949.

35. MAHLER, MARGARET S., ROSS, JR., J. R., and DEFRIES, ZIRA. Clinical studies in benign and malignant cases of childhood psychoses (schizophrenia-like). *Am. J. Orthopsychiat.*, **19**:295-305, 1949.

36. OSMOND, H., and SMYTHIES, J. Schizophrenia: a new approach. *J. Ment. Sci.*, **98**:309-315, 1952.

37. PIOUS, W. L. The pathogenic process in schizophrenia. *Bull. Menninger Clin.*, **13**:152-159, 1949.

38. POTTER, H. W. Schizophrenia in children. *Am. J. Psychiat.*, **12**:1253-1270, 1933.

39. PUTNAM, MARIAN C., et al. Case study of an atypical two-and-a half-year-old. Round Table. *Am. J. Orthopsychiat.*, **18**:1-30, 1948.

40. PUTNAM, MARIAN C., RANK, BEATA, and KAPLAN, S. "Notes on John I. A case of primal depression in an infant," in *The psychoanalytic study of the child.* Vol. 6, New York: International Universities Press, 1951.

117

41. RANK, BEATA. Adaptation of the psychoanalytic technique for the treatment of young children with atypical development. *Am. J. Orthopsychiat.*, **19**:130-139, 1949.
42. RANK, BEATA, and MACNAUGHTON, DOROTHY. "A clinical contribution to early ego development," in *The psychoanalytic study of the child*, Vol. 5. New York: International Universities Press, 1950.
43. REICHARD, SUZANNE, and TILLMAN, C. Patterns of parent-child relationships in schizophrenia. *Psychiat.*, **13**:247-257, 1950.
44. ROSEN, J. N. The treatment of schizophrenic psychosis by direct analytic therapy. *Psychiat. Quart.*, **21**:3-37, 1947.
45. SHEIMO, S. L., PAYNTER, JANE, and SZUREK, S. A. Problems of staff interaction with spontaneous group formations on a children's psychiatric ward. *Am. J. Orthopsychiat.*, **19**:599-611, 1949.
46. SHULMAN, A. J. The etiology of schizophrenia. *Psychiat. Quart.*, **24**:515-531, 1950.
47. SULLIVAN, H. S. The modified psychoanalytic treatment of schizophrenia. *Am. J. Psychiat.*, **10**(o.s. 88):519-540, 1931 (and other papers).
48. _____. Therapeutic investigations in schizophrenia. *Psychiat.*, **10**: 121-125, 1947.
49. SZUREK, S. A. Some problems in collaborative therapy. *A.A.P.S.W. Newsletter*, **9**:1-7, 1940.
50. _____. Notes on the genesis of psychopathic personality trends. *Psychiat.*, **5**:1-6, 1942. Reprinted in S. A. Szurek & I. N. Berlin (Eds.), *The antisocial child: his family and his community.* Vol. 4, the Langley Porter Child Psychiatry Series. Palo Alto, Calif.: Science and Behavior Books, 1969.
51. SZUREK, S. A., JOHNSON, ADELAIDE, and FALSTEIN, E. Collaborative psychiatric therapy of parent-child problems. *Am. J. Orthopsychiat.*, **12**:511-516, 1942. Reprinted in S. A. Szurek & I. N. Berlin (Eds.), *Training in therapeutic work with children.* Vol. 2, the Langley Porter Child Psychiatry Series. Palo Alto, Calif.: Science and Behavior Books, 1967.
52. SZUREK, S. A. The role of clinicians in the treatment of juvenile delinquents. *Fed. Probation*, **7**:30-33, 1943. Reprinted in S. A. Szurek & I. N. Berlin (Eds.), *The antisocial child: his family and his community.* Vol. 4, the Langley Porter Child Psychiatry Series. Palo Alto, Calif.: Science and Behavior Books, 1969.
53. _____. Child therapy procedures. *Psychiat.*, **7**:9-14, 1944. Reprinted in S. A. Szurek & I. N. Berlin (Eds.), *Training in therapeutic work with children.* Vol. 2, the Langley Porter Child Psychiatry Series. Palo Alto, Calif.: Science and Behavior Books, 1967.

118

54. _____ . Dynamics of staff interaction in hospital psychiatric treatment of children. *Am. J. Orthopsychiat.,* **17**:652-664, 1947.

55. _____ . Some principles of child guidance practice. *A.A.P.S.W. Newsletter,* **16**:116-122, 1947.

56. _____ . Remarks on training for psychotherapy. *Am. J. Orthopsychiat.,* **19**:36-51, 1949. Reprinted in S. A. Szurek & I. N. Berlin (Eds.), *Training in therapeutic work with children.* Vol. 2, the Langley Porter Child Psychiatry Series. Palo Alto, Calif.: Science and Behavior Books, 1967.

57. _____ . Some impressions from clinical experience with delinquents. In K. R. Eissler (Ed.), *Searchlights on delinquency.* New York: International Universities Press, 1949, pp. 115-127. Reprinted in S. A. Szurek & I. N. Berlin (Eds.), *The antisocial child: his family and his community.* Vol. 4, the Langley Porter Child Psychiatry Series. Palo Alto, Calif.: Science and Behavior Books, 1969.

58. _____ . An attitude towards (child) psychiatry. Part II. *Quart. J. Child Behav.,* **1**:36-54, 1949. Reprinted in S. A. Szurek & I. N. Berlin (Eds.), *Training in therapeutic work with children.* Vol. 2, the Langley Porter Child Psychiatry Series. Palo Alto, Calif.: Science and Behavior Books, 1967.

59. _____ . The family and the staff in hospital psychiatric therapy of children. *Am. J. Orthopsychiat.,* **21**:597-611, 1951.

60. _____ . Some lessons from efforts at psychotherapy with parents. *Am. J. Psychiat.,* **109**:296-302, 1952. Reprinted in S. A. Szurek & I. N. Berlin (Eds.), *Training in therapeutic work with children.* Vol. 2, the Langley Porter Child Psychiatry Series. Palo Alto, Calif.: Science and Behavior Books, 1967.

61. _____ . Concerning the sexual disorders of parents and their children. *J. Nerv. Ment. Dis.,* **120**:369-378, 1954. Reprinted in S. A. Szurek & I. N. Berlin (Eds.), *Learning and its disorders.* Vol. 1, 1965, and *The antisocial child: his family and his community.* Vol. 4, the Langley Porter Child Psychiatry Series. Palo Alto, Calif.: Science and Behavior Books, 1969.

62. TIETZE, TRUDE. A study of mothers of schizophrenic patients. *Psychiat.,* **12**:55-65, 1949.

63. WEXLER, M. The structural problem in schizophrenia: therapeutic implications. *Int. J. Psycho-Anal.,* **32**:157-166, 1951.

64. _____ . The structural problem in schizophrenia: the role of the internal object. *Bull. Menninger Clin.,* **15**:221-234, 1951.

65. YAKOLEV, P. I., WEINBERGER, M., and CHIPMAN, C. C. Heller's syndrome as a pattern of schizophrenic behavior disturbance in early childhood. *Am. J. Ment. Defic.,* **53**:318-337, 1948.

66. HERSKOVITZ, H. H., Chairman. Childhood schizophrenia. Round Table, 1953. *Am. J. Orthopsychiat.*, **24**:484-528, 1954.

SECTION THREE

STAFF INTERACTION

INTRODUCTION

The development of a therapeutic milieu requires the development of a staff who can collaborate effectively in the service of the child and family. Such staff development and integration occurs primarily through the repeated efforts of senior psychiatric and nursing staff members. This senior staff has learned some of the problems involved when the majority of patients on the ward are less severely disturbed.

The same senior staff, in subsequent experience with psychotic children as the whole population of the ward, continues to develop further their own understanding of their interaction with children, with their families, and with each other. They are then better able to help other new staff members to develop the most effective methods of helping seriously disturbed children.

The impact of the seriously disturbed child on the staff and their efforts to work together in a therapeutic fashion for the benefit of the child and toward their own further growth and understanding is described in the following papers.

CHAPTER 8

STAFF PROBLEMS WITH A SPONTANEOUS PATIENT GROUP*

S. L. Sheimo, M.D., J. Paynter, R.N., and S. A. Szurek, M.D.

When we speak of impulse to such and such action, of tendency to such and such behavior, of striving toward such and such goal, or use any of these words which sound as if you, a unit, have these things in you as if they can be studied by and for themselves, we are talking, according to the structure of our language and the habits of common speech, about something which is observably manifested as action in a situation. The situation is not any old thing, it is you and someone else integrated in a particular fashion which can be converted in the alembic of speech into a statement that "A is striving toward so and so from B."

Harry Stack Sullivan [1]

This concept has been helpful in dealing with the problems that have arisen around the formation of spontaneous groups in a children's psychiatric ward. As Sullivan would say, the staff, whether nurse, attendant, or psychiatrist, becomes a participant observer [11, 12].

Redl [2], Bettelheim and Sylvester [3], and others have reported upon the dynamic processes within groups of disturbed children in the preadolescent age range. Bender[4] speaks of the destructive and disintegrating effects such spontaneously formed groups may have on ward management and on the therapeutic program. The destructiveness of these groups often tends to invite their suppression by the staff. Even

---

*Reprinted by permission from *The American Journal of Orthopsychiatry*, **19**(4), October, 1949, 599-611. (Copyright, The American Orthopsychiatric Association, Inc.)

when suppressed, they may develop as secret or underground activities. Stewart and Axelrod [5], as well as Bender [4], report efforts with group therapy programs to meet these problems. Such programs, however, in our experience, often fail to prevent such spontaneous group formations and their destructiveness.

Since the opening of this children's ward in the fall of 1944, at which time there were more aggressive than neurotically inhibited children in the ward population, many spontaneous groups have been organized, often in direct opposition to the nurses and attendants. At one point in the history of this children's ward, the group members actually feared disapproval and punishment from one of its dictatorial leaders more than from the nursing staff in charge. Many efforts at curbing such activities were tried, such as attempts to forbid organization of such groups, restriction of the privileges and even the temporary isolation of the leaders, as well as directed group therapy programs. The turnover and change of staff were constant. Sutton [6], too, experienced and reported this problem of frequent resignation of nurses on such a children's psychiatric ward.

Partly as a result of these earlier experiences, the policy of admitting the impulsively aggressive child gradually shifted to that of admitting primarily the more inhibited, withdrawn child. Even so, there were usually two or three children of the more uninhibited type on the ward. Just prior to the initiation of this study, a small group began to form, with Leo, age nine, one of the more uninhibited, aggressive boys, as its leader. As will become evident later, it soon developed that here was another natural "central person"[1] who was destined to be a "dictator." The problems presented to the nursing staff by the troublesome behavior of the group which formed around him soon became frequent subjects of discussion at the daily ward staff conferences [9].

UNEXPRESSED STAFF DISAGREEMENT

In one of these conferences the senior psychiatrist suggested that perhaps more could be learned about these groups if the staff's reactions to them were not merely efforts at suppression. This might be a means of discovering the needs satisfied by such spontaneous formations [8]. The part the staff played in such activities might also be better understood and the forces within such groups used more therapeutically. One of the senior psychiatric nurses and the psychiatric resident undertook to observe and record events during the months that followed. The psychiatric resident, who was relatively inexperienced, spent much time on

---

[1] Redl [7] uses the term "central person" as synonymous with leader.

the ward becoming acquainted with the children and discussing some of the problems more informally with the nurses, especially with the two senior nurses.

In several subsequent staff conferences the details of the proposed study were gradually evolved. Rules and limitations within which the organization could develop would be kept at a minimum. Other factors in the group formative process, such as its purpose, leadership, and activities, would be determined by the various forces within the group itself. The staff would interfere only when it became necessary to protect the group or individual members from their own aggressive, destructive impulses—whether directed toward themselves or others. When necessary, this would be done not for the purpose of directing the group's activities, but to help the members decide what would be best for the group as a whole. This would involve giving them an opportunity for *developing* democratic procedures so that it would not be necessary to protect the group from all the effects of their own totalitarian or autocratic regime.

Some of the staff were hesitant and found it difficult to agree fully with this conception. One of the nurses actually expressed resentment toward the program and at times resorted to stricter disciplinary measures. The other senior nurse expressed a feeling of reluctance and hopelessness. She remarked that she had learned from her earlier psychiatric training that such impulsive, aggressive children ("psychopaths") could not be helped to change basically in personality organization, but could only be controlled by a strict routine.

During the six-month period covered by this report, there was a group of sixteen children which remained relatively constant. Of this group, eleven were boys, age range five-and-one-half to twelve; five were girls, four of whom were between eight-and-one-half and twelve; and one was an adolescent girl, age sixteen. Since we wish to emphasize in this paper the processes within the group of patients and between the group and the staff, we shall not present a formulation of the psychopathology in any given patient.[2] This group of children will be roughly divided into two general types: (*a*) the uninhibited type—the impulsive or aggressive child— and (*b*) the inhibited type, i.e., the more withdrawn, the anxious, neurotic child, or the more obviously psychotic child. In the group of sixteen

---

[2] Likewise, the concurrent treatment of the parents, a factor which also affected the events here reported (and which is an equally important part of the therapeutic program), will not be included because of considerations of space. For example, at this time the therapist of Leo's mother was having special difficulty in relieving her anxieties and conflicts.

children on this ward, twelve were of the inhibited type and four were
of the uninhibited type.

GROUP FORMATION

The group whose activities are here recorded, with Leo as its leader,
avowedly became organized for the "benign" purpose of playing "cowboys and robbers." It was a small group composed of an "elite" of four
to six children within a matrix of an unorganized majority consisting of
the remainder of the ward population. The more permanent members,
i.e., the "elite," were as follows: Philip, age eleven, an inhibited, intelligent boy, was usually, although reluctantly, first lieutenant. Donald, age
seven, an uninhibited, aggressive boy, was completely subservient to
Leo and often the scapegoat of the group. Ned, age twelve, a passive and
rather isolated but highly intelligent boy, occasionally left the group,
but gradually gained in prestige, eventually becoming first lieutenant.
George, age twelve, was an aggressive, impulsive boy, who was actually
larger and stronger than Leo but never manifested the latter's qualities
of leadership. No group ever formed around him; he was in and out of
the group frequently, but he was the only one whom Leo feared. When
in the group, he was used by Leo as his strong man for difficult tasks,
and was allowed reluctantly by Leo to share in leadership honors. George
often asserted himself against Leo, who distrusted him because of his occasional willingness to betray group secrets to the nurses. Percy, about
eight years old, was the most obviously divided in his loyalties between
the group and the staff. From the point of view of the group, he was a
"stooge," and hence was frequently ejected. These roles in the group
were illustrated about this time in a play centered around a rhythmic
dance and produced under the supervision of the physical education
director [10].

Efforts to Deal With the Group

Prior to the staff discussions leading to the new plan of handling Leo
and his group, the activities and influence of this group had spread over
the twenty-four hour period. Members were chosen, excluded, or ejected
at Leo's will. All group members were expected to share any blame or
punishment arising from Leo's activities. If any member disagreed with
his ideas, he was threatened with ejection from the group, and even with
physical punishment. Though the members often expressed their discontent to the nurses, they were unable to do so directly to Leo or to defy
him at this time. When any of the members were reprimanded and

disciplined, Leo would immediately take up the issue and go about the ward loudly proclaiming "One for all and all for one."

After the effort to suppress Leo's activities and gang, and after the first discussions regarding the new plan, another group was formed, with encouragement from the evening nurse, for "social and entertainment purposes." Ned was elected president, and Elaine, age eleven, often a vigorous vocal opponent of Leo, was elected vice-president. Leo refused to join this group but attempted to coerce Ned, with threats of bodily harm, into ejecting Elaine and then appointing him vice-president. At this point Nurse A[3] stepped in and suggested that Ned call a meeting of the group and discuss the "Leo-Elaine situation." Ned said he was afraid to oppose Leo's wishes. Consequently, the nurse stated that she would hold a meeting of the group, and Leo agreed to permit the boys to attend.

Nurse A was uncertain whether any active participation from the subordinate members would ensue. Her purpose in holding the meeting was to give each member an opportunity to express himself freely, and to give the group an experience in democratic procedures. She started out by explaining how a leader in a democratic society is chosen, how each member within a group has freedom to voice his approval or disapproval and to vote for the person he prefers. The person with the most votes then becomes the leader. At first the group members reacted indifferently and apathetically, but this changed as the meeting progressed.

George spoke up first in the meeting, saying that it did not matter who was originally elected leader because Leo would continue to be the "power behind the throne." He supported this statement with numerous examples of Leo's underground activities after the gang had been officially disbanded, or when there was no nurse around. Percy immediately took this up, expressing not only strong feelings of resentment and opposition toward Leo, whom he acknowledged as a good leader in some respects, but also pointing out very accurately that the submissiveness of the others would operate to make any democratic procedures futile. When asked for his opinion, Ned hesitantly agreed with Percy. Thus, Leo, denying every criticism, was attacked from all sides by members within the group. Finally, Philip, who up to this point had been unable to voice any opinion, asked, "Why do we need a leader anyhow?" and suggested, "Let's just all play together." Everyone except Leo agreed, and the meeting was adjourned.

This experience was discussed in considerable detail in staff conference. Nurse A remarked that she felt discontented with her role in the

---

[3] For the purpose of identification, the two senior nurses who were primarily concerned in this group experience will be referred to as Nurse A and Nurse B.

meeting, that perhaps she had been too passive in it. Was she getting satisfaction from seeing Leo attacked from all sides? It was suggested that apparently Leo had some positive qualities, because he was inevitably placed in the position of the leader in any group, and the rest of the members themselves had remarked that no one was as good as he.

EFFECT ON LEO

For a week following the meeting, Leo was sullen, resentful, and defiant. Tension on the ward increased, and Leo was constantly getting into trouble and annoying the nurses. This reached an intensity unbearable to Nurse A, who released verbally much of her annoyance and resentment toward him; but afterwards she was able to say to Leo that she felt that he was unhappy and that it was perhaps the result of the meeting. She admitted her mistake of acquiescing in the others' attack on him and not actively recognizing his positive qualities. She praised him for them, but told him firmly that what she did not approve of was the *type* of leadership he provided for the group. Thereupon Leo began to cry and said he felt he was all alone, that no one cared for him, that everyone, nurses and boys, was on George's side, and that everyone was against him. The nurse then was able to be warm toward him while maintaining her position in regard to his impulsive behavior.

Following this episode between Nurse A and Leo, it was observed that the group immediately reorganized, with Leo again the central person. The general tension and annoyance in the ward atmosphere were reduced to a minimum, and even though Leo remained the leader, there seemed to be a greater readiness on the part of George and Percy to voice their disapproval and feelings toward him. Leo, on the other hand, became less threatening and retaliatory in response to such opposition, and would occasionally come to the nurses for help in settling some of his group problems, and especially to obtain their aid in controlling George.

Slowly the group began to include more of the children from the general ward population. For about two months the activity of the group centered around a fort built of orange crates and placed in the ward playroom, and much fantasy play was observed. Two of the girls were nurses, while the boys were cowboys, fighting imaginary battles and returning to the fort wounded so as to be treated by the "nurses." One evening the group indulged in an active "war" against the nurses [staff] instigated by Leo to settle a mild personal grievance with them. Each child was asked which side he wished to be on. Except for two of the psychotic children, all chose to be on Leo's side. Several apologized for their choice. Percy sent a note to Nurse A before the attack saying, "I love you but I have to kill you." The group had prolonged "powwows," planning the attack upon the nurses. The battle lasted about an hour, with the staff indulging in "roughhousing" with the "Indians," who finally captured the nurses and attendants. Such activity, with greater constructive features and freedom, occurred more frequently when Nurse A was in charge.

The Triangular Situation

At this time the pet cat was in heat, and the children became interested in having her mated. This situation led to much interest and inquiry in regard to the origin of babies, and also led to some fantasy play around Elaine and George getting married, and Elaine having a baby because she was "in heat."

Much of the activity now consisted of collecting various articles about the ward which were carried as "treasures" to the fort. These treasures consisted at first of cowboy and war equipment brought from home, then of articles from the ward supplies for their first aid kits and some food, especially fruit. Most of the treasures, particularly the most prized items, were concentrated in the hands of the leader and his current first lieutenant, George. All items collected by the group members were turned over to Leo, and he, in turn, distributed the articles he did not want to the other members. At this point Nurse A stepped in, suggesting and urging that there be a more equal distribution. Leo argued that he and George collected most of the articles, so equal distribution was unfair. The nurse then suggested that all be given equal opportunity as well as responsibility for contributing to the fort stores.

However, when other members became responsible for contributions, some of the treasures began to include more of the essential ward equipment, which was taken from supply rooms on the ward. Upon discovering this, and because some of the fruit was spoiling, Nurse B intervened and asked that all the food and essential ward equipment be returned to its proper place. She forbade the collecting of any ward equipment. Conflict between children and nurses then increased. Stealing and concealing replaced overt collection and open hoarding. The more essential the article of ward equipment, the more likely it was to disappear. As a punishment, Nurse B ordered all stores, both ward equipment and personally owned articles, confiscated for a week.

Just about this time, the hospital supply clerk, after a visit to the ward, observed that if the children should ever have access to matches, the fort would become a fire hazard. This possibility caused the nurses some concern. The children then began to steal matches from the pockets of nurses and attendants, and from the nurses' station, keeping these matches hidden in the fort. This was discovered by Nurse B who, in consultation with the supply clerk, examined the fort and then definitely decided that it was a fire hazard, that the nurses could not take this responsibility, and that it was inadvisable to have the fort on the ward. She therefore asked the group to move their fort activities out of doors.

Beginning of Rebellion

Following this, Leo became more defiant and abusive toward the members of the group, while the group seemed to become more submissive and enslaved by their leader than they had been for some time. There was a marked increase in their aggressive, destructive behavior. They refused to allow any except the most loyal group members to frequent the outdoor fort; they continued to steal ward equipment and material which even included some patients' charts. The fort was now located in a secluded wooded spot in the hills behind the hospital, in close proximity to the University power plant. During this time there were repeated efforts on the part of the senior nurses to inspect the fort, to recover essential ward equipment, and to forbid such activity. After each attempt the children became more aggressive. Complaints began to come in from the superintendent of the power plant and the medical school business manager via the medical superintendent of the hospital. It was reported that some of the boys were throwing rocks through the windows of the power plant and attempting to roll a large ball of wire through the windows into the plant, which could cause a short circuit. Fears for the safety of the children were expressed by the research foundation, which was housed behind the power plant and had many pens behind a fence in the open for dogs and other animals. They feared that the children might be bitten by some of the animals and possibly infected with diseases being studied by the research staff.

However, not all of the children's activities were destructive. For instance, a garden was planted. Underbrush was cleared to enlarge the space for the fort, and an old tub was prepared for use as an aquarium. But destructive incidents seemed to predominate. On one occasion, on a trip to a nearby park, the group attempted to hold up a strange boy and take his money for the purpose of buying equipment.

Tension among the staff grew. The children seethed with rebellion. Staff conferences centered around possible reasons for this aggressive behavior. The staff had sensed for some time that something was wrong and had made efforts to discover what it was and to correct it. The psychiatrist suspected that some issues between the staff and children had not been completely settled. Repeated staff discussions failed to relieve the tensions. Complaints of destructive acts from persons outside the immediate ward personnel increased. Some decisive action had to be taken.

The senior psychiatrist, with Leo and George and some of the staff, explored the fort in the hills, noting its relationship to other buildings on the University campus. He told the boys of the complaints made to him and expressed some annoyance with their behavior, but told them he would try to intercede with his superiors and other complainants in order to save the fort. He then discussed the situation with the superintendent of the hospital and the superintendent of the power plant. The latter stated that he was frankly concerned that the children might get hurt as well as damage some vital machinery, and that the group seemed to be running around without adequate supervision. (This impression might have been due to the fact that nurses on this service do not wear uniforms on duty.) The director of the research laboratory was insistent that the children be kept away from the open cages because of the danger of infection from the experimental dogs. The psychiatrist did not wholly agree that this danger was great, but because complaints from this source continued, he felt he could not press for permission for the children to continue using the path, which ran immediately beside the pens and was the only route to the fort.

Beginning Resolution

Consequently, he called a meeting with Leo and Ned and told them, in the presence of Nurse A and the psychiatric resident, of the position in which the activities of the group had placed him in relation to his superiors in the hospital and others in the campus community. He told them that he wanted them to have fun and had tried to save their fort, but although he very much regretted it, the matter was now out of his hands and restrictions would have to be placed on their activities. He expressed his annoyance with them and said that he felt they did not need to act this way, that they could behave differently and still have fun, although he admitted that the attitude of the staff might in part account for some of their behavior. He promised that the staff would try to discover and to modify what it was in themselves that contributed to the disturbance.

In reaction to the senior psychiatrist's comment concerning staff attitudes, and in order to give all the group members a chance to talk and learn about the restriction of their activities, Nurse A and the psychiatric resident called a meeting of the whole group and presented the situation to them. They expressed essentially the same feelings as those of the senior psychiatrist and told the children that until such time as the staff felt that they could be trusted, they would have fewer of the liberties and privileges they had thus far enjoyed.

Following these sessions, the aggressive and destructive behavior on the part of the group subsided. Their activities began to take on a predominantly constructive form. They concentrated on the garden in the neighborhood of their outdoor fort and did more planting, weeding, and watering. They planned to use the vegetables for a party for their parents at the end of the school year. They "camped" in sleeping bags on the ward. Projects developed around the production of a play for the parents, which the group members themselves expressed a desire to present at the end of the school year.

With this change in attitudes all around, Leo's tyranny really came to an end, although his leadership continued. There was frank and open disagreement or criticism of him by his followers. Hostile expressions occuring in reaction to staff attitudes became more verbal. The tension of the staff decreased.

DISCUSSION

In retrospect, as we formulated this report, it became clear to us that the problems of the staff in respect to the spontaneous group formations actually increased following the suggestion of the senior psychiatrist that the staff's methods of dealing with such groups be modified. Although the plan was intended to further therapeutic ends, the result of the suggested modification of previous staff methods, which had worked to some degree at least in controlling difficulties, proved actually to be at the same time somewhat destructive and disintegrating. It became evident that the plan was applied before it had been thoroughly thought out in all its implications. To understand why this was true, it is necessary to go back a little way into the past history of the ward and reconstruct briefly the relations between staff members prior to the new plan. There was already a smoldering and submerged conflict between Nurse A and Nurse B which had its beginning in the early history of the ward. Nurse A was originally one of the senior nurses in charge of the children's ward when there was, as previously mentioned, a predominance of aggressive patients causing much disturbance on the ward and in the rest of the hospital. In order to meet these difficulties, Nurse B was placed in charge and made senior to Nurse A. Nurse B was rather self-assured and decisive. She tended to be firm and at times strict and suppressive. She was at the same time constantly on the lookout for recreational privileges for the children, for gifts of toys and equipment from likely donors, and the ward routine was considerably enlivened and enriched by her efforts.

During this period Nurse A, although often not in sympathy with some aspects of Nurse B's methods, tended to conform and submit to her attitudes. However, at times Nurse A would partially retire from active participation in the handling of aggressive children or groups of them. The differences between these two personalities were frequently evident in staff conferences. Nurse A was more intuitive, more capable of empathy with neurotic children, and consequently better able to report the details of the behavior of such children. She was able to suggest the probably subjective feelings not only of the children, but of herself and of the staff as well. Nurse B would frequently dismiss the activities of the day with "Everything is all right. They act just like normal boys." If Nurse A reported some episode which seemed to the psychiatrist a change in the emotional state of a child, Nurse B often quickly remarked that this had been true for a long time. Their competition for preferred status with, and approval by, the senior psychiatrist was indicated in many other ways.

The senior psychiatrist's plan served to increase this conflict between the two most experienced members of the nursing staff, which began to assume the proportions of a definite rift and resulted in a more open division in the rest of the staff. It may be that the senior psychiatrist, although aware of these previously existing tensions in the staff, both underestimated their degree and failed to foresee the disintegrating effect of his suggestion. The plan was frustrating to Nurse B who, being unsympathetic to it, was also confused by it. She tended thereafter to retire from her previous active supervisory control and in effect passively to resist and to deprecate Nurse A's efforts. In this way she expressed indirectly some of her resentment toward the senior psychiatrist for what perhaps seemed to her a depreciation of her methods and judgment, and also of her status with him.

On the other hand, the plan served as an encouragement to Nurse A, who liked the less authoritarian attitude implied in it. However, for several reasons she felt some lack of confidence in applying it. Her previous training and her experience of having had relatively little success with such children made her dubious as to whether the aggressively uninhibited or "psychopathic" patient would respond to treatment, or whether his behavior patterns could be changed. Her status in relation to Nurse B, and her inhibited rebellion against the latter, increased her anxiety and hesitation in carrying out the plan, despite her eagerness. Nurse B's continuing doubt and partially inhibited deprecation of the whole idea further increased these conflicts of Nurse A. The psychiatric resident, eager for more active participation in the work, and recognizing the research possibilities in the plan, perhaps tended by his enthusiasm to increase the pressure on Nurse A to go ahead despite her reluctance. At the same time, because of his relative inexperience, his subordinate status, and his overidentification with the senior psychiatrist, he was unable to be sufficiently helpful to either of the nurses, although even more aware than the senior psychiatrist of the rift in the nursing staff. Although he listened to the complaints and doubts of both, he was more of a passive observer than an active participant in the early course of events.

This rift between the senior nurses was reflected in, and increased, a divisive alignment of the junior nursing staff and attendants. They became divided in their loyalties according to their own personal inclinations. Some of them were more comfortable with Nurse A, while others were more at ease with Nurse B. The schedule of work was arranged so that each of the senior nurses was in sole charge of the ward for a continuous period of three or four days. This arrangement increased the confusion of staff attitudes. Neither of the senior nurses had, on her days in charge, junior nurses and attendants who were all wholly sympathetic to her. This alternation of regimes also contributed to the inconsistency of attitudes to which the patients were exposed. It was obvious that the patients sensed the differences and conflicts and utilized them for their own ends. For example, they expressed their fear of Nurse B to Nurse A, while Nurse B complained to the psychiatric staff that the children were more excitable, and the junior nurses and attendants more upset, after Nurse A had been in charge.

Lack of space does not permit us to demonstrate in detail what we consider to be a definite correlation between the conflicts within the staff just described and the behavior of the spontaneous group formation previously narrated. A few examples must therefore suffice.

After an initial period of happier and more constructive activity on the part of the group under Leo's leadership, following the tentative inception of the new plan by Nurse A, increase of hostile aggressive activity ensued. It will be recalled that the children initiated and enjoyed construction of the fort on the ward and the open collection of treasures in it. Nurse A considered unimportant the displacement of some articles of ward equipment and accepted the hoarding of food and fruit sympathetically. Her attitude was in part an expression of her inhibited rebellion against the authoritative and overly restrictive tendencies of Nurse B, as well as of her sympathy with the plan of giving the children greater freedom. The food naturally began to spoil, and the waste was an offense to Nurse B's personal attitudes toward waste of food. The displacement of ward equipment violated her sense of good ward management and her nursing principles. Her prohibiting the collection of all treasures, and confiscating even personal belongings among these treasures for a whole week, expressed not only the limits that needed to be applied to reduce the inconvenience to the staff, but also represented some of her inhibited resentful tensions. In reaction, the gang began to steal, and they stole even more essential articles of ward equipment. The ukase of Nurse B aroused further resentment and associated anxiety in Nurse A. The subsequent increase in unruly behavior of the gang, which was usually greater on her days in charge, was a result of her anxiety, while simultaneously giving vicarious gratification to her resentment against Nurse B.

The operation of similar dynamics between staff tensions and reactive destructiveness of the group was evidenced in what followed as a result of the concern about the fort as a fire hazard, and its removal from the ward to the hill behind the campus. Nurse A's lack of concern about matches (because in her experience they were usually returned to her without any accidents), and Nurse B's anxiety about them, expressed the complicated attitudes between them previously described. The stealing of matches increased, justifying the removal of the fort from the ward by Nurse B. This increased the hostility of the gang and at the same time enlarged their theater of operations. Their aggressive, destructive activity against the campus community and against the larger community around the hospital evoked, in turn, the complaints of the campus authorities. These were, of course, visited upon the responsible head of the children's ward, namely, the senior psychiatrist. Thus the train of events initiated by the senior psychiatrist's suggestion came back to him in full circle with a kind of poetic justice. The prematurity of his suggestion, his underestimation of the intensity of staff tensions which his suggestions released, and his failure to deal effectively with these tensions in staff conferences during the course of ensuing difficulties were the "sins" for which he was "punished." They made it necessary for him to act directly and decisively in an effort not only to meet the real difficulties with the campus and local community created by the behavior of the children, but also to heal the rift in the attitudes of his staff. His handling of the leaders of the group tended to close the ranks of the staff behind him in relation to the group. His firmness and frank resentment combined the unhesitating decisiveness of Nurse B with the desire of Nurse A to give the children greater freedom. As a result of his attitude, Nurse B's skepticism was justified and her resentment appeased, while Nurse A's vacillations were reduced and anxieties regarding the destructiveness of frank expression of anger by a therapist toward patients were somewhat allayed.

A further opportunity occurred for the resolution of the conflicts within the staff about this time. The senior psychiatrist was away for ten days, and Nurse B went on a five weeks' vacation. During this interval problems caused by the behavior of the group had to be met by Nurse A. In moments of greatest uneasiness she made an effort to get relief through discussions with the psychiatric resident. Although in general he supported her, he tended to encourage her to make her own decisions. In reaction to this, and perhaps because of his relative inexperience, Nurse A was able to express more frankly her resentment to him. She would say, for example, "What are you trying to do—act like a psychiatrist?" After such discussions she was able to return to the problem of the children and the subordinate staff and act more firmly and decisively. The successful solution of such problems during this period tended to increase the self-confidence of both toward each other and toward the patients.

Our conclusion from this effort at formulating our experience is that no study of the dynamics of a group or of an individual patient on such a ward is complete without the study of the dynamics of staff interaction as well. It has already been reported by others [11, 12] that the behavior of the therapist, or, in our case, of the staff, needs to be an integral part of the report of clinical experiences. In this sense we agree with Sullivan that no observer can avoid being a participant of that which he observes. Furthermore, we would agree with him that for a more complete understanding of events in a psychiatric sense, it is necessary for the observer, with equal alertness and self-scrutiny, to observe his *own* participation.

* * * * *

ADDENDUM, 1970

The reasons for including this paper in a volume which is largely devoted to the development of an inpatient psychiatric service primarily for psychotic disorders of preadolescent children may be of interest.

The study described herein was performed within a few years after the present director assumed his duties in February 1946. During this period the majority of the patients on the ward were not psychotic. Hence, the kind of group formation described has not been seen by the staff in subsequent years, when the majority of the patients on the ward were seriously withdrawn and markedly isolated from one another. In describing some of the events of those years, this paper constitutes a bit of the history of the development of the inpatient practices and of the experience of the staff of this service.

The study was performed because at that time the problem described was a recurrent one for the staff and because it was hoped that something could be learned to improve the staff's way of dealing with the more destructive and more malintegrative influences of the group behavior on the individual patient's benefit from hospitalization. Due to

136

the dearth of psychiatric staff at that time, relatively few of the children had any individual psychotherapeutic work offered to them. Therefore, the effort to apply more clearly delineated principles to the work with the group of patients was an expression of the hope that under these circumstances some directed, therapeutic influences that were more consistent with psychodynamic theory underlying individual therapy might be made available.

The study further demonstrated to the staff the importance for its therapeutic effectiveness of two inseparable factors: (*a*) that of the degree of their individual self-awareness in professional work with the patients; and (*b*) the need for constant assessment of the response of patients to the attitudes and behavior of staff members toward one another. It made clear that transference-countertransference phenomena (more complicated than those in the dyadic situation of individual therapy because involving a number of patients and staff on the ward) *were* present and needed recognition and specific identification. These transference-countertransference phenomena required resolution for the formation of a therapeutic milieu in which patients could progress in the solution of their own conflictful personal problems.

The importance of alertness to such intra-staff processes, of course, had been, was being, and continued to be repeatedly stressed beyond this specific study in many conferences and reviews of treatment about the daily events on the ward, in which the behavior of the patients was constantly reviewed in the context of the staff's efforts. In this experience with patients who were less severely disordered than those who are psychotic, all the efforts with the staff proved to be valuable, and were even more important in the later years when the entire population of the ward was made up of psychotics. The study described here gave a particularly clear example of phenomena that often occur beyond those more explicitly recognized in formal staff group conferences—phenomena not often identified in the publications of the time on inpatient psychiatric work with children.

The conclusion from this study and from the other references, implicit and explicit in the discussion portion of this paper, is that this transactional [13] mode of thought about clinical problems is as fruitful for therapeutic decisions in inpatient work with a group of patients as it is in individual psychotherapy.

REFERENCES

1. SULLIVAN, H. S. Conceptions of modern psychiatry. *Psychiatry,*3: (24), 1940.

2. REDL, FRITZ. Group psychological elements in discipline problems. *Am. J. Orthopsychiat.,* **13**:77-81, 1943.

3. BETTELHEIM, B., and SYLVESTER, E. Therapeutic influence of the group on the individual. *Am. J. Orthopsychiat.,* **17**:684-692, 1947.

4. BENDER, LAURETTA. Group activities on a children's ward as methods of psychotherapy. *Am. J. Psychiat.,* **93**:1151-1173, 1937.

5. STEWART, K. K., and AXELROD, P. L. Group therapy on a children's psychiatric ward. *Am. J. Orthopsychiat.,* **17**:312-325, 1947.

6. SUTTON, HELEN A. Some nursing aspects of a children's psychiatric ward. *Am. J. Orthopsychiat.,* **17**:675-683, 1947.

7. REDL, FRITZ. Group emotions and leadership. *Psychiatry,* **5**:573-596, 1942.

8. BUXBAUM, EDITH. "Transference and group formation," in *Psychoanalytic study of the child.* Vol. I. New York: International Universities Press, 1945, pp. 361-364.

9. SZUREK, S. A. Dynamics of staff interaction in hospital psychiatric treatment of children. *Am. J. Orthopsychiat.,* **17**:652-664, 1947.

10. VAN VLEET, PHYLLIS. Rhythmic activity—a project in group therapy with children. *Am. J. Orthopsychiat.,* **19**:79-86, 1949.

11. SULLIVAN, H. S. Therapeutic investigations in schizophrenia. *Psychiatry,* **10**:121-125, 1947.

12. _____. Notes on investigation, therapy, and education in psychiatry and their relations to schizophrenia. *Psychiatry,* **10**:271-280.

13. DEWEY, JOHN, and BENTLEY, ARTHUR. *Knowing and the known.* Boston, Massachusetts: Beacon Press, 1949.

CHAPTER 9

DYNAMICS OF STAFF INTERACTION*

S. A. Szurek, M.D.

PSYCHIATRIC NURSE-PATIENT INTERACTION—A THESIS

The dynamics of individual therapy, i.e., the processes in the situation of a therapist and child, have received much attention, thought, and experimentation. Group therapy, that is, the situation of several patients and one therapist, has similarly been the subject of an increasing number of studies and clinical efforts.

At a recent psychiatric meeting (of the American Psychiatric Association, Chicago, May 1946) there was a round table discussion on a topic entitled, "The Psychodynamics of Residential Treatment of Children." During this discussion several participants suggested that in addition to direct individual treatment in play or interview sessions with the child, and in addition to concomitant therapy of the parents, there was much to be learned about what went on between other adults and children in a residential treatment center or psychiatric hospital ward for children. It was suggested that the counselors, nurses, and attendants in such situations might constitute, by virtue of the time they spent with such patients and by virtue of the care they gave to them, a valuable therapeutic resource. Perhaps still too frequently, for various reasons avoidable and unavoidable, that part of the staff personnel which has most personal contact with the hospitalized psychiatric patient has not participated as

---

*Reprinted by permission from *The American Journal of Orthopsychiatry,* **17**(4), October, 1947, 652-664. (Copyright, The American Orthopsychiatric Association, Inc.)

fully[1] as it might in clinical conferences or informal discussions with supervising and resident psychiatrists and other professional members of staff. Their recorded observations of the behavior of patients and their technical assistance in medical procedures and custodial functions have long been utilized, or at least required. The extent to which personnel attitudes affect the patient's emotional state is a matter of general clinical experience[2] even outside a psychiatric ward or hospital. The deliberate use of the relationship between patient and nurse by the physician for therapeutic purposes is probably as old as the art of nursing. But its frank acknowledgment as a therapeutic adjunct in psychiatric literature[3] and discussions and the study of its dynamics and relative importance in the treatment of the patient are relatively infrequent [4].

The influence of discussions between psychiatrists and nurses in one such clinical setting upon the behavior and progress of the patient in the hospital impressed the participants so strikingly that some of these experiences led to mutual recognition of its value and more conscientious use. One of the nurses said in effect quite spontaneously early in this experience, "Let us talk about this child's behavior at ward rounds. It seems as if when we talk about such problems they disappear."

Because of what appears to be a wider applicability of such an approach, the recording of several excerpts from this experience was considered of some value. Obviously, none of the samples of psychiatrist-nurse-patient interaction is an isolated and discrete incident having no connection with the growing complex relation between them. They are rather indicative only of the latter, and perhaps are those parts of it most easily described.

SETTING

The circumstances of these examples of staff interaction may be of interest. The ward, with a bed capacity for sixteen children under twelve

---

[1] Rowland [1, 2] describes the relatively closed caste system characteristic of the social structure of a mental hospital's employees, emphasizing in particular the closer contact of the nurses and attendants with patients. There is also discussion of types of interaction processes and of prevalent attitudes of conflict between these staff members and the patients.
[2] Kimber [5] places stress on the importance of psychiatric nursing as the treatment needed by most hospitalized psychiatric patients.
[3] Reichert [3], in addition to Kimber, is among the few psychiatrists who call attention to the therapeutic possibilities of the attendant-patient and nurse-patient relationship. From personal communication the writer is aware that Sylvester and Bettelheim at the Orthogenic School, Chicago, are also interested in this problem. See also [7] and [6].

140

years of age, is on the fourth floor of a psychiatric hospital located on the urban, medical campus of the State University. The remainder of the hospital's 100-bed capacity is devoted to the care of adult patients. On the children's ward itself, in addition to a day room, playroom, and two individual rooms for isolation purposes, and a dining room serving also as a schoolroom, is the office of the psychiatrist-director of the service where the staff gathers for almost daily morning discussions. Those attending include the nurse in charge, two to four psychiatric resident physicians, the Fellow in psychology, the psychiatric social worker assigned to the children's service, and the psychiatrist responsible for the service. Frequently the school teacher, the occupational therapist, other nurses, and attendants are invited to participate.

Contextual Reporting by Nurse

Discussions are generally begun by the nurses who are asked by the psychiatrist to tell of any events which appeared important to them in the previous twenty-four-hour period. Whether or not anything is evoked by such a general question, each patient is then named by the psychiatrist as another question to elicit comments about progress, general behavior, physical condition, or about some special attitude and problem previously discussed. A deliberate effort is made to encourage each participant of the conference not only to describe what has been observed and heard from others about bits of the patient's spontaneous behavior, but also to express surmises as to its meaning, as well as the overt and subjective response to the patient. Especial effort is made to elicit as many details about the incident or behavior reported as possible: all persons involved and their attitude and behavior throughout; as exact chronological order of events as possible; the connection, if any, to such events as letters, gifts, or visits of relatives; medical procedures and the subsequent behavior of the patient in reaction to the adult or adults in question.

The emphasis is placed on simple, nontechnical verbal descriptions. The psychiatrist now and again encourages further elaboration by repeating a phrase, or by suggesting several alternative motivations or feeling tones implied in the description of the patient's behavior for the reporter to choose from or to add his own interpretations. In all such discussions the implications made clear and explicit are: (a) that the patient's motivation is often made evident not only by observing all possible details, but also by noting the feelings evoked; (b) that the nurse or attendant is not only "the eyes and ears" of the doctor and often his best medicine, but is often the only person who may be able to understand and deal effectively with the child's attitude at the moment; and (c) that perhaps the most important clues as to treatment may become manifest in such incidents.

After all possible elaboration has been made by the nurse, attendant, or teacher, the others of the staff are free to add their remarks before the psychiatrist responds with his comments. His comments are not only in the nature of possible interpretations of the psychodynamics, if these have already not become clear in the foregoing discussion, but are also frequently comments of approval or satisfaction at the manner of handling problems. When the meaning and purpose of the patient's attitude are not clear, a frank admission of ignorance is coupled with expressions of encouragement to observe further, and of confidence that persistent study may reveal the answers to problems. Sympathetic acknowledgment is made of the difficulties experienced in tolerating the drain upon one's emotional reserve in certain types of trying occasions; the difficulty, for example, of restraining an impulse to respond at times with frank resentment and impatience.

The psychiatrist also explicitly assumes responsibility for a difficult choice in management, but this is done as a last resort. Wherever possible, suggestions or clues for dealing with problems are sought from the nursing staff. Modifications may be added by others in the conference as well as by the psychiatrist. In this manner an interpretation or a decision is often the achievement of the entire group, requiring only the agreement and approval of the psychiatrist. Any anxiety, uncertainty, indecisiveness, and even discouragement of any member of the group also obtains ventilation, dilution, and often relief, especially when the psychiatrist himself leads in giving frank and full verbal expression to any such feeling he himself or others in the conference may have. Occasional individual discussions of a nurse or attendant with the psychiatrist add further opportunities for the discharge of uncomfortable feelings not only toward some patient, but also toward other members of the staff. There are probably many other nuances, processes, and effects of such frequent verbal interchanges not easy to isolate for description. Perhaps some such interindividual processes in the staff may be suggested and their effects on the behavior and feelings of the patients be in some measure revealed in the examples which follow.

PROBLEMS IN EATING

Eating, nutrition, and food habits are generally matters for considerable concern to nuring personnel, reinforced perhaps by principles of their professional training.

142

Case 1. A girl of eight years, among other symptoms, had for weeks picked at her food, eating little despite urging and coaxing of the nurses. She had lost eight pounds in two months, which concerned the nurses who described at conference the patient's food habits and their own efforts to modify them. In this discussion the psychiatrist suggested not only several possible meanings of the symptom in terms of the patient's previous relation to her mother, but also that in this instance it might be better to give the child absolute freedom to eat as much or as little as she wished. Assuming the responsibility for the experiment's failure and the patient's continued loss of weight, the psychiatrist expressed confidence that the natural appetite and hunger of the child could be relied upon in the known absence of organic disease.

For three days following this conference, the patient watched the nurses continually throughout meals, manifesting obvious surprise at their acceptance of untouched plates without comment or concern. She began to eat on the fourth day, increasing the amount gradually until at the end of two weeks she was eating a full meal and gaining weight.

The first impulse to sympathize with or to reassure an uneasy patient—so often a part of the so-called common-sense attitude of nurses—when tempered by discrimination based upon a more precise comprehension of the psychopathology involved, may help toward resolution of the particular conflicts.

Case 2. A malnourished, underdeveloped, shy girl of fifteen repeatedly complained to the nurses about the teasing of several preadolescent boys. They chanted so insistently that another boy or the male resident physician was her boyfriend, that the patient wept angrily and was very restless and agitated. In the conference discussion, her ambivalent interest in sex, men and boys, as well as her great conflict regarding her status, became evident from the reports of several observers. The psychiatrist suggested that instead of consoling the patient, as previously, the nurses admiringly comment on the boy's good looks and otherwise give evidence of accepting her adolescent strivings. Within a few weeks not only did the patient become much more relaxed generally, but she began to use lipstick and nail polish and asked for a permanent wave. Incidentally, the teasing of the boys decreased considerably.

PROBLEMS OF DESTRUCTIVE-PSYCHOTIC BEHAVIOR

The repeated and detailed discussions of the staff's experience with disordered behavior of psychotic degree and intensity may be of crucial importance in its treatment.

Case 3. A boy of seven, whom we shall call Dan, had been a difficult nursing problem for about four months prior to the inception of the daily staff conferences. He avoided contact with other children, stayed in his own room, screamed for nurses when he needed to go to the bathroom, or waited until no other children were about and dashed into it. There he remained until removed by the nurse. In his own room he scribbled on the walls, tore his bed linen, threw articles out of the window, and, although previously thoroughly toilet trained, often urinated on the floor. On several occasions, after playing with water in the bathroom, he succeeded in flooding the room and corridor. After such exploits, upon the approach of the nurse, the patient often injured himself severely. For weeks there was an ulcer on his lip from his biting it, self-inflicted bruises and abrasions on his legs, and lacerations on his arms where he had bitten himself. There were large, discolored swellings on his head from bumping it against walls and objects, and "black eyes" from punching himself. At such times he shrieked and screamed continually for two or three hours, often covering his head with a pillow.

If Dan's attention could be obtained at such times by the adult, he complained of a pain in his finger or obsessively began to ask many questions. He had filled the bathtub to see how many gallons it would take to fill it. How many gallons would it take to fill the whole bathroom? How many to fill the ward? How many to fill the whole hospital? Or, how much did the doctor weigh? Did the nurse weigh more than the doctor? Which doctor on the ward weighed most? How much does a balloon weigh? How much does a bubble weigh? Or, on other occasions, what hurts more—to bite your finger or have a door slam on it? During this time, for about four months, he had been receiving individual play therapy from a woman therapist twice a week in hourly periods.

The most marked change in behavior prior to the conference discussions of Dan's symptoms was a decrease in the frequency of the screaming spells. For the first two and a half months these occurred repeatedly during the day and two or three times at night, lasting one-half to two or three hours. In the last six weeks of the first four-month period there was a gradual decrease until nine consecutive nights occurred without screaming.

On the first night of duty of a nurse new to the ward, screaming so severe and prolonged recurred that not only the children's ward but the entire hospital was disturbed, and the patient had to be removed to another part of the hospital. The new nurse's embarrassment and concern was relieved in a discussion with the psychiatrist. She was told that the patient's screaming was a very difficult symptom to deal with, and not only other children but the rest of the patients in the hospital might on such occasions be disturbed. The psychiatrist in charge took the responsibility for meeting the complaints of other services for such occurrences, which are neither preventable nor uncommon in mental hospitals. It was suggested she do what she could to calm or soothe Dan without removing him from the ward and without too much concern about the other patients for the time being. The following night Dan screamed again but it was much briefer in duration and ended in his whispering in response to the calm firmness of the nurse. Although he woke during the following three nights he whispered to get the nurse's attention and told her his wishes directly. Only once after this, about a month later, did Dan scream at night. He stopped when the nurse approached and whispered that his mother was going to skip a visit to him.

As previously mentioned, discussions at daily staff conferences with the nurses began about four months after Dan's admission. His behavior was their chief concern. The psychiatrist acknowledged repeatedly how confusing and trying Dan's behavior must be, and said that any adult faced with the provocative exploits of such a child would sometimes become quite angry. For various reasons the adult in attendance on a psychiatric ward might attempt to suppress the anger. The exhibition of self-injury that occurred after destructive or mischievous acts would necessarily arouse in the adult some guilt, anxiety, vacillation, and eventually a sense of futility and helplessness in dealing with the child.

The obsessive questions appeared to the psychiatrist as anxious efforts on Dan's part to distract the adult from consequences he feared, and not necessarily only as evidence of a precocious scientific curiosity, as suggested by his father. On other occasions the same questioning appeared to be a distorted and covert expression of a hostile impulse since efforts at answering the questions led only to further and more absurd questions. In any case, if the adult was left baffled with anxious annoyance at the patient's behavior, there was no immediate settlement of the issue.

The psychiatrist commented that he could not suggest what others might do under such circumstances because they might have different feelings in reaction to Dan's behavior, but he himself would have the impulse fully and frankly to express feelings of annoyance, resentment, or disapproval. He could then feel freer, with more genuine interest in Dan's welfare, to restrain him firmly from any physical self-injury, saying also that he did not wish the boy to suffer or hurt himself, nor to exaggerate either the offense or the adult's resentment. Obsessive questioning would be brushed aside till the child clearly understood all that the adult felt. If eventually Dan's attention were secured, he might be helped to reduce his guilt and restore his self-esteem by making some sort of restitution, e.g., helping the adult to clean up any mess, etc.

On one or two occasions, during a walk through the ward, opportunities occurred for the psychiatrist to demonstrate some of the things about which he had spoken to the nurses and residents. He once firmly but gently restrained Dan from self-inflicted blows, examined his lip, and left his questions unanswered, and asked Dan to tell about why he was frightened or angry.

After several discussions the nurses spoke of the relief to their sense of frustration with Dan, and of their feeling that a definite attitude had been outlined. After a few incidents in which they settled issues, a marked change in the child's behavior became evident in two weeks. His disturbed periods became less frequent and shorter, self-punishment was less extreme and within a month disappeared. By the end of two months Dan attended school, showed much interest in other boys on the ward, and expression of his disappointments or of his wishes became more direct. The obsessive questioning gradually became relatively rare. It is not claimed that Dan's disorder was cured by this means, but only that he became much more accessible. Therapeutic hours with his therapist became more productive, and his parents, also seen in therapeutic interviews, were more hopeful. The mother, especially, was somewhat better able to manage the boy during visits with him away from the ward.

PAINFUL BOWEL MOVEMENTS AS A PROBLEM

It is not surprising that physiological functions of patients, and perhaps especially those of the gastrointestinal tract, which are well known to be susceptible to modification by psychological influences, should be affected by staff discussions. This point, however, may be further emphasized by citing the following episode.

Case 4. Tom, age eight, had been so withdrawn all his life that he had spoken only two or three words, and then only under marked emotional stress. He had spent about a year and a half prior to his admission here in two children's psychiatric hospitals. Later performance tests proved his intellectual capacity was within the average range. When enraged by very minor thwartings, he sat on the floor digging his fists into his eyes, thumbs in his mouth, drooling saliva, and rebuffing anyone who came near him. He was slovenly in dress, in eating, and in toilet habits, soiling and wetting himself frequently.

On admission to the ward and for a few weeks later there were protruding hemorrhoids, with fresh blood in the stools. Nurses expressed concern about this and asked if laxatives, fruit juices, or other dietary changes should not be instituted. Discussion ensued at the conference of the probable role of the patient's inhibited and self-directed rage in the appearance of the rectal symptoms. The psychiatrist presented examples from previous clinical experience with constipated patients, in which lack of anxiety on the part of the therapist, and his expressions of firm confidence that bowels do not move without medical urging, had successfully ended constipation. The contribution of nurses and physicians to continued constipation and to the patient's anxiety about it in their insistence on a daily bowel movement, and the frequent use of laxatives in hospitals was also pointed out. He suggested that the staff wait until the patient and staff became better acquainted.

Following this conference one of the nurses remarked to another staff member how reassuring the attitude of the psychiatrist was. Thereafter the nurses were able to show their sympathy to the boy during his painful bowel movements. The bloody stools, which occurred every two or three days in the first two weeks after admission, gave way to bloodless ones within a week, and to normal daily movements within fourteen days. One resident physician later facetiously remarked that as the nurses relaxed, apparently the bowel also relaxed.

SELF-DESTRUCTION AS A PROBLEM

Intercurrent increases of inhibited resentful tension on the part of one or more members of a staff is occasionally dramatically expressed in sudden emergence of a self-destructive symptom in a patient. Its treatment includes not only attention to the patient, but also to the staff.

Case 5. About two months after admission Tom suddenly began an upward flipping of the nail of his middle finger against his right cheek, coupled with a marked prolonged inspiration. This stereotyped act was so persistent that he was brought to the morning conference. A broad area of the cheek along the corner of the mouth and nose extending up toward the eye was markedly reddened and swollen. The flipping was frequent and automatic, interrupted only when the nurse embraced the child and put him on her lap. Discussion revealed only that it had appeared in the previous twenty-four to thirty-six hours. No one could relate any recent change or event of interpersonal significance in Tom's experience on the ward. The psychiatrist suspected some increased hostile tension in the staff toward him but contented himself with the remarks that the boy was in many respects obdurate, difficult to like and care for with his slovenliness of personal habits and tendency to rebuff adults. It was agreed that a soothing lotion and a light dressing be applied to the cheek, and as much individual attention be given the child by those nurses or attendants who most enjoyed being with him, in short shifts if necessary, so that none might feel burdened beyond endurance.

On the following morning the child was again presented to the conference with the cheek now crusted and even more inflamed. He had permitted the dressing to remain and the finger flipping had decreased during the day shift, but he had so repeatedly torn off the dressing during the late afternoon and evening that it had finally been left off, while the flipping continued unabated. Still no clues as to the source of the difficulty were apparent. The psychiatrist expressed his discouragement that neither he nor the staff was reaching or influencing the source of the tension. A resident psychiatrist suggested a soothing ointment and a lighter dressing more firmly attached. He remarked that despite the symptom, the child was easier and friendlier with the staff, to which the nurses agreed. After this conference a nurse reported privately to the psychiatrist that one or two members of the staff found it difficult to be with Tom and had expressed their dislike and disgust. He accepted this information with some discouragement, but hoped that these staff members would express their resentment of the boy to one another.

On the following day the inflammation of the cheek had improved and within a few days subsided completely. It was not established whether this change occurred as a result of the discussion. It seems probable, however, that the psychiatrist's frank expression of his own discouragement with himself and with the staff was an important factor in the changes in attitudes of the rest of the staff toward the problem.

THE PROBLEM OF THE HOPELESS DIAGNOSIS

Attitudes of the staff toward prognostic implications of the diagnostic titles given to the condition of a patient were found to have an important bearing upon the patient's progress and behavior.

Case 6. An eleven-year-old girl, with a history of marked withdrawal and very queer behavior since very early childhood, had previously been diagnosed as schizophrenic and admitted to a hospital, where she remained for months without improvement. Following admission, she remained much of the day in the first month near or on her bed, whispering, clapping her hands, self-absorbed, often grimacing, dancing rather grotesquely, or assuming queer postures and positions. Sudden eruptions of intense rage in which she kicked out windows and doors, broke dishes, alternated with pulling up her dress, removing underclothing, and urinating on the floor. Infrequent, large, and apparently painful bowel movements were deposited on the floor in corners or elsewhere. Open genital and anal masturbation was frequent. Nurses only later were able to admit that they felt there was little hope for the child, and showed much less spontaneous interest in her than in other less disturbed patients.

Finally, one morning a nurse expressed perplexity about how to deal with a new variation of the masturbatory activity. The child was reported as frequently dancing toward a nurse, masturbating and chanting with glee, "Janie is playing with her vulva, yes? To put your hands in your vulva is bad! The doctor will cut you off! Going to put your hands in your vulva anyway!" Then laughing, she ran back to her bed in the corner. Although the child was reassured by nurses that she would not be "cut off," the behavior continued. The nurses reported that the fascinated curiosity of other children in Janie's masturbation had been dealt with with calm explanations that Janie was sicker than they were. The children accepted this explanation with a decrease of interest in her.

The psychiatrist expressed ignorance as to the complete genesis, motivation, and meaning of this type of masturbation. However, he was impressed that the patient, whatever the total complex of impulses being expressed, was moving away from her corner, and perhaps a little out of her autistic world toward a real person—the nurse. He suggested that the nurse might say on such an occasion, "Oh, I'm sorry, Janie, that I've been busy and haven't had the time to spend with you." Then she might add that she now had time to play with her, or that she was busy but would be free shortly.

There was further discussion about the possibility that withdrawal, perhaps a defensive measure as a result of unhappy experiences with people, did not signify that the withdrawn child was actually or wholly unresponsive to the real feelings and attitudes of others. No one could say with certainty what all the factors were which produced the schizophrenic picture in either children or adults. There were an increasing number of clinical reports of favorable results of persistent efforts of therapists to establish durable affective contact with schizophrenic patients.[4] Perhaps the global discouragement of such patients induced discouragement in the people around them, and a vicious cycle tended further to fix the disorder of the patient. It was a question of trying to understand, and perhaps only occasionally of getting a glimpse of what such a patient felt and expressed in an extremely distorted or fragmentary manner, and then responding to it. In any case, frank expression of one's own feelings toward such a person—even if at the moment resentful or impatient—might give opportunity to the patient to experience a continuity of affective contact with others. That is, the expression of the adult's anger might have two effects: (a) the patient might have the

---

[4] See Fromm-Reichmann [8 and 9], especially the latter, for summary of psychotherapeutic efforts with psychotics by various therapists, and for references to literature on this subject, also [10].

experience that the adult was not anxious about showing resentment toward the child because it implied confidence that the child could tolerate it; and (*b*) the child would experience the adult's continuing, friendly, freer interest after expression of the resentment. In either or both instances there would be no rupture of affective contact between the two as is likely to occur when the adult struggles with some inhibited resentful feelings and is therefore unable to feel friendly interest in the child. It might then be an experience for such a child that she was not excluded, estranged, hopelessly misunderstood, and given up by others as perhaps she already tended to feel toward herself.

It was frankly admitted that such an attitude would probably not bring immediate results or that it might fail altogether. The staff was invited to participate in an experiment. The absence or the relative absence of prompt affective response on the part of such a child to the adult's offer of contact would probably continue to be a discouraging factor. On the other hand, this attitude on the part of the nurses toward the patient might also provoke demands of such intensity or outbursts of rage upon slight frustration that these reactions might also evoke uneasiness, dismay, and a tendency in the nurse to withdraw from the patient.

Three or four days after this discussion the nurses spontaneously and with evident satisfaction reported that "the idea worked." On the first day after the conference Janie stopped the gleeful masturbation immediately upon the response of the nurse, as suggested in the conference. The number of such masturbatory episodes in front of nurses decreased sharply, and in its place the child began to call the nurses by name for various requests. Gradually she began to approach nurses more and more actively, seeking satisfaction in play and acceding to requests to help clean up after urinations or defecations on the floor. Periods of self-absorption in dancing, posturing, or whispering to herself were more and more replaced by activities with nurses. She was able to eat in the dining room with other children with fewer outbursts of rage and destructiveness. Exposing her genitals, urination and defecation on the floor gradually decreased markedly in the following months. Eventually Janie remained for longer periods in the schoolroom and began to participate in the work. Whereas in the first few weeks of her residence she was generally observed standing alone ten to twenty feet apart from the group during recess out of doors, she was more often seen trying awkwardly and tentatively to play ball with the nurse and other children.

As in the instance of the previously described psychotic boys, it is not suggested here that the disorder was in any basically significant degree improved by such experiences. Janie is still far from well. Individual therapy both with the patient and the parents is clearly necessary, and has been started. But it is also evident that the child is more accessible, obviously happier on the ward and, one may perhaps assume, having a much more integrating experience in the hospital than she might otherwise have. At the time of this writing Janie has been in the hospital over ten months, and menses have been established. At the very least, one may say that progression in the direction of deterioration or increase of affective withdrawal has not occurred.

An additional observation made in the course of this type of experience with the staff of nurses and attendants was a certain cumulative effect of such conference discussions upon their attitudes toward patients. The progressive training or growth in therapeutic capacity was manifested in several ways. There appeared greater freedom and spontaneity, which was reflected not only in conference discussions but also in responsiveness to patients. During discussions the staff tended to report more completely the relations between patients, and between themselves and patients. The reports were instances of interpersonal interaction and sequences of interpersonal events rather than the previously prominent descriptions of one patient's actions or symptoms as if *in vacuo*. There was an increased tendency to express something of what the child appeared to feel and to what events or characteristics of others, including themselves, the child seemed to be reacting. Expressions such as "I had the feeling that the boy was afraid . . .," or "It seemed to me as if so-and-so was angry about . . .," or "I guess maybe I wasn't too certain . . ." were heard more often.

The nurses were able openly to object to the opinions of other members of the staff and to maintain their own positions with reasoned arguments or with additional observations against the objections of others. Spontaneous suggestions for dealing with particular problems of particular children were more frequently offered. Their responses became more precise therapeutically. On the one hand, it was evident that there was a more conscientious effort to understand the meaning and real purpose of a child's action or attitude and to deal with it; on the other, there was a greater frankness, directness, and simple honesty about their own reactive feelings toward the child. The latter was exemplified by the nurse telling a boy, after patiently listening to his obsessive questioning about apparently irrelevant matters, that she still did not understand what he wanted or was concerned about, that she wanted to understand and help, but could not help feeling a little annoyed, impatient, or baffled. Such responses often led to some resolution of the issue or greater frankness on the part of the child. Space permits only brief illustrations of the nurses' efforts to understand and deal with the actual motivations or reasons for a patient's anxiety or symptomatic acts:

In one instance, a seven-year-old boy was screaming and complaining of various pains and aches. The nurse, instead of indefinitely attempting to quiet and comfort him, asked what he was really worried about, and eventually obtained the statement that he did not know whether his mother was going to visit him that day. The nurse telephoned the mother, received a definite reply, and communicated it to the boy, which relieved his tension and screaming promptly.

In another instance, a schizophrenic girl of eleven suddenly kicked a little retarded, epileptic girl who had been sitting on a nurse's lap. Instead of reacting with reproof or restraint to this hostility, the nurse asked the older child if she, too, wished to sit on her lap. The younger child, she was told, had been there for some time and would not mind going to play; if she wished, she too could take her shoes off and come and sit. The schizophrenic child, for the first time since her admission, responded promptly, took off her shoes, and cuddled contentedly for some time on the nurse's lap.

TOTAL STAFF MOBILIZATION IN SERIOUS PROBLEMS

Occasionally, with very difficult clinical problems, this more complete staff collaboration appears to be a more effective therapeutic approach:

A sixteen-year-old girl, of dull average intelligence, from a deprived, rural background, had been disabled for almost a year by paralysis of the entire right leg and left arm. Repeated, careful, complete examinations revealed no organic disease. She had been in the hospital for about seven months, and efforts at individual psychotherapy under sodium amytal and sodium pentothal sedation were without positive results. Her initial rather resentful unresponsive attitude gradually gave way to mutism toward the hospital staff and her family. She made no spontaneous effort to move about for her needs, nor to care for herself, and refused to participate in occupational therapy or in entertainment such as movies. She was indifferent about her future and about returning home.

At the beginning of her eighth month of hospital residence she was transferred to the children's ward despite her age, as a last experimental effort at treatment. Limitation of space does not permit more than a few brief comments regarding the staff's experience with this patient. It must suffice to say that after numerous conferences in which details of her behavior and the reactions of individual nurses to her were repeatedly discussed, the first marked change in attitude and behavior appeared. After much deliberation, and after inclusion of nurses and attendants from all three shifts in discussions and decisions, there emerged an attitude of encouraging confidence in the girl coupled with increasing firmness toward her and greater expectation of her. Within two and a half months the patient moved about with the help of a chair for all her needs, dressed and cared for herself, and she spoke to all members of the staff. She became much more cheerful and responsive, began to read, and for the first time enjoyed visits from her family and was eager to make visits to her home. She began to move her paralyzed hand and foot slightly upon urging. Further treatment was interrupted when her parents decided to take the patient home, insisting they could themselves complete the treatment which had been started.

DISCUSSION

As a participant in these experiences I have no settled convictions about the significant dynamisms operating in the group behavior described, nor confidence that efforts at abbreviated formulations of such processes would be very complete or satisfactory to others. Perhaps readers of this attempt at communicating our experience will be better able to supply these for themselves, or suggest aspects to the writer which are not evident to him. Perhaps a few concluding comments may indicate and emphasize those factors which have seemed important.

The inclusion of the nursing staff as very significant collaborators in the therapeutic process is not only a logical consequence of the premise that all interpersonal influences are important in the therapeutic process, but is also a clear and unambivalent expression and application of this general principle. The serious importance accorded to the nurses' role certainly increases their sense of participation in and consequent enthusiasm for a common effort. Ambivalence toward one another regarding status, and possession of esoteric knowledge and skill between nurses and other clinicians of the staff, at least have an opportunity to be reduced. Coordination of efforts with the patients of individual therapists and with the rest of the staff as to tempo and goals becomes more possible.

Within the limits of more or less unalterable (by these discussions) personality traits of individual nurses, such group discussions offer a greater prospect that the patient's problems, symptoms, or impulses will meet with a uniformity of attitudes from all the staff. This often results in a greater security for the patient with a consequent more rapid change in his self-attitudes. Similarly, within these same limits, something of the therapeutic principles and attitudes learned in individual treatment—even though probably very diluted—may become incorporated into more of the patient's whole experience in the hospital.

In all of this, one can isolate for particular attention the factor of the relief of the anxiety of the entire staff. Open expression in group discussion by the psychiatrist of the more or less common but suppressed or repressed reactions of the staff to the child's symptoms—about which the staff frequently has some shame, disgust, guilt, or even fascination—certainly tends to reduce tensions. Perhaps it may also increase somewhat their tolerance for themselves and hence for the patients.

Another aspect, or perhaps it is only another way of saying the same thing, is that the immature, regressive, and ego-alien impulses of the children tend to be accepted with less defensive anxiety and resentful efforts at suppression by the staff, and with greater indulgence of the regressive needs. When the psychiatrist admits and accepts the difficulty of tolerating with relative equanimity the regressive or hostile trends of patients, the staff's expectation of itself may be reduced to more comfortable and realistic proportions. This necessarily results in greater patience toward such impulses and in calmer firmness. The greater patience, however, does not permit overindulgence to regressive trends to the point of further fixing them. Implied in such attitudes of tolerance and firmness is a confidence in the patient's eventual ability to learn other attitudes, which is often a powerful encouragement to the progressive tendencies of the personality. None of these factors or aspects is new to any therapeutic situation, but their operation between the patient and a larger number of persons in the hospital appears to be the significant addition.

Another result of such closer collaborative relation between the nursing and attendant personnel on the one hand, and the other clinicians on the other, is that overburdening a particular nurse or attendant beyond her emotional capacity for a given symptom or for a given patient may be less likely. When a nurse or attendant is found to experience particular difficulty with a certain patient, measures may be taken to reduce her difficulty. A discussion between psychiatrist and charge nurse usually decides whether the problem is to be dealt with (*a*) by the charge nurse directly, (*b*) by an individual conference with the psychiatrist and the nurse in question, or (*c*) by reducing the time such a nurse will be asked to spend with the child she finds difficult. The attempt is to help the nurse, if possible, in resolving her conflict if she wishes to do so. In any case, she is relieved of further responsibility with regard to the patient, immediately if necessary, and permitted to return to the problem of her relation with the patient when she is ready. There are, of course, limits to this possibility, namely, the number of patients in residence and the staff available to care for them. When the limit is reached and pressure upon the nurse cannot be alleviated, she herself may ask for transfer to another service. Such requests are always granted with no invidious implications as to her general professional capacity.

It is certain that many other aspects of this problem have not been elucidated and discussed in this study. It is hoped that what has been touched upon may stimulate further explorations and more publications of the experiences of others in this field of increasing clinical importance.

REFERENCES

1. ROWLAND, HOWARD. Friendship patterns in the state mental hospital: a sociological approach. *Psychiatry,* **2**:3, 363-373, 1939.

2. _____ . Interaction processes in the state mental hospital. *Psychiatry,* **1**:3, 323-337, 1938.

3. REICHERT, ARNOLD H. Morale and the attendant: a note on personnel problems in hospitals for the mentally disordered. *Mental Hygiene,* **28**:4, 632-638, 1944.

4. DEVEREUX, GEORGE. The social structure of a schizophrenia ward and its therapeutic fitness. *J. Clin. Psychopath. and Psychotherapy,* **6**:2, 231-265, 1944.

5. KIMBER, W. J. T. Social values in mental hospital practice. *Brit. J. Ment. Sci.,* **85**:354, 29-44, 1939.

6. SZUREK, S. A. Child therapy procedures. *Psychiatry,* **7**:1, 9-14, 1944.

7. GILBERT, RUTH, and SUTTON, HELEN. A children's psychiatric service. *Am. J. Nursing,* **43**:570-572, 1943.

8. FROMM-REICHMANN, FRIEDA. A preliminary note on the emotional significance of stereotypes in schizophrenics, *Bull. Forest Sanitarium,* Des Plaines, Ill., **1**:17-21.

9. _____ . Remarks on the philosophy of mental disorder. *Psychiatry,* **9**:4, 293-308, 1946.

10. KNIGHT, ROBERT P. Psychotherapy of an adolescent catatonic schizophrenia with mutism: a study in empathy and establishing contact. *Psychiatry,* **9**:4, 323-339, 1946.

CHAPTER 10

THE UNIQUE ROLE OF THE CHILD
PSYCHIATRY TRAINEE

Irving N. Berlin, M.D., and Adolph E. Christ, M.D.

The trainee in child psychiatry who is involved in an inpatient or day
care setting is beset by many problems, perhaps the most ubiquitous of
which is that of finding a unique role for himself. He discovers that nurses,
teachers, occupational therapists, and the like, who spend most of their
day with the child, have more information and in some instances a more
intimate relationship with the patient than he is likely to have. Each
worker feels that his interaction with the child is the most vital to his recovery. The child psychiatry trainee, having lived through similar feelings
early in his adult inpatient work, is again beset by uncertainties about
how much his few therapeutic hours with the child are worth in contrast
to the time and effort of his collaborators. When he finds that other
child-care personnel are also involved on a daily basis in helping parents
learn to interact more effectively with their child, he often wonders what,
in fact, he has to contribute that is his and only his [7–9]. We have come
to believe that in addition to the psychotherapeutic role, the synthesizing
or integrating role is a potentially unique one for the trainee. We will describe our efforts at delineating that role somewhat later.

The concepts to be discussed here have concerned teachers of child
psychiatry and directors of child psychiatric inpatient settings for many
years [1, 2, 14–18, 20, 21]. We have tried to analyze our experiences,
consider many of the issues raised by our trainees, and synthesize our
formulations for our own benefit and to stimulate discussion with others.

The specific tasks that the trainee should master can be roughly classified as follows: (*a*) assessment of psychopathology in the child and parents; (*b*) evaluation of emotional level of development of the child,
especially in terms of degree of ego development, needed to plan a

therapeutic milieu program; (c) assessment of cognitive development of the child, in Piaget's terms [11, 23], to help plan the steps in educational experiences to promote mastery and cognitive growth; and (d) psycho-therapeutic work with child and parents.

The assessment of parental pathology, defenses, and ego strengths, which helps one decide how to assist parents to provide a facilitating milieu for their child, is a collaborative task for the trainee and ward staff. In addition to the trainee acting as collaborator and team member, he is expected to provide leadership. One of the recurring miracles is that many trainees do manage to master these tasks and find their unique role in the process. It also reassures the teachers and helps them expect more of the impossible from their students.

PSYCHOTHERAPY WITH THE CHILD

Psychotherapeutic work with the child and family enables the therapist to gradually identify and isolate the areas of nuclear psychopathology and to define those in which the child and family are most ready to engage therapeutically. As the therapist can share the psychotic experience or empathically understand the child's feelings, he may become aware of the child's ambivalent fear of involvement with and investment in another person. Such fears result from serious deprivation of nurturance and are expressed in the psychotic behavior. Similarly, the therapist may understand the child's terror about communicating feelings, especially expression of angry, sexual, sensual, and tender feelings experienced from and toward another person. Guilt, rage, hate, love, fear, strong desires for nurturance, and fear of retaliation from adults for direct or symbolic expression of negative feelings are all present. The resulting admixture makes understanding the meaning of behavior as well as the therapeutic work difficult.

With even the most primitive child, the therapist must learn as his first task to follow the child carefully in play therapy. Later he may need to focus actively and sometimes forcefully on the emerging nuclear conflicts. This may be done by clarifying one aspect of the emotional interaction between them. The therapist tries in various ways to describe both verbally and nonverbally his state of feeling and his perceptions of the interactions so that the child, from repeated experiences, finds a dependable base for his interactions. Diagnostic understanding of nuclear conflicts comes not only from direct observations of child and parents, but also from data gathered in a careful evaluation of the family events that preceded the illness. There is no need to stress the importance of the data that slowly takes shape from the past history of each family member and reveals their resultant integrative and conflictful capacities for living. The interactions of family members in response to specific stresses presented by the child's emerging pathology and his response to therapeutic efforts give further clues that help clarify nuclear conflict areas. As the family members are involved in a search for ways to meet each other's needs, clarification and beginning resolution of these core conflicts result in gradually increasing sensitivity to mutual needs and a greater repertoire of satisfying interactions. In the child this results in a greater readiness to move beyond the areas of fixated or regressed emotional and cognitive development.

THE THERAPIST'S ROLE AS A TEAM MEMBER

In his role vis-à-vis the other team members, the trainee has a twofold task. The first is to share his growing insight about child and family with the other team members, thus alerting them to the possible meaning of the child's behavior as it is continually observed in the milieu. It helps them focus on using each experience with the child to contribute to the clarification and refinement of the meaning of the child's behavior. Increased understanding and awareness begin to provide a different, more integrative and responsive milieu experience for the child.

The trainee's second function is to facilitate a collaborative interchange with the ward staff so that their interactive behavior with the child, parents, or child and parents together, leads to a better understanding of the family. It is no easy task to integrate and synthesize data so that the behavior of the child or parents as observed on the ward and in psychotherapeutic work can be understood as an expression of their circular psychopathological conflicts rather than as oppositional or malicious.

Senior child psychiatrists must first provide examples of such integration of data and help the trainee and ward staff experience its usefulness. This is particularly true in the interpretation of the often anxiety-producing behavior of the parents in their interaction with ward personnel. As such behavior becomes understandable to the staff, therapeutic handling of interactions with child and parents also becomes important in altering the behavior and attitudes of each. The material that results from all such therapeutic interaction is considered available to the psychotherapist in fostering insight and conflict reduction in his patients. As part of the therapeutic contract parents and child are helped from the beginning to understand and agree to the exchange of observations of the ward team with the psychotherapist. The trainee's transition from having a theoretical understanding to providing practical examples of how the staff might use these interactions therapeutically around specific activities is usually not achieved until some time in the second year of child psychiatry fellowship. Hence, the responsibility for development of strategies on the basis of such complex understanding rests with the more experienced psychiatric social workers, psychologists, chief nurses, and senior child psychiatrists, until the trainee can assume this function with his own cases.

FACILITATING EMOTIONAL DEVELOPMENT

The therapist's role in facilitating the emotional development of the child is twofold. First, he needs to enlist the collaboration of all the ward staff in elucidating elements of the child's present stage of development. He then encourages the staff to utilize their knowledge and insight to help the child achieve the very next developmental steps. Thus, when a child being cared for by a new staff member indicates a need to be fed or cuddled, the experienced staff members and trainees can describe from their experiences the sequences that might be expected to occur as the child works through this particular stage and is ready to move on. Nurses can be particularly helpful by describing in case vignettes how their own involvement for a time precluded recognition of the child's readiness to move on, because they were enjoying the feeding or cuddling so much themselves. The trainee needs to develop skills that facilitate other staff members' contributions to the learning of all the staff. How a particular child may be helped to take the next step requires close and free collaboration, sharing of information, and freedom to alter the plan as new data are gathered and assessed in the team effort. The capacity of the trainee and other staff members to predict sequences of behavior and direction of growth makes it easier for inexperienced staff to recognize readiness for change and thus to be helpful to the child.

Close collaboration between staff and psychotherapist is essential, since a child may sometimes function on different levels with milieu staff and therapist. Thus, in psychotherapy the more primitive core of the child's nuclear conflicts may still be worked on after he has progressed through several successive stages of psychosexual development, especially in terms of ego function with the ward staff.

How are these sequences learned by the fellow? We have found that most trainees are deficient in applicable knowledge of the emotional developmental stages of the child. In lectures, seminars, and journal seminars they learn the theoretical framework of emotional maturational stages [3–6, 10–13, 19]. They are, however, still a long way from using this theoretical framework to understand the observed behavior of the normal, neurotic, or psychotic child.

Furthermore, we find it is very difficult for the trainees to separate out in a behavioral sequence those aspects that represent regressive pathological distortions from those due to fixation. Essential as this differentiation is for the therapist in play therapy, it may become crucial at times for the ward staff. Understanding the conflictful components of behavior that have resulted in the symptoms permits corrective inter-action. However, in developmental arrest an environment must be created that is suitable for emotional growth and development at the emotional level of the child, and which facilitates the next steps beyond it. For ex-ample, destructive behavior may be symptomatic of unconscious conflict and may engage the adults in a characteristic way for that child and fam-ily. However, the child's striving for autonomy and independence indi-cates not only conflict but the need to be helped toward greater self-direction. He needs to be given choices, or he gets drawn into severe power struggles [22]. Thus, when Sandy, a four-year-old psychotic boy, initially hit himself and others at every opportunity, this could be under-stood historically in terms of conflicts from experiences with his harsh, punitive father and helpless, nonnurturant mother. The ward staff were alerted to interrupt his assaultiveness by restraining him until his experi-ences with the staff and playing out his terror and anger with the thera-pist made it possible for him to relate to others with verbal demands and abusiveness, which slowly merged into permitting physical closeness.

Jenny, at age five, however, began to lash out at everyone as she began to emerge from autistic isolation and frozen immobility. She slowly reacted to the warmth, nurturance, and cuddling of the nurse and to the patient engagement of her therapist, who used her inert hands in his to mould clay. The violent striking out was seen as a developmental phase combining assertiveness and testing of her world as she slowly lost her fear. Jenny was helped to channel her anger into more effective use of large and small muscles. Thus, with each outburst she was given a choice of clay to pound, paint to splash, or wet sand and flour to mash. These were her first vehicles for discharge of feelings and later opportu-nities to select areas for mastery in clay modeling and building. Each outburst was viewed as an opportunity to provide Jenny with alternative ways of asserting herself and of selecting the vehicles for learning and mastery. With the development of large and small muscle skills and greater independence and initiative, she was then able to take her place in the ward kindergarten group.

When the staff understands the child's behavior in terms of efforts to master developmental tasks, they are quickly able to recognize any new signs of increasing maturation and to foster independence and auton-omy with rapid reduction of the destructive behavior. They are also less disturbed by the sometimes necessary brief periods of regressive behavior. The child psychiatry fellow can achieve such learning through repeatedly observing someone else attempting this differentiation. Thus, he slowly acquires competence in classifying levels of the child's emotional development, in translating the theory and applying it to concrete behavioral examples given by the ward staff, and in involving the staff in planning ways to help the child develop.

When sequential development is not specifically fostered, the child's conflicts may be reduced, but he often fails to mature. The milieu may in this way iatrogenically produce a new conflict area. Thus Frank, a six-year-old autistic boy, very gradually was able to move out of his shell and to communicate in clearly heard words rather than frightened, barely audible whispers. The self-rocking stopped and echolalic sing-song TV commercials were more audible as he responded to the nurturance and encouragement of ward staff and engaged in the playroom in alternately feeding the baby doll and then, with gradually increased vigor, smashing it to the ground. For several months the repetitive verbalizations were clear and strong. He moved with confidence and could be persuaded to join in group activities, though on the periphery. Parents reported greater vigor in speech and movement, with occasional single word commands for food or a toy. Then he began to fade into his old soft, hardly audible speech, moved about less, appeared awkward, and became isolated. Close analysis of this phenomenon brought into focus staff contentment with the first behavioral changes without any clear plan to assess where he was in terms of ego development and to work toward the next step to help him move toward more age-appropriate behavior. Our second and planned efforts had to overcome the massive withdrawal and then utilize his readiness at each developmental stage to provide opportunities for relationships, learning, and mastery appropriate for the next stage via nurses, nursery school, occupational therapy, dance therapy, and so on. This time the milieu facilitated continued progress rather than the prolonged plateau that usually ends in regression.

EFFORTS AT COGNITIVE ASSESSMENT

We now come to the area of cognitive development of the child. Using Piaget's model [11], we observed that most of the severely disturbed psychotic children who require hospitalization operate in the sensory-motor or pre-operational stages of development. The task of the therapist is to involve a collaborative team of teacher, occupational therapist, nurse, and psychologist in an attempt to clarify the thinking level of the child. Does he have an inkling of causality? Does he recognize the permanence of the object? How much and when can he structure his environment? Is he capable of using any make-believe or imagination? Are there any areas where he can distinguish between self and others? Can he find the thread that relates several behavioral sequences? These are but some of the questions to which therapist and staff must address themselves if they are to make teaching of the child possible. The major task of teaching while the child is on an inpatient or day care unit is to help him acquire those precursors to academic skills that will enhance his satisfaction in learning and eventuate in his being able to learn and participate in the school situation after his discharge.

The therapist's role in this area is to stimulate the recurrent analysis of the child's cognitive level. Thus, the psychologist's evaluations and the teacher's observations must be correlated with other staff observations and data from the psychotherapeutic work. Often such an assessment takes many weeks of close observation and careful testing and retesting of the parameters of the child's cognitive functioning. Sometimes a child's disruptive behavior will not be an expression of psychopathology as much as an expression of utter frustration because the environment is making intellectual demands on him for which he is not ready.

Another task of the therapist is to serve as a stimulus to the other members to collaborate with him in the exciting discovery of methods and techniques that will teach the child such things as the differences between self and others, pretend play, phantasy, and reality, and to help him understand that hitting a child and getting hit back by that child are related. They must also find ways to help the child begin to experience object constancy.

Still another task of the therapist is to encourage and help the teacher and nurse to relay their experiences to the parents. His intimate knowledge of the parents' psychopathology, resistances, and defenses allows the therapist to clarify with the teacher and nurse the best possible methods by which this can be done. Should parents be observers and participate in some activities with other children, or are they ready, with help, to be engaged with their own child in ward activities? How is all this learned? Usually the fellow is totally unprepared for this task.

The greatest problem in the trainee's learning about cognition is in structuring the day care program in such a way that he is not left out of this process. Usually the teacher, occupational therapist, and nurse bring these areas up with the ward director or the psychologist when the trainees are not present. In part it is out of his province—hence it does not require his involvement. Since this material is not taught elsewhere in a general or child psychiatry program, he must learn it in this setting. Since it does not deal with psychopathology or psychotherapy, he may prefer not to be involved in an area for which he is so ill-prepared. Besides, until he learns about cognitive development, he feels anxious and vulnerable and requires support from senior staff members.

This is an area of particular importance to the child psychiatry trainee. It adds a dimension for understanding and discussing the child that enhances his contacts with educators, either as a therapist of the schoolchild or as a school consultant. A major collaborative effort, particularly on the part of teachers, psychologist, chief resident, and ward director, is required to discuss the cognitive aspects of the child's problems in meetings where the trainees participate, in order to clarify these concepts and make them familiar to the trainee. The senior child psychiatrists must then repetitively help the fellows carry out observations and engage in discussion until these concepts are useful and familiar to the trainee.

One final unique area in the role of the child psychiatric trainee is responsibility for planning termination of the day care experience for child and family, with transition to outpatient treatment and involvement in other community resources such as school. The intense involvement of the ward staff with a severely disturbed child that is so necessary for the child's improvement demands that the trainee maintain sufficient objectivity to help the ward staff make the termination a therapeutic experience.

THE SYNTHESIZING ROLE

The trainee uses his psychotherapeutic work with the child and parents to provide additional data for understanding the degree of psychopathology and emotional and cognitive levels of the child, as well as to facilitate overall planning for the next steps toward which the team should work. As the trainee learns to assume the synthesizing role, he is faced with examining data from all sources and trying to integrate them for himself and for the team. He must similarly learn to gently explore and uncover the data available in the observations of team members and himself to explain a crisis and to help resolve it. This learning process occurs with some difficulty and discomfort. As has been indicated, it requires the model of a senior child psychiatrist who demonstrates the process to the trainee and whose involvement in this process decreases as the trainee gains experience and competence.

Another aspect of the child psychiatry fellow's work with the child differentiates him from his collaborators. He begins to use his growing understanding of psychopathology and psychotherapeutic methods not only to contribute to the child's general gains, but also to consolidate each step of the growth occurring in all aspects of the therapeutic milieu efforts with the child and parents. Thus, interpretive behavior, comments, and play therapy activities timed in terms of the overall movement may serve to focus sharply and resolve conflicts at a moment when symbolic mastery is possible. With the very sick child, he may be the only one who can permit himself to share the child's psychosis as a way of understanding the conflicts and slowly begin to find methods of conflict resolution. This is another aspect of the synthesizing role.

Thus, Phil, a seven-year-old child whose oral sadistic behaviors were gradually reduced in ward activities and in school, with increased mastery through a variety of living and learning tasks, did not make full use of his energies. He could not move on to the next step in conflict resolution until, in the light of this progress, an old theme in play was reintroduced by his therapist to permit symbolic playing out of a conflict. The therapist brought out alligator and frog puppets that had been abandoned months before. In the ensuing five play therapy sessions, biting, chewing, and swallowing of the frog were increasingly free and voracious as the therapist first made the appropriate sounds and verbalizations for both puppets. Finally the child joined in, and then took over with increasing freedom. This was quite different from the violent, anxious, and desperate play of some months back. In the last of these hours he, as the alligator puppet, restored the frog he had just killed to life with a grand gesture. Subsequently the child's capacity to learn, to pay attention, and to experience pleasure noticeably increased on the ward, and his teasing and aggressive behavior decreased at home.

A similar consolidative function occurs in work with parents. The variety of therapeutic efforts by all team members, and the parents' experiences, both successes and problems in dealing with the child and their efforts in psychotherapy, are synthesized in terms of their past history and their intra- and interpersonal conflicts. Well-timed interpretive comments often permit the parents to move to the next step in their work.

In summary, the specific tasks of the child psychiatry trainee are to learn to use his growing knowledge and competence to synthesize all the data provided by every team member, to define the psychopathology of the child and parents, the emotional and cognitive levels, and to help evolve a collaborative therapeutic program step by step for his patients. Most important, his psychotherapeutic engagement with child and parents provides the base for all his learning.

REFERENCES

1. BERLIN, I. N. A history of challenges in child psychiatry training. *Ment. Hyg.*, **48**:558-565, 1964.

2. _____ . Some implications of ego psychology for the supervisory process. *Amer. J. Psychother.*, **14**:536-544, 1960.

3. BRIDGES, K. Emotional development in early infancy. *Child Develop.*, 3:324-341, 1932.

4. BRUNER, J. S. *The process of education.* New York: Vintage Books, 1960.

5. _____ . *Toward a theory of instruction.* Cambridge: Belknap Press of Harvard, 1966.

6. _____ and OLVER, R. *Studies in cognitive growth.* New York: John Wiley & Sons, Inc., 1966.

7. CHRIST, A., CRITCHLEY, C., LARSON, M. & BROWN, M. The role of the child psychiatric nurse. *Nursing Outlook,* **13**:30-32, 1965.

8. _____ & GRIFFITH, R. Parent-nurse therapeutic contact on a child psychiatry unit. *Amer. J. Orthopsychiat.,* **35**:589-593, 1965.

9. _____ & WAGNER, N. Prevention of iatrogenic factors in child residential treatment. In J. Masserman (Ed.), *Current psychiatric therapies,* Vol. 6. New York: Grune & Stratton, 1966, pp. 46-54.

10. ERIKSON, E. *Childhood and society.* New York: W. W. Norton & Co., Inc., 1963.

11. FLAVELL, J. *The developmental psychology of Jean Piaget.* Princeton: D. Van Nostrand Co., Inc., 1963.

12. FREUD, S. *Three essays on the theory of sexuality.* London: Imago Publishing Co., 1949.

13. GESELL, A. & ILG, F. *Child development.* New York: Harper & Brothers, 1959.

14. GREENWOOD, E. Role of psychotherapy in residential treatment. *Amer. J. Orthopsychiat.,* **25**:692-698, 1955.

15. ITTELSON, W. Some factors influencing the design and function of psychiatric facilities. Progress Report of the Department of Psychology, Brooklyn College, 1960.

16. PAVENSTEDT, E. The nursery school, day care center, and developmental studies. *J. Amer. Acad. Child Psychiat.,* **5**:349-359, 1966.

17. REDL, F. The concept of a "therapeutic milieu." *Amer. J. Orthopsychiat.,* **29**:721-736, 1959.

18. ROBINSON, J. Planning institutional programs for children. *Quart. J. Child Behav.,* **3**:233-239, 1951.

19. SPITZ, R. A. *A genetic field theory of ego formation: its implication for pathology.* New York: International Universities Press, 1959.

20. SZUREK, S. A. & BERLIN, I. N. Teaching administration in the training of child psychiatrists. *J. Amer. Acad. Child Psychiat.,* **3**:551-560, 1964.

21. _____ . The question of therapy for the trainee in the psychiatric training program. *J. Amer. Acad. Child Psychiat.,* **5**:155-165, 1966.

22. WHITE, R. Competence and the psychosexual stages of development. In M. R. Jones (Ed.), *Nebraska symposium on motivation.* Lincoln: University of Nebraska Press, 1960, pp. 97-141.

23. WOLFF, P. The developmental psychologies of Jean Piaget and psychoanalysis. *Psychol. Issues,* 2(1), Monograph No. 5. New York: International Universities Press, 1960.

SECTION FOUR

PSYCHIATRIC NURSING ON A CHILDREN'S WARD

INTRODUCTION

The nurse in this setting is the key figure in the therapeutic environment of the children's ward. Her self-awareness as a means of understanding the child and being able to work with him therapeutically is an important element in the success of the transactions with him. This awareness of self, of the child's needs, of the messages conveyed by his behavior, and of the meaning of the verbal and nonverbal communications of other staff members, are vital to the effective and integrated work of the nursing staff.

How such awareness is used in a wide variety of activities is described in the following papers.

CHAPTER 11

NURSING IN HOSPITAL PSYCHIATRIC THERAPY FOR PSYCHOTIC CHILDREN*

M. J. Boatman, M.D., J. Paynter, R.N., C. Parsons, R.N.

HISTORY OF NURSING PROJECT

The staff of the Children's Service of the Langley Porter Neuropsychiatric Institute evolved from their first fifteen years' experience certain concepts concerning the nature of the nursing skill needed in providing a therapeutic living environment for hospitalized psychotic children. They also developed a number of hypotheses pertaining to the methods by which such skill can be attained by the professionally trained nurse. Early in 1960, with the aid of a three-year National Institute of Mental Health Project Grant,[1] this staff undertook to provide a more adequate clinical test of these hypotheses than they had previously been able to achieve. Inherent in this clinical test would also be the more precise refinement of the hypotheses as well as the clinical demonstration and further development of the concepts they embodied.

This paper will discuss these concepts and hypotheses, describe something of the experience in which they evolved, and indicate the nature of the current work in the first year of the project.

*Reprinted by permission from *The American Journal of Orthopsychiatry,* 32(5), October, 1962. (Copyright, the American Orthopsychiatric Association, Inc.)

[1] This work was partially supported by the National Institute of Mental Health Project Grant OM-234, entitled "Nursing in Hospital Psychiatric Therapy for Psychotic Children."

SETTING AND STAFF[2]

The relatively small fourteen-bed Children's Ward is on the fourth floor of the Institute, which is located on the side of a steep wooded hill in an urban, middle-class residential district, and which faces a heavily traveled street. A small outdoor play area is on the grounds, and there is a large public park within walking distance. All of these factors have implications for the clinical program and the nursing care for the children. These include some limitations of activities, concern for the children's safety when off the ward, and the staff's awareness of the problems created by the impact of the children's behavior on the community.

The entire ward program is under the close supervision of the senior psychiatrists. Individual psychotherapeutic work with children and parents is largely carried out by the six psychiatrists in training for child psychiatry. Senior social workers and psychologists contribute to the program. The basic ward staff consists of eleven psychiatric nurses, five psychiatric technicians (trained attendants), one elementary school teacher, and one quarter-time occupational therapist. Recently there have been two graduate nursing students, one studying for a master's degree and the other doing post-master's work. Since March 1960, there have been two project nurses.

TREATMENT PHILOSOPHY

All facets of the ward program are outgrowths of the experience and the philosophy of the Children's Service staff during the past fourteen years [1-14]. The attempt has been to develop a program in which every aspect of the care of the psychotic children who were hospitalized would be a precise and integral part of the total psychotherapeutic endeavor.

About six years ago it became apparent to the senior staff that the next step in their overall clinical research, training, and treatment program needed to be an intensification of the development of the nursing skills in providing a twenty-four-hour therapeutic environment on the ward. Factors that contributed to this recognition were: the nature of the ward population; the more precise delineation of certain concepts concerning the therapeutic goals and the nature of the skill needed by the staff; and the staff's achievements and difficulties in attaining these goals.

---

[2]For a more complete description of the setting, staff, admission criteria and treatment hypothesis see Chapter 4. Many details have been omitted here to minimize repetition.

Concepts of Care

For approximately the past eleven years, the population of the ward has been made up almost entirely of the most severely disturbed of the many psychotic preadolescents seen by the staff. These children not only show psychotic behavior but show it seriously and persistently at all levels of functioning. Although sometimes disconcertingly sporadic and shifting in its manifestation, such symptomatic behavior persists almost continuously in one form or another throughout each child's day.

The staff's experience, from continuous efforts to understand the needs of and to achieve an adequate psychotherapeutic program for these psychotic inpatient children, led them to place increased emphasis on several of their original assumptions. These included the following concepts. (*a*) Every staff person needs to behave at all times in that precise manner which may help the child, first, to reduce his disorder (i.e., his internalized conflict), however manifested at a given moment or in a given activity; and second, to provide opportunities for the child to develop more integrated behavior at whatever level is timely for his own maturational and emotional capacities. (*b*) The degree to which hospitalization of a psychotic child is a positive part of the psychotherapeutic program depends in large measure on the degree to which the nursing staff can achieve the above goals in moment-to-moment, twenty-four-hour care of the child. This is particularly true in the areas of the necessary daily activities of living such as rising, dressing, toileting, playing, eating, going to bed, and sleeping. (*c*) The skill required by the nursing staff in the attainment of these goals must be based in knowledge and understanding—of psychopathology, of childhood, and of the goals themselves—and must encompass the ability to apply effectively this knowledge and understanding. This skill therefore includes the exercise of spontaneous intuitiveness and technical proficiency and the ability to make prompt independent clinical judgments consistent with the psychiatrist's therapeutic aims.

CONCEPTS OF SKILL

Approximately six years ago, as a result of continuous observation and reflection with the senior nurses, the senior psychiatrists formulated even more specifically their concepts as to the nature of the skill needed by the staff in this setting, as follows. (*a*) Any destructive activity of the child—although symptomatic—requires firm, nonretaliatory, promptly protective restraint that is gentle and continuously personal. Furthermore, this restraint needs to be so applied that it leads the child toward reduction of projected fears about his own sensual wishes for contact; in short, so that it leads to the child's greater relaxation, self-confidence, and trust in the staff. (*b*) Sensual self-gratifications of the child, which are not destructive, and which often appear following restraint of the type described, need to be so understood that they will not be suppressed by any action of the staff. (*c*) Any regressive behavior by the child, such as self-absorption and withdrawal, needs to be so understood that the staff will be able to remain attentively but nonintrusively available so long as this contributes to the child's reduction of his anxiety, or to help the child redirect his activity if and when it leads to mounting anxiety in himself. (*d*) Any emerging spontaneity and interest shown by the child needs to be so promptly recognized and attentively followed that timely but noncoercive encouragement may be offered. (*e*) Any efforts of the child to learn and master skills of self-care or other satisfying activity needs such timely offer of help as is necessary to reduce self-frustration and to provide repetitive opportunities for achievement. (*f*) In addition, in all aspects of the work, each staff member needs to discriminate his own role in the child's experience so clearly, and obtain his own satisfactions in it so fully, that he in no way needs to interfere with the child's relationship to his own parents, with the work of the individual psychotherapist of the child or parent, or with any other staff person's contribution to the therapeutic environment. In other words, all this requires that kind of collaboration with other staff members that can be described as an integration of the entire staff in the work toward a common therapeutic goal.

Both prior and subsequent to the more precise formulation of these concepts, as much attention as staff number and time permitted has been given to the development of the nursing staff. The senior staff's accumulating observations have led them to a number of preliminary conclusions concerning several aspects of these experiences, including the assessment of nursing skill, what distinguished those persons who attained it most thoroughly, some of the assets and deficiencies that the professionally trained nurse had for the work, and what some of the major difficulties were in attaining more satisfactory nursing staff development.

Assessment of Development of Nursing Skills

They have found a number of sources of information to be useful in their assessment of the skill of each member of the nursing staff. Evaluations from these various sources usually corroborate each other and are often confirmed by the subsequent steps in the person's development. The staff makes direct observations of the nurse's manner of interacting

with the child on the ward. They review and interpret formal and informal reports from other staff members concerning all aspects of her
work, both clinical and administrative. They review observations and
reports concerning a given child's current behavior and overall progress
(weighed carefully in the light of all clinical data about the child's disorder and events in his life extraneous to the nurse's contacts with him).
They review her own verbal and written reports concerning her observations of and work with the children. Attention is given to such factors
as the degree of her understanding of and the appropriateness of her
responses to the children's behavior; the clarity and completeness with
which she describes clinical sequences; the objectivity with which she
includes descriptions of her own behavior and attitudes as they relate to
the clinical sequences; and the accuracy with which she can judge the
effectiveness of her own and others' interactions with the children.

The staff estimates from all the above sources the degree to which
she can maintain focus on the clinical task, particularly at times of
tension on the ward; the degree to which she can contribute to and
participate in the clarification and understanding of clinical problems;
the manner in which she utilizes supervisory experiences; how she con-
ceives of the use of authority, her own and others'; how ready she is to
gain job satisfactions from her own developing competence rather than
from slavish dependence on the senior staff.

Attributes of the Skilled Nurse

Those members of the nursing staff who have achieved considerable
skill in caring for psychotic children have seemed to be distinguishable
in certain ways. They were, for the most part, from the group of professionally trained psychiatric nurses. They stayed on the ward for a
period of years. They were persons to whom the most experienced of
the senior nurses and/or psychiatrists were able to offer individual supervisory time, at least at critical periods. They were eventually able to use
such individual supervisory time as was available for thoughtful reflection
concerning the meaningfulness of their own behavior in interaction with
the children.

The senior staff has found that the modern-day, truly professionally
trained nurse has certain particular assets for work in this hospital treatment setting. She has learned to accept responsibility for working with
physicians and other professional persons when the health, even the life,
of another human being may depend on her participation in the collaborative job. She, like the physician-psychiatrist, has been trained to react
with professional skill and attitudes toward necessary physical contact

with patients. She is, in part, prepared for extreme dependent needs of patients expressed simultaneously in emotional and bodily ways, e.g., in such body language as saliva play, head-banging, soiling, and wetting. She, like the psychiatrist, has a medical background that enables her to continue to provide all necessary care of the child even during episodes of illness, injury, and complicated medical procedures. Such continuity of care by the same persons during both physical health and illness has been found to be helpful to hospitalized psychotic children. She, like other professional persons, has an intellectual awareness of bodies of knowledge that she can draw upon and the capacity to utilize them critically. She, like persons of the other major disciplines, has an identification with the particular ethos of her own profession. Such professional identification has been found to be a necessary prerequisite for the development of ever-increasing professional skill in the long-term program. In addition, such professional identification and experience in collaborating with physicians are important in the development of the kind of skill considered necessary, i.e., skill that implies such thorough grounding in general principles that these become an integral and spontaneously available part of total behavior. As long as adequate staff support is available, the nonprofessionally trained workers sometimes react to the children with more intuitiveness and spontaneity than the inexperienced nurse. They are, however, seldom able to become truly thoughtful about the interactions, and rarely develop skills that can be promptly applied with precision in new or in crucial and trying situations.

The senior staff has also found the professionally trained nurse to be insufficiently prepared for work in this setting in some ways. She does not have adequate knowledge and understanding of the special needs of childhood, nor does she have sufficient knowledge and understanding of psychopathology. She does not possess the necessary technical knowledge needed for skillful guidance of progressive learning by children who have difficulties in the mastery of simple tasks of childhood such as self-care, motor skills, and adequate speech. She does not have sufficient personal experience with or understanding of intense emotional reactions such as those that are so inevitably and so forcefully brought out in herself and others by the persistent negative, hostile, regressive, and sexually sensual behavior of psychotic children.

Certain difficulties have repeatedly or continuously prevented the senior staff from providing as thorough and consistent a program of inservice preparation of nurses as their experience indicated was potentially possible. A relative shortage of personnel in relation to the constant pressure of staff jobs to be done on the ward and in the Institute has prevented them from having sufficient time to offer enough of the nurses the desirable continuity and frequency of individual supervisory sessions with experienced supervisors. It has made it impossible to develop an adequate program of guided study and discussion for the nursing staff. This relative staff shortage and its consequences have also contributed to some of the nurses leaving the ward prematurely. These include nurses who were needed to fill urgent jobs elsewhere in the Institute, as well as those who found work with psychotic children too distressing in the absence of adequate supervision. We are not referring here to those few who had no interest in or were unsuited for learning to work with the children. Even the in-service program that has been developed is repeatedly disrupted by the special needs created by the slow though steady influx of new nurses—junior staff who rotate during a period of orientation to psychiatry and to the Institute, some graduate students, and replacements for staff members who leave.

Supervision in Development of Skills

Throughout the country there is a general lack of recognition that the acquisition of professional skill in this exacting area of nursing requires a considerable degree of experience on the part of the supervisor, a very considerable length of time on the part of the nurse, and a relatively high degree of consistency and frequency in the contacts between the two. On this ward as elsewhere, any major change in existing staffing patterns to provide for these requirements has been impossible in the absence of adequate clinical demonstrations to draw on in the justification of budget requests.

From the foregoing observations and conclusions, it can be seen that the staff feels that some of the nurses have achieved considerable skill in the care of some children much of the time. However, neither the nurses nor the psychiatrists have been content with its consistency; with their understanding of the precise clinical application of skill involved and its variability; with the length of time it took them to achieve what skill they have; or with the degree of their success in conceptualizing and communicating what they have learned so that nurses or other workers on the ward might be helped to learn more rapidly.

Several years ago it became increasingly apparent to staff that any more thorough and meaningful program of clarification and application of methods by which nursing skill could be developed would require additional persons who could participate in it long enough to be effective, and who were not completely subject to the day-to-day service demands.

NIMH PROJECT

Convinced of the current local and general importance of further understanding of the nature and development of psychiatric nursing skill with hospitalized psychotic children, the senior staff began to consider the need for additional monies to provide a small group whose primary task would be to pursue this goal within the existing clinical program. When they heard that the National Institute of Mental Health was interested in supporting clinical projects designed to develop and demonstrate improved methods of care in special areas, they thought that the project they had already conceived might well be an appropriate one. A three-year project entitled "Nursing in Hospital Psychiatric Therapy for Children" was approved, and on March 1, 1960, it was initiated.

Aims of Project

Five aims of the project to be carried out with a few professionally trained nurses were defined, as follows:

1. To establish a demonstration program of in-service preparation of nurses in the skill needed in providing a therapeutic living environment for hospitalized psychotic children.
2. To test, in this clinical program, the senior staff's hypotheses that such skill can be developed by the professionally trained nurse through:
   a. Adequate clinical practice for two or more years;
   b. Individual supervision which:
      (1) is provided by an experienced nurse supervisor;
      (2) is adapted to the needs of the individual nurse;
      (3) is concerned with every aspect of the work;
      (4) affords her opportunity to increase that kind of self-awareness which is essential to becoming a true practitioner capable of professional performance in new and stressful clinical situations;
   c. Guided study and discussion of factual knowledge and technical competencies in those areas where she is insufficiently academically prepared;
   d. Participation in the recording and review of her own clinical work and progress.
3. To refine these hypotheses more precisely.
4. To gain more definitive knowledge concerning various aspects of the clinical application of nursing skill.

5. To establish the groundwork for the development of nurses as experienced supervisors and research collaborators in this expanding area of child psychiatry.

With the aid of the total Children's Service staff, three persons have major responsibility for the project. The Project Director is the Assistant Director of the Children's Service and the psychiatrist who has direct responsibility for the clinical administration of the ward. The Project Co-Director is the Superintendent of Nursing Services of the Institute. The principal Nurse Investigator, under the direct supervision of the Project Director, is responsible for the implementation of the work.

Developing Project

The plan calls for the annual addition of two nurses, relatively or totally inexperienced in children's work, who are able and willing to commit themselves to two or more years of the planned program of study, clinical work, and intensive supervision. Factors also considered in selection are of course the same criteria for selection used in appointing all nurses at the Institute. These include a review of the applicant's past school and work performance and a personal interview to assess her motivations, her capacity for evaluating her own strengths and weaknesses, and the nature of her interest in or apprehensiveness about the prospective job as she sees it.

In the current first year of the project, one nurse selected for it has had five years of nursing experience in adult psychiatry, and another was a new graduate. Each was assigned primary responsibility for the nursing care of a six-year-old schizophrenic child. This differed from the assignments of the ward nurses in that the project nurses had more flexibility as to the time they spent with the children. For example, they were encouraged to participate in ward activities only as they felt it would be meaningful to their particular assignment. Part of this clinical assignment was to help the child participate in all aspects of the ward program, including such structured activities as occupational therapy [13], rhythm groups [12], and nursery school.

It quickly became apparent that the project nurses were insufficiently prepared for understanding the goals and methods appropriate to the special activity areas. They found themselves feeling clumsy and self-conscious in rhythm-dance groups, inadequate and bored in occupational therapy sessions, and irritable in the classroom.

Part of the project plan had been to provide seminars in areas where the nurses' knowledge proved insufficient. Mutual discussions around the clinical experiences noted led to the decision to begin this part of the work with their participation in a modern dance group, followed by attendance at a two-week workshop in dance. Informal seminars were arranged with the occupational therapist and the educational psychologist. As the nurses' attempts to understand their children became more intensive, a seminar in psychopathology was begun with the Project Director.

In addition to these special seminars, they attended the ward's daily clinical conferences. They contributed both informal and carefully prepared reports of their clinical observations and work in those conferences that pertained to children assigned to them. Like all the nurses, each of them met once a week with the psychiatrist who was the therapist of the child assigned to her.

Individual Supervision of Nurses

From the beginning, particular emphasis was placed on the individual supervisory sessions each of them had three times weekly with the Principal Nurse Investigator. They were encouraged to use the time to increase their self-awareness of their own reactions and motivations, as well as to gain more precise understanding of the children and their therapeutic needs.

As anticipated, one of the most difficult parts of the program was the preparation of the detailed daily records. Each nurse prepared a daily process recording of her work with the child. Immediately following each supervisory session, both the nurse and the Principal Nurse Investigator prepared a summary of what they thought had occurred in the conference. Although these recordings were not used in the supervisory sessions, the Principal Nurse Investigator used them to help her understand the nurse and her progress.

DISCUSSION

It is too early in the work to draw any definitive conclusions. However, it is the staff's impression that the methods employed are proving to be effective in the progressive development of skill by the project nurses. In fact, they seem to be developing skill more rapidly, more thoroughly, and more steadily than staff nurses did with their more limited supervision, or master's students with their more limited clinical experience.

The informal seminars have certainly proved to be very helpful. The two nurses are already outstanding on the ward in their lack of self-consciousness in the child-group activities. They seem to have gained a real sense of the potential therapeutic benefit the children may gain from increased pleasure, awareness, and mastery of body skills. They have begun to take a creative part in planning as well as in utilizing occupational therapy and nursery school activities, both at structured times and in informal play. In recent weeks, when the ward program was disrupted at times by some major reconstruction work, these nurses have spontaneously assumed leadership at critical moments. At such times, they appeared to be more flexible and more attuned to *all* of the children's needs than were many of the staff nurses.

The staff has been interested to note that the project nurses have in no way escaped the periods of deep discouragement that have been almost universal for new nurses on this ward. It is apparent, however, that the project nurses have been able to find more ready and more constructive ways of understanding and learning from these periods than have most other nurses. The staff feels that this may be primarily the result of the frequency, continuity, and nature of their individual supervisory sessions. However, more valid assessment of this awaits added time and study, since multiple factors influence this aspect of their development. These include such consequences as are inevitable from being "special" and from feeling morally committed both as to the endeavor and to the length of time committed to it.

The authors have attempted to describe this staff's slowly evolving concepts concerning the nature of nursing skill needed in providing a therapeutic living environment for hospitalized psychotic children. They have indicated their hypotheses as to how such skill may be attained by the professionally trained nurse. They have indicated the nature of a beginning three-year project to demonstrate, study, and further develop these concepts and hypotheses. It is of course their expectation that further reports delineating the results of the project will follow this preliminary presentation.

REFERENCES

1. BOATMAN, MALETA J., and S. A. SZUREK. A clinical study of childhood schizophrenia. In Don D. Jackson (Ed.), *The etiology of schizophrenia.* New York: Basic Books, Inc., 1960, pp. 389-440.
2. ENG, MARIETTA, GEWERTZ, JOANNE R., and BOATMAN, MALETA J. A creative rhythmic movement group for psychotic children in a psychotherapeutic program. Unpublished paper read at Annual Meeting of American Orthopsychiatric Association, 1959.

3. ENG, MARIETTA, and BOATMAN, MALETA J. The occupational therapy program on a ward for psychotic children. In *Proceedings of the American Occupational Therapy Association 1960 annual conference.* New York: American Occupational Therapy Association, 1961, pp. 33-36.

4. REID, JOSEPH H., and HAGAN, HELEN R. A descriptive study of the program of the Langley Porter Clinic, Children's Inpatient Service. In *Residential treatment of emotionally disturbed children,* New York: The Child Welfare League of America, Inc., 1952, pp. 200-221.

5. SHEIMO, S. L., PAYNTER, JANE, and SZUREK, S. A. Problems of staff interaction with spontaneous group formations on a children's psychiatric ward. *Am. J. Orthopsychiat.,* **19**:599-611, 1949.

6. SZUREK, S. A. Some observations on the dynamics of staff inter-action in hospital psychiatric treatment of children. *Am. J. Orthopsy-chiat.,* **17**:652-664, 1947.

7. _____. Remarks on training for psychotherapy. *Am. J. Orthopsy-chiat.,* **19**:36-51, 1949. Reprinted in S. A. Szurek & I. N. Berlin (Eds.), *Training in therapeutic work with children.* Vol. 2, the Langley Porter Child Psychiatry Series. Palo Alto, Calif.: Science and Behavior Books, 1967.

8. SZUREK, S. A., SHEIMO, S. L., and PAYNTER, JANE. Problems encountered in dealing with handicapped and emotionally disturbed children. *Am. J. Occup. Ther.,* **3**:303-307, 1949.

9. SZUREK, S. A. The family and the staff in hospital psychiatric therapy of children. *Am. J. Orthopsychiat.,* **21**:597-611, 1951.

10. _____ Some lessons from efforts at psychotherapy with parents. *Am. J. Psychiat.,* **109**:296-302, 1952. Reprinted in S. A. Szurek & I. N. Berlin (Eds.), *Training in therapeutic work with children.* Vol. 2, the Langley Porter Child Psychiatry Series. Palo Alto, Calif.: Science and Behavior Books, 1967.

11. _____. Childhood schizophrenia: psychotic episodes and psychotic maldevelopment. *Am. J. Orthopsychiat.* **26**:519-543, 1956.

12. SZUREK, S. A. and BERLIN, I. N. Elements of psychotherapeutics with the schizophrenic child and his parents. *Psychiatry,* **19**:1-9, 1956. Reprinted in S. A. Szurek & I. N. Berlin (Eds.), *Training in therapeutic work with children.* Vol. 2, the Langley Porter Child Psychiatry Series. Palo Alto, Calif.: Science and Behavior Books, 1967.

13. SZUREK, S. A. The roots of psychoanalysis and psychotherapy. *A search for principles of general psychotherapeutics.* Springfield, Ill.: Thomas, 1958.

14. _____. Playfulness, creativity, and schisis. *Am. J. Orthopsychiat.,* **29**:667-682, 1959.

CHAPTER 12

ONE NURSE'S RELATIONSHIP WITH
A PSYCHOTIC BOY*

Deane L. Critchley, R.N., M.S.

EDITORS' NOTE, 1970

This detailed review of the interaction between one child and his assigned nurse is an example of the kind of descriptive summaries of each staff person's work which we strive toward. Miss Critchley was one of the few post-master's graduate nursing students whose academic program permitted her to spend most of her time in clinical work, collaboration, and close supervision on the ward. Her program was, therefore, much like that of the nurses in the project described in Chapter 11, and her experiences contributed to the early phases of that program.

This paper is a result of my experience in working with a hospitalized eleven-year-old psychotic boy over a nine-month period during post-master's study in psychiatric nursing. It focuses on one aspect of this work—the nurse's contribution to therapeutic work with the child within a specific research effort in a particular clinical setting. No attempt has been made to describe the total psychotherapeutic effort with the child and his family.

Because of the then-existing academic schedule within the University of California School of Nursing Master's Program, a post-master's year was decided upon to provide a more intensive, consistent clinical experience.

*Reprinted by permission from American Nurses Association, Inc., in Monograph 16, *Phases in Human Development: Relevance in Nursing,* 1962. (Copyright, American Nurses Association, Inc.)

Those in charge of my program and I felt that spending a relatively long period of time in clinical work primarily with one child would best help me achieve two objectives: clarification of the fundamental principles of caring for disturbed children; and further development of the nursing skills I would need to be a contributing member of the professional team. This paper describes a part of my work during this time and shows how an intensive continuous nurse-patient relationship can be a major contribution to the total psychotherapeutic program for hospitalized emotionally disturbed children.

This experience was obtained on the fourteen-bed ward for psychotic children at the Langley Porter Neuropsychiatric Institute, San Francisco. Since the staff of the Children's Service does not consider the severity of a child's disorder as the sole basis for admission to the hospital, most of the children on the ward have severe psychopathology, with the diagnosis of schizophrenic reaction, childhood type.

PHILOSOPHY OF INPATIENT WARD

Since 1946 one of the staff's main clinical research efforts has been to test the hypothesis that psychotic disorders of childhood are of psychogenic origin [2, 7, 8; see also Chapter 9; 9; see also Chapter 18; 10, 11]. One implication of this hypothesis is that in addition to the psychiatrist's specifically psychotherapeutic work with the child in the playroom, other staff members working with the child could, if prepared, contribute to the reduction of his disorder. Each staff person could also provide opportunities, geared to the child's own maturational and emotional capacities, that would help him develop more integrated behavior. To achieve these goals, the nursing staff's responsibility is to utilize the child's moment-to-moment twenty-four-hour care—in such areas of daily living as rising, dressing, toileting, eating, going to bed and sleeping, as well as in play activities, school, and occupational therapy [4; see also Chapter 15]. This kind of attentiveness is often more readily achieved if each child has a staff person available to him. While this staff-patient ratio has never been entirely possible on our ward, it has been a constant objective; at present a staff member is available to each child for some portion of each day.

More specifically, the nursing staff attempts to achieve these goals in the following ways [1; see also Chapter 11]:

1. By responding to the child's destructive behavior firmly but non-retaliatively to keep him from hurting himself or others, by attempting to strengthen his trust in the staff and thus allowing him to gratify his wishes for contact in a more relaxed and pleasurable manner.

2. By understanding the sensual needs of the child so that when they appear in nondestructive ways, they will not be suppressed by any action of the staff.

3. By understanding the child's regressive behavior such as self-absorption and withdrawal and remaining attentively available as long as his activity seems to be reducing the anxiety, but helping to redirect his activity if it leads to increased anxiety.

4. By promptly recognizing and following the child's emerging spontaneity and interest, offering timely noncoercive encouragement and help when he tries to learn and master self-help skills or other satisfying activity, to reduce his frustration and provide repetitive opportunities for achievement.

5. By understanding the roles of various people in the child's experience so that his relationships with others—such as a parent, a psychotherapist, or other members of the nursing staff — are in no way interfered with but are, in fact, supported and reinforced through working toward a common therapeutic goal.

Operational Methods

The foregoing philosophy and objectives formed the framework within which I worked. Although my role as a post master's student was new both to me and the ward, I had had my clinical experience on this same ward while working toward a Master of Science Degree in psychiatric nursing.

Because my program was geared toward providing maximal learning opportunities, my only staff responsibilities were those directly connected with and part of the therapeutic care of my assigned patient, whom I will call Kelly Collins. I attended the various ward conferences in which the staff presented experiences with the parents and children, and current problems were discussed. Weekly conferences with the child's therapist gave me an opportunity for exploring my own feelings about particular problems as they arose in working with Kelly and for constantly clarifying my role within the therapeutic goals of the clinical work. These meetings served to keep us both aware of the daily and weekly experiences of Kelly and his family. I had individual conferences with my nursing supervisor three times a week, and learned to translate the philosophy of the service into concrete practices for working with Kelly, and with the other children, in the daily routine of living. These supervisory conferences helped me to explore my feelings regarding problems involving Kelly, other children, or staff members, particularly any feelings that might interfere with learning the necessary professional skills.

PSYCHIATRIC CASE SUMMARY

Kelly was a full-term, 8 lb. 12 oz. infant delivered without complications following an uneventful pregnancy. Breast-feeding was stopped
after three weeks because of his mother's insufficient milk supply and
painful nipples. At four weeks he developed severe vomiting, and his
weight dropped to ten ounces below his birth weight. At three months
he underwent surgery for correction of pyloric stenosis. At four months
his parents left on a two-day vacation, returning to find that Kelly had
developed eczema. He was hospitalized frequently, and his arms were
splinted to prevent scratching. During one of these hospitalizations,
asthmatic breathing was noted. At eight months an obvious asthmatic
episode occurred. The family had moved five times within six months.
The father had had four jobs, and the parents seldom saw each other.

When Kelly was two-and-one-half-years old, a brother was born. His
parents remarked at the time Kelly seemed "like a newborn baby." His
development was slow. He did not sit alone till thirteen months or crawl
till fifteen. He was between two-and-one-half and three years when he
began to walk; began to feed himself at two years but was not weaned
from the bottle until age three-and-one-half. Toilet-training, started at
three years, was unsuccessful. At age five he made a few sounds but
spoke no words. His parents stated that he ignored them and also other
children; he spent most of his time in self-preoccupied bizarre behavior.

Kelly was first seen at the Langley Porter Institute at the age of five
for psychiatric study. He did not seem to recognize anyone, including
his parents; his only response was a blank expression. He ate continuously but was not overweight. He rarely vocalized. He soiled and wet.

Physical examinations were unremarkable except for slight asthmatic
chest rales. Laboratory studies, including electroencephalogram, chest
and skull X-rays, and bone-age determination, routine blood and urine
tests, were all negative.

Psychological tests indicated that he functioned at the level of a child
about half his chronological age. It was not clear whether his retardation
was primarily due to permanent intellectual defect, functional factors, or
a combination of the two. However, Kelly's past history, his autistic behavior, and his occasional flashes of alert and purposeful behavior strongly
suggested to the psychologist that the retardation was due to his severe
emotional problems. Although she could not say so with certainty, there
was a good possibility that his intelligence was normal.

At the close of the study, the psychiatrist felt that psychotherapy
might help toward resolving Kelly's many emotional difficulties and
clarifying the nature of his disorder. The child's parents insisted that he

was defective but agreed to a trial. Kelly and his parents were seen weekly on an outpatient basis. In the course of therapy Mrs. Collins developed carcinoma of the breast which metastasized. During her terminal illness four years later when Kelly was nine, the family discontinued therapy.

At that time, Kelly had been seen for 158 playroom hours. According to this therapist's record, the child was diminutive, aloof, physically active and alert though aimless. Kelly uttered a word or two from time to time but there were no real verbal exchanges with the therapist. The child spent much of his time in ritualistic footstamping while holding his penis.

Shortly after therapy was discontinued, Mrs. Collins died. Five months later Mr. Collins requested inpatient care for Kelly, and a psychiatric re-evaluation was arranged. The re-evaluation revealed that Kelly was essentially unchanged since his initial study, although the psychological tests indicated some improvement over the previous rating. Kelly was described as a rather appealing, thin, tense boy. During sudden outbursts of overtly anxious behavior he stiffened and trembled. He restlessly circled the room, often pinching his penis hard or grinding his pelvis against the sink. He dumped crayons, clay, blocks, etc., so quietly and slowly that it was difficult to realize he was actually "wrecking" the playroom. When this behavior was stopped by the therapist, the child spent much time quietly and deliberately putting things back. He did not speak but frequently let out a high-pitched interrupted squeal.

On physical re-examination all findings were within normal limits except for retarded bone age.

The psychiatric staff had reservations about admitting Kelly for several reasons. The family's lack of progress in outpatient therapy, Mr. Collins' indecisiveness about participating in therapy, Kelly's age and his persistent and intense symptoms—all suggested a very bleak prognosis. However, the staff offered a trial of psychiatric inpatient treatment for Kelly. The father agreed to this plan which included weekly appointments with the psychiatrist for himself.

Previous Nursing Efforts

Kelly had been on the ward for eleven months before I began working with him. During that period two different therapists and several nurses had worked with him, due to circumstances beyond the staff's control. He was described as an extremely isolated child largely preoccupied with his own body in such activities as repetitive footstamping, rhythmic head and body movements, frequent open masturbation, wetting, and sometimes soiling and smearing the feces. His vocalizations were loud and unintelligible; he used few words; and he often wheezed.

Efforts to make contact with Kelly were unsuccessful. If a person approaching him reached out a hand, Kelly would cringe as if about to be struck, say excitedly, "Go potty," and dash out of sight. This response occurred so frequently and persistently that the nursing staff felt both rejected and discouraged. At other times he made erratic, impulsive, aggressive overtures towards the staff and other children. Only in retrospect was the staff able to recognize and correlate his increased frenzy with an attempted friendly overture or an invitation to join a group's activity.

Kelly began to show his conflict about self-gratification, especially through contact with people, in more openly self-degrading ways. It reached the point where Kelly took a cracker someone had offered him, stepped on it, and ate the crumbs while the person watched helplessly. He swallowed such things as bobby pins and paper clips. Anything movable and small enough, including pieces of his clothing, might be thrown out the window or flushed down the toilet. He wheezed oftener and the severity frequently called for medication which was not always effective. He began to wet his pants three to four times a day and also at night; he still made numerous trips to the toilet not only to void but to isolate himself, to masturbate, to play in the toilet, and on occasion to flush the toilet with his head in the bowl. The nurses, who had become anxious about Kelly's opinion of them as well as of himself, often discussed his case at ward conferences.

He gradually began to express his feelings more clearly, first showing anger and disappointment—when his father missed a visit or arrived late, when a planned outing was canceled or postponed, when he felt rejected by his nurse who was working with another child and unable to grant his request immediately. Kelly would then yell loudly and angrily, kick furniture, bang doors, and hit out at whoever was at hand to help him. He often had a temporary episode of asthmatic wheezing at these times. But sometimes he showed pleasure, too, smiling smugly when praised for a bit of coloring or for his ability to follow a step or finger game. He began to try out more words, uttering them explosively. When looking through a book with his nurse he would point to objects and try to name them, obviously expecting her to confirm or correct him. He became openly, though ambivalently, eager for affection from his nurse and from other staff members. He would approach to sit on their laps, ask for a hug, or just stay near them. But he could tolerate their nearness only briefly before he tried to hit out or turn a hug into a stranglehold or hair-pulling.

MY WORK WITH KELLY

This was essentially Kelly's condition when I began to work with him.

His reaction to the news that I would be his nurse was typical of his continuing ambivalence about trusting adults. He hugged me very tightly, perhaps to say, "I'm glad you want to," and then pushed my head sharply against the wall, perhaps to say, "I don't know how much my nurse you'll be."

In helping Kelly through daily routine my first goal was to know and understand him and to show him he could trust me. I thought that I should be there when he was troubled as well as when we had things to do together just for fun. While I was trying to understand him, it was easy to accept his wetting and his messiness since, for me, this seemed the reasonable therapeutic approach. It became more and more apparent as I got to know him better that this behavior, particularly the wetting, was directed specifically at what I meant to him. Often on my return to the ward he would be near the entrance. He began to greet me more often with a direct "Hello"—and also with wet pants. Eventually, every time I left him for a coffee break, to look after another child, or to attend a conference, he either wet himself shortly before I returned, or when I approached, he stood in front of me and deliberately wet.

At first I felt guilty about leaving Kelly, rationalizing that his wetting seemed justified, no matter how good my reason for leaving. But I soon realized that a disproportionate amount of our time was spent in changing his pants, especially when there were so many other things to do.

My discouragement increased. I was able to discuss my feelings in supervisory conferences and finally felt more free to discuss the problem of wetting in a ward staff conference. The discussion made it clear to me that the staff believed Kelly's wetting was a way of telling me he was angry when I left him. It also revealed that Kelly had been unable—and up to this point I had been ineffective in helping him—to express himself in a more *open and direct* way. In the face of his anxiety, this was his way of expressing himself at the moment. Nevertheless, the wetting was self-deprecatory in that it was an ineffective and self-defeating way of showing his feelings. I felt that I was participating in his self-depreciation by accepting wetting as his expression of disappointment and anger and the wish for more contact with me. After two more such episodes I was able to act decisively, but I, too, had become angry and disappointed.

On finding Kelly wet when I returned to the ward, I lost my temper. I told him angrily that I was "sick and tired" of spending all our time together changing his pants. There were many things we could do that would be fun. No matter how mad he might be at my leaving him, wetting was a poor way of showing his feelings since we both knew he could tell me more directly. As I spoke, Kelly's behavior shifted to the kind of directness he feared. He began to yell loudly and angrily, perhaps to comply with my request to "be more direct." His deviousness had perhaps been a protection against the rage that appeared. He came at me kicking and hitting wildly. I held him firmly until he calmed. As we both relaxed, I said I wouldn't let him hurt himself or me and I thought he could now tell me in words how he felt. "You know I like you" I added, "or I wouldn't get angry about your treating us both so badly by wetting when you're mad at me." There was no further need to restrain him, and he cuddled against me. After a few minutes I suggested that we change his pants. He took my hand and we went to his clothes locker; for the first time he changed his clothes with little assistance or delay. From then on Kelly was dry for longer and longer periods during the day, even though I was not always with him, until he rarely wet his pants while awake. This improvement continued throughout his stay on the ward. Even the night wetting was only occasional.

This experience enabled me to be more often direct and honest with him without becoming angry. I do not think that my expression of long-suppressed anger was the helpful part of this experience; it merely let me be more direct and deal more honestly with him. If I had been more certain of myself earlier, the same result might have occurred without suppression of my feelings and the subsequent outburst.

One other major crisis also pointed up the absolute need for clarifying my own feelings. Midway in Kelly's and my relationship, his father, for reasons beyond the scope of this paper, decided to try to place him in a state hospital for retarded children. The time came closer for Kelly's father to take him to the hospital to find out whether he would be accepted. I was reluctant to discuss the trip with Kelly because I wasn't sure that his father had mentioned it. I felt this information should come first from his father. In retrospect, this points up the need for close collaboration between the psychotherapist and the nurse, which was at the moment prevented by problems arising from unresolved feelings about Mr. Collins' wish to move Kelly.

About two weeks before the scheduled trip, Kelly became quite irritable; he often refused to join in activities and when induced to do so soon withdrew into a brooding silence or struck out wildly at me with little apparent provocation. I am sure I knew that Kelly must have had some idea about the proposed change in hospitalization, and that his behavior was a response to my own feelings. I was upset about the plan because his progress over the months seemed to indicate that he was not defective and could improve much more. I also realized that I had become attached to Kelly and I would miss him. This in turn made me more uneasy; I interpreted it as overattachment and therefore inappropriate for an objective, detached professional nurse. Outwardly I reacted with extreme anger toward the father for "doing this to Kelly." I thought Kelly had a right to feel angry and resentful. In my anger toward Mr. Collins, I felt unable to share the responsibility of handling Kelly's feelings. It was Mr. Collins' problem—let him solve it. This proved an ineffective method as Kelly was acting out particularly with me, pulling my hair, wetting his pants, and wheezing so severely that he often required medication. We were both miserable.

Overcoming Emotional Barriers

After a particularly harrowing morning which ended with both of us furious, I burst out with, "Are you so upset because of your father's plan to take you to another hospital?" Kelly looked at me directly then immediately walked away, saying, "Go potty." We walked to the bathroom in silence. He began to sob loudly and suddenly rushed at me with clenched fists. I began to cry and, holding him, told him how angry and hurt he must be with me and how sorry I was. I said I didn't want him to go to another hospital, and if he went, I would miss him. I admitted that I had been angry with his father, but his father had the right to choose what he believed would be best for both of them.

After this, Kelly and I both seemed more able to accept our feelings: I could contemplate his possible departure much more calmly, and he was less angry. He seemed sad and depressed at the prospect of leaving, but did not express himself toward me as he had done earlier. His irritable, regressive, destructive behavior ceased, and he could listen calmly when I talked about his possible change. I told him what the hospital would be like and what he might see and do there. I also said that no definite decision had been made, and we could still do many things together.

Kelly did not seem particularly upset by his visit to the other hospital. He was refused admission because the doctors considered his disorder primarily psychotic and their program was not applicable. After this incident, I never again questioned the need to be constantly attentive to Kelly and his behavior.

Kelly's response to my directness and my increased understanding of his behavior in different situations clarified for me what the senior staff meant by an attitude of hovering attentiveness. This close attention was primarily an attempt to prevent his surprisingly quick destructive behavior. I had used repetitive and persistent restraint and redirection of his destructive behavior in areas such as rising, dressing, toileting, eating, play, and going to bed. I was constantly on the alert to prevent his dumping, messing, or in some way destroying whatever he was working with and thus destroying his pleasure in the activity.

An example of our early interactions was the morning routine. I sat next to him at breakfast, watching every move in an attempt to keep him from throwing or spilling food. Next we would wash and brush his teeth. At first it took two people to clean his teeth—one to hold him and one to brush. Persistent urging was necessary to get him to do anything more than turn on the water. He would dabble his hands, brush the towel, and leave. I consistently offered Kelly the choice of brushing his teeth himself or doing it for him. When he indicated that he wasn't ready to do it himself, I expressed regret and my hope that he might do the brushing the next day. He gradually allowed me to brush his teeth without assistance at times, and even offered active help. But at other times he attempted to throw the toothbrush out of the window or down the toilet, or clamped his teeth on it and pulled out the bristles. I told him this behavior did not seem to be satisfying or helpful to him, and that I would help until he could brush his teeth alone and have the fun of doing this and other things for himself.

Gradually, Kelly seemed to have less conflict about satisfying his own bodily needs and was better able to allow himself the satisfaction of learning and doing, such as assuming more responsibility for self care. He participated more freely in school, occupational therapy, and other activities. He would tell himself in words what to do, following the directions I had previously given him. I simply had to stand by as he carried out these activities. After a disappointment, Kelly often returned to earlier modes of behavior. He would repeat my verbal directions, e.g., "Brush your teeth," as if for reassurance, but could not carry them through without some assistance from me. If I was able to recognize and voice his feelings for him and offer gentle physical guidance, he relaxed and completed the activity.

As he developed increasing confidence in himself and trust in me, he began to reach out for more independence and initiative. He would ask to go for a walk, saying, "Where we going?" lead me to the front door and indicate that he wanted it opened by "key for" (his version of a staff member's question "What do you want the key for?"). His speech became understandable although it was often explosive and unclear. When on a walk he would indicate that he wanted to go "dis way," pulling my hand. We both enjoyed these walks and outings. Kelly often commented spontaneously on the things he saw, pointing and vocalizing in a way with which I had become familiar. Sometimes he started to sing a favorite song or nursery rhyme, expecting me to join in. If I did not, he would tug at my chin as if to move my lips. He rarely lapsed into his previous self-preoccupied behavior while off the ward.

Kelly's verbalization increased markedly. Only after working with him for about seven months did I realize how unintelligible his speech was to the rest of the staff. When other staff members misunderstood what he was saying, and they often did, he became angry and upset because his requests were not met. I urged him to slow down and introduced verbs and pronouns into his phrases, which became a game. There was progressively greater carry-over so that at times Kelly would look at me with a grin, saying in a singsong voice, "I want to go potty," instead of, "Go potty." His increasing trust in people was shown by his open acknowledgment that he wanted to be with others, and identification of himself, the staff, and the other children by name.

Integration in Total Program

Reports of the school teacher and the occupational therapist revealed that Kelly's increased freedom was also evident in other settings. In school Kelly at first functioned better when alone with the teacher, initially for only a few minutes at a time, and then for longer periods. He slowly became more interested in learning, at first mainly in music. As his participation in this activity increased, he was found to have almost perfect pitch and an excellent sense of rhythm. With encouragement, he began to pick out melodies on the piano and learned simple tunes.

As his satisfaction increased, he seemed eager to know more about everything. He learned to recognize and write the alphabet and numbers. He played for long periods with me and later with others, writing his name in tinker toys, constructing varied and complex structures with an Erector set, looking through books, pointing out words, and naming objects with obvious pleasure.

Kelly's participation in occupational-therapy activities, which included crafts, rhythm, and dance, progressed with his work in school and on the ward. By the end of the ninth month of my work with him, Kelly had progressed from destroying his materials, or standing in a corner of the O.T. shop masturbating, to open interest in the craft projects and concentrated attention on handling the tools and following directions. Though he still rarely used a tool without some token assistance from me, such as my hand over his when he held a hammer, he tried to do the work correctly and finish the project at hand. His lingering ambivalence about his work was sometimes indicated by his apparent disregard for a finished article; he often threw it away, lost it, or let some other child destroy it.

Ending the Work

Toward the end of this period, Mr. Collins decided to place Kelly in a private program for emotionally disturbed children. This time I found it easier to help prepare Kelly and myself for the change in various ways. When we were engaged in daily routines, I would say that he would do these same things wherever he went and that someone would be there to help him. When he became upset I mentioned that if he felt and behaved this way elsewhere others would keep him from hurting or being hurt. I tried to stress the positive aspects of his leaving as well as what we could do together in the meantime.

The last month before his expected departure was a difficult one. Kelly did not maintain his level of achievement in all respects but he did not regress to the behavior described before the previous near-departure. His therapist was on vacation and Kelly saw his father infrequently during this month. He was aggressive toward the staff and other children and toward himself. He pulled hair, hit and kicked, and tore his clothes. However, this behavior seemed a more open and direct means of communicating his feelings than wetting and frequent asthmatic attacks. He had a few episodes of wheezing, usually at night. Kelly sometimes isolated himself when I was away, lying on his bed or sitting on the toilet masturbating. He would respond to someone's approach by saying "Go potty," but was easily diverted into some other activity. He continued to seek out people, sometimes acting aggressively but more often teasingly; he more often attempted to be close to people than to withdraw. On the last two days before his expected departure, he was able to say "I go to _____," naming the hospital.

Kelly did not leave at this time. I continued to work with him until his father placed him in another state hospital some fourteen months after the nine-month period described here, and he continued to improve in the interim. At the other hospital he has been receiving tranquilizers and frequent medication for his asthma attacks which have become more frequent and severe. He is more preoccupied with self, and his verbalization has decreased. Although wetting, self-destructive, and aggressive behavior have reappeared, his overall behavior is still more integrated than when he was first admitted to the Langley Porter Neuropsychiatric Institute.

DISCUSSION

This paper describes nine months of intensive nursing care of a psychotic child in an inpatient psychiatric treatment center for children. The goal of treatment was resolution of the child's internalized conflict and freeing of his energies for progressive learning. This goal was based on the hypothesis that childhood schizophrenia is psychogenic and results in the distortion of basic sensual impulses, which are expressed in frustrating, self-defeating, and destructive behavior. The child's disorder is believed to have stemmed from early experience in living with people who were themselves in conflict. It was felt that the child's disorder could be reduced by his work with people free or becoming free from similar conflicts within themselves. This hypothesis is described in greater detail by Boatman and Szurek [2].

Kelly's conflict manifested itself in all areas of expression, seriously interfering with his ability to experience any satisfaction. For example, his wish to be near people was often distorted into an anxious, hostile impulse expressed through nearly suffocating hugs and hair-pulling. And after eagerly accepting food, he would throw it on the floor and stamp on it before eating it. Again, after finishing with some degree of pleasure a project in occupational therapy, he often threw it away on his way back to the ward.

The child's ambivalent distorted behavior at times made it difficult to determine his actual wishes. A nurse who is constantly attentive to the behavior of such a child will be more likely to identify his needs and help him achieve as much pleasurable gratification as possible. She can also be more helpful if she constantly strives to recognize and understand feelings aroused in her by the child. Strongly angry and retaliative feelings have a tremendous influence on her behavior with the child. For example, my own angry feelings about Kelly's wetting and my anxiety about them, as well as the staff's criticism of my handling of this situation, interfered with my ability to be more helpful to him.

I now believe that my anxiety about being angry and implications of this anger for me personally were more disruptive to my work with Kelly than the anger itself. After I began to resolve my feelings about it, I could express my anger and my reasons for it more clearly and directly to Kelly. This experience may have reassured him about expressing his own anger with less intense anxiety. Resolving conflicts about feelings aroused within oneself is one of the difficult problems faced by the nurse working with disturbed children [3, 5].

Recognizing and understanding one's feelings is important in working not only with the child but also with other staff members. Learning to communicate relevant material, an inherent part of the work with hospitalized disturbed children, is difficult for any new staff member. Certain problems arising from the very nature of the work are encountered by all staff members learning to work with disturbed children. These problems were perhaps further complicated by my being the first graduate nursing student to have post master's clinical experience on the ward. Staff members were at times discouraged and angry because they could not spend as much time and energy in working with their assigned children as I did with Kelly. These feelings sometimes focused on one aspect of his behavior or on my apparent ineffectiveness in dealing with his behavior. Although it is impossible to say whether these feelings were present among staff members all the time, it seemed that I found them difficult to deal with only when I was in conflict about some aspect of my work with Kelly or his therapist. It was at these times that I found it most difficult to discuss my feelings or those of other staff members. As I became more certain of my goals for Kelly and possible ways of achieving them, this problem with other staff members decreased sharply. As the nurse learns more about the problem at hand, communication with other staff members is enhanced and it becomes easier to attend to intrastaff problems while continuing to help the child.

Supervision is an important area in work with disturbed children. My weekly conferences with the child's therapist were necessary and useful to examine Kelly's behavior within the context of his relationships with significant people in his life—his family, his doctor and nurse, other children, and staff members. Equally important were my three weekly conferences with my nursing supervisor who was aware of the nurse's problems when working with emotionally disturbed children. This supervision not only shortened the often tiring and discouraging learning period, but also aided me toward helping Kelly and understanding myself and my relationship with him.

In most hospital settings the proportion of nurses to children does not permit the intensive work described in this paper. And far too few skilled nurses are available to give individual frequent supervision to help other nursing personnel learn aspects of the work involved in caring for disturbed children. Such supervisory skills are developed through learning the necessary nursing skills and acquiring greater self-understanding. Nevertheless, I believe the principles presented here are applicable to nurses working with disturbed children in most settings [6].

At the Langley Porter Neuropsychiatric Institute, staff members are increasingly convinced that intensive continuous nursing care can be a major contribution to the total psychotherapeutic program for each hospitalized child. Since the experience described in this paper, the staff has continued to explore ways of providing such experiences for more children and of helping more nurses learn the necessary skills to carry out the intensive care.

REFERENCES

1. BOATMAN, MALETA J., PAYNTER, JANE, and PARSONS, CORRINE. Nursing in hospital psychiatric therapy for psychotic children. Paper accepted for publication in the *Am. J. Orthopsychiat.*

2. BOATMAN, MALETA J., and SZUREK, S. A. A clinical study of childhood schizophrenia. In Don D. Jackson (Ed.), *The etiology of schizophrenia.* New York: Basic Books, 1960, pp. 389-440.

3. BLOCH, D. A. Residential treatment for disturbed children. *Nursing Outlook,* **5**:636 (November 1957).

4. ENG, MARIETTA C. The occupational therapy program on a ward for psychotic children. *Proceedings of the 1960 annual conference.* New York: American Occupational Therapy Association.

5. GODBOUT, ROSE and PETRICK, ARLENE. The child and the nurse. *Nursing Outlook,* **6**:460 (August 1958).

6. SUTTON, HELEN A. Some nursing aspects of a children's psychiatric ward. *Am. J. Orthopsychiat.,* **17**:675 (October 1947).

7. SZUREK, S. A. Psychotic episodes and psychotic maldevelopment. Childhood Schizophrenia Symposium, 1955. *Am. J. Orthopsychiat.,* **26**:519 (July 1956).

8. _____ . Dynamics of staff interaction in hospital psychiatric treatment of children. *Am. J. Orthopsychiat.,* **17**:664 (October 1947).

9. _____ . The family and the staff in hospital psychiatric therapy of children. *Am. J. Orthopsychiat.,* **21**:597 (July 1951).

10. _____ . Playfulness, creativity and schisis. *Am. J. Orthopsychiat.,* **29**:667 (October 1959).

11. _____ . Some lessons from efforts at psychotherapy with parents. *Am. J. Psychiat.,* **109**:296 (October 1952). Reprinted in S. A. Szurek & I. N. Berlin (Eds.), *Training in therapeutic work with children.* Vol. 2, the Langley Porter Child Psychiatry Series. Palo Alto, Calif.: Science and Behavior Books, 1967.

CHAPTER 13

NURSES AS CHILD CARE WORKERS[*]

Maleta J. Boatman, M.D.

EDITORS' NOTE, 1970

This paper was written for and read at the Annual Meeting of the American Association for Children's Residential Centers, November 1963. As is indicated, it was largely through the stimulating yearly discussions with this relatively small group of persons, all very interested and involved in residential treatment for emotionally disturbed children, that the author became aware of the relative lack of use of registered nurses in such programs. Aside from the prohibitive cost of nurses' salaries, there seemed to be considerable doubt that trained nurses were the persons who were likely to be willing and able to offer disturbed children the help they needed in the twenty-four-hour milieu.

This paper describes somewhat different experiences of finding some professionally trained nurses to be most capable of such work, at least in our center for seriously disturbed children with the kind of staff supervision we provide.

If you were to enter the small Children's Ward at the Langley Porter Neuropsychiatric Institute looking for the persons who were responsible for providing the round-the-clock care of one of the children, you would find them by asking for "Johnny's nurse" or for the "charge nurse." If you were a physician specialist called from the adjacent University

[*]This work was partially supported by the National Institute of Mental Health Project Grant, No. 5-R11-MH-234-3, entitled "Nursing in Hospital Psychiatric Therapy for Psychotic Children."

hospital as a consultant regarding a child's acute illness or injury, you might look about at the tousled young women clad in gay sweaters and skirts or slacks and ask, "Where in the world *are* your nurses?"

NURSES OR OTHER CHILD CARE WORKERS

Until about ten years ago I had taken this state of affairs for granted—that is, that one would usually *hope* to find registered nurses, who might or might not look like nurses, on any unit that provided twenty-four hour treatment for emotionally disturbed children. Since then, a series of experiences, one of which has been membership in this American Association for Children's Residential Centers, has led me to a clear awareness that my assumption was incorrect.

There are many recurrent basic questions about who the child-care persons should be as well as about how many are needed, how much they should be paid, how they should be trained, how long they should be kept on the job, and how their duties can best be defined.

This lack of clarity and of agreement about the professional background and training necessary for child care workers probably reflects two factors: (*a*) residential treatment is still in an experimental stage and it is therefore too early to have answers to some questions; (*b*) to the degree that answers may exist, they can be understood only in the context of the total operation of some particular center.

I would like to tell you a little bit about the Children's Ward at Langley Porter Neuropsychiatric Institute, with particular emphasis on our experience with nurses as child care workers. I am going to assume that most of you know something of our setting, facility, auspices, and treatment concepts, and start by giving you a picture of what our staff and patients are like at this point in time, 1963.[1]

STAFF AND PATIENTS

The basic staffing pattern and alterations in its numbers and proportions have been more of an externally imposed reality than a clinically determined factor. As a training and research Institute established early in this mid-twentieth century, it has not been easy to add staff, but it has been *easier* to add: trainees rather than faculty; personnel for short-term carefully designed research rather than clinicians; specialists in new areas rather than more or better trained personnel already present. As in most hospital psychiatric inpatient facilities, over-all clinical-administrative

---

[1] For a detailed description of all of these aspects, see Chapter 4.

direction has been given to psychiatrists from the start, and administrative and professional leadership in the patient-care areas has been given to professionally trained nurses. Throughout the Institute, the Nursing Service provides patient care with a staff composed of a ratio of two registered nurses to each nonprofessionally trained worker. Under California Civil Service Classifications, these are known, respectively, as Psychiatric Nurses and Psychiatric Technicians. When the Institute's Nursing Service positions are entirely filled, which they seldom can be, the Children's Ward has a nursing staff of fifteen: one Senior Psychiatric Nurse; five to six Psychiatric Nurses; three to four Junior Psychiatric Nurses; and five Psychiatric Technicians. Although we have tried unsuccessfully to budget for senior supervisory positions and to enlarge the total number of positions in the nursing staff, we have never seriously considered trying to alter its basic composition. Some of the desired positions have been temporarily available in the last four years through sources that I will mention later.

Other positions concerned primarily with the children's inpatient work are: one occupational therapist; one speech therapist; and one elementary school teacher from the Special Education Division of the city's school system. The four to six full-time child psychiatry trainees provide most of the psychotherapy for hospitalized children and their parents. The immediate clinical-administrative responsibility for the ward resides with the child psychiatrist, who is the Assistant Director of the Service—that is, with me.

As a result of many factors, our ward usually has twelve or thirteen young and severely disturbed psychotic children, four to fourteen years of age, who are hospitalized for long-term intensive psychotherapy, and who stay from one to seven or more years. The other one or two children are usually hospitalized for intensive diagnostic study or treatment-planning, and stay from three weeks to two or three months. Parents as well as children are seen regularly by a child psychiatrist. One criterion for a child's staying for therapy beyond a period of brief service is the parents' willingness to try to use their individual appointments as psychotherapy for themselves. There are no set visiting hours. Most children go home most weekends. In recent years, some have been day-patients only.

NURSE AS PART OF TREATMENT TEAM

The nurse becomes part of the treatment during the several weeks of outpatient study, at the point at which hospitalization is considered. Parents and child are invited by the psychiatrist to see the ward and talk with the charge nurse. If admission for inpatient study is likely, the child will spend some time with the particular nurse who will help him most during his first days on the ward. The nurse also talks with the parents about their child, the ward program, and what clothes and spending money he may need. This is sometimes a very important part of reducing the child's and parents' fears and is an integral part of the establishment of the therapeutic atmosphere for all of them. The following vignette illustrates the nurse's work.

Tim was a thin, mute, withdrawn, autistic six-and-a-half-year-old who had been separated only once for part of a day from his forty-five-year-old mother. He still wore diapers. Fatigued and depressed, his mother was eager but anxious about trying an inpatient study. The fifty-year-old father was critical of her need for a rest, since their other two children were grown. In planning Tim's admission, the nurse, Miss K., told him and his parents that they might visit or call at any time, but explained the children's day so that they could plan which times would interest them most and be most convenient for all concerned. She asked how many diapers Tim had been using and suggested that mother bring training pants as well. Although Miss K. expected to use only the pants and told the parents that this was her hope, she knew that absolute assurance without personal experience would present herself, Tim, and the mother with an unwise challenge. She explained that she and mother could decide better together after a week or two whether he would need one or both. Although mother was clearly frightened and threatened by this and each subsequent innovation, she was able to accept and begin to participate in the efforts presented in this clear, firm, but non-critical, non-coercive way by Miss K. It also seemed to us that Tim was freer to respond with less prolonged fear to these new opportunities for more integrated behavior than if he and his mother had heard them as efforts to wean him away from her.

Psychotherapeutic Nursing Care on Admission or Study

At the actual time of admission of a child, his assigned nurse is made free for the day to spend almost all her time with him. She helps him and his parents put his clothes away and tries to be sure that questions about laundry, the parents' next visit, when the child will first go home, his spending money, and so forth are clear. If the parents are vague, she tells them of the staff's efforts to tell the child with certainty and accuracy what he may expect, and asks them to let her know as soon as they have been able to decide about the particular situation in question. She tries to gauge the degree of participation she needs to have in the family's first farewell, remaining only unobtrusively available if possible. More often she needs to help the parents say a definite goodbye rather than slipping off. If so, she explains that we feel it is better for the child to show distress at their leaving rather than to find himself uncertain of their departure. In subsequent hours she tries to gauge how much to show the child, when to invite him into ward activities, how much privacy to allow him, and so forth by watching him closely for signs of mounting anxiety or tentative interest. Before she leaves for the day she helps him become acquainted with the afternoon and evening staff, and tells him clearly when he may expect her return. It is her job to alert the other staff members to special problems and help he may need with regard to toileting, eating, or bedtime.

Although the psychiatrist would have discussed these things with her prior to and on the day of admission, it can be seen that she needs to use a good deal of initiative in timing her efforts, making clinical observations, and finding those responses that hopefully will be precisely coordinated with those attitudes that are considered psychotherapeutic in this particular program.

Importance of Nursing Background

During the inpatient study period of several weeks, the nurse may need to use all her skills in combining the child's psychotherapeutic and diagnostic experiences. Procedures planned by the psychiatrist may range from a simple physical exam through an electroencephalogram and dental check to such major things as pneumo-encephalogram. The nurse's knowledge of the procedures involved and her ability to help in the medical care attendant on them are of great help to her in making them as unfrightening as possible. In some instances it has appeared as though the child's trust in the staff grew more rapidly around some such procedure than around other experiences.

The nurse's capacity to care for the child during illness, injury, or medical procedures continues to be an important contribution, however long the hospitalization. The following vignette illustrates this.

Sarah was older than most of the ward children when she was admitted for the second time. Psychotic since infancy, she had gained speech and developed isolated skills that indicated superior intelligence and artistic sensitivities. Seriously handicapping phobias and compulsions had taken the place of more destructive and regressive symptoms as her reaction pattern to traumatic events. Shortly before father's ill health and mother's need to go to work had necessitated rehospitalization, the efforts of the mother, who was perhaps overly concerned with nutrition, to help the girl with adolescent acne and serious tooth decay had resulted in a phobia of sugar, chocolate, and butter. As readmission became likely, Sarah also developed a compulsion to spit half-chewed food back into her plate. The nursing staff felt repelled by her thin, tense body and by her whining, grimacing, food-spitting aloofness. They felt baffled and angry at her affectless ignoring of their overtures and her retaliative tantrums when they slacked their efforts to relate to her. They felt inadequate and began to suspect the senior psychiatrists of personal favoritism rather than re-search interests in the continued work with the family. When it seemed that their psychotherapeutic knowledge and skill and the psychiatrists' and charge nurse's efforts to be helpful might prove insufficient, Sarah developed acute appendicitis, virus pneumonia, and infectious mono-nucleosis in rapid succession. The technicians felt even more inadequate than before, but the nurses had renewed feelings of competence and nurturance. Uncomfortable and frightened, Sarah was likewise accepting of pain-relieving contact. Despite her repetitive panic over eating and drinking, the nurses became patient, firm, and imaginative. At the end of two months of illness in bed, Sarah had gained seven pounds in weight and had developed a continuing openly trusting and eager relationship with her nurse.

INDIVIDUAL NURSING IN ACTIVITIES

Until a few years ago we had seen the nurses' major areas of effective-ness to be those of free play and of the daily necessities of living (physical care, bathing, eating, and toileting). Their primary relationship to school and O.T. was to see that the children got there and to be available to handle behavior outbursts. A few fortuitous occurrences led us to suspect that it might be helpful if an assigned nurse could participate on a one-to-one basis with her child patient in activities planned and presented by the skilled specialists. Our nursing staff of fifteen could not be stretched enough to care for children twenty-four hours a day, seven days a week and still explore this possibility with enough consistency to be conclusive.

Four years ago we found several ways to try this hypothesis more thoroughly. On several occasions the University of California School of Nursing had a graduate particularly interested in children's psychiatric nursing. One of our former very experienced nurses returned to help pre-pare and eventually to carry out an NIMH grant request concerned with nursing skills and in-service training. Under the supervision of this nurse, we have now had a total of ten nurses from these projects who were able to spend four to six hours a day with an assigned child, for nine months to three years. The incidental resultant of increases in staff numbers has also permitted more of the regular staff nurses to have increased time with individual patients. As the nurse moves with her child from school to free play to lunch and wash-up to O.T., she takes with her her acute knowledge of the youngster's needs and his ways of communicating them. The teacher and the occupational therapist have found that the children gain skills more readily than before. The nurses find themselves better able to help the children relate one experience to another. It has made it possible to provide group experiences for children who were still too isolated and fearful to relate in any meaningful way with peers.

Emergence of Peer Groups Through Individual Work

Pat, David, and Tom are seven, eight, and nine. It is not uncommon these days to see them dashing down the corridor outside the ward and laughing together at the ward door like any three mischievous little boys. When Miss M. rounds the corner from the school room several seconds later, joking about their having run and hidden from her, no stranger would be surprised, but we are elated. This is new in the last few months, for previously each of these boys has been aloof from each other and from all other children. Six months ago each would have been animated only if closely engaged in activity with the nurse who had been working with him for two to three years. Eight-year-old Pat, for instance, was a silent, grimacing or blank-faced child of five-and-a-half when Miss M. joined the staff, two months after his admission. He glided away from any approaching person, looked directly at no one, played only with minute pieces of toys in repetitive secret manipulations of them, screamed in terror if cornered by a more aggressive child, and struggled frantically to escape from any adult who tried to cuddle him. Miss M. accompanied him everywhere during each day for several months before she learned to recognize his quick sidewise glance at a toy as an indication that he would be interested if she played with it, telling and showing him what it could do. It took a year of relating all he saw to their other common experiences such as, "Look, Pat, the green car in the school book is just like your daddy's," before he began to let his eyes rest on her face or on the object at hand. It was seven months after he glanced at a roller skate that he was first skating. In the interim however, he had touched one, thrown one, rolled one, been pulled while sitting on one, and watched Miss M. skate. A year ago he had begun to say words to the speech therapist after Miss M., and he had played at making hollow sounds into a tinker toy can. In O.T. he would hammer wood if Miss M.'s hand rested lightly on his. In school he would point to the word card if Miss M. was sitting next to him. In the playground he would take turns with David and Tom on the slide, although none of them would hold hands with any but a nurse for a circle game. This spring, their nurses found they could sometimes encourage them to continue their parallel play while one or two of the nurses helped set up another activity at a distance from them. When this year's vacations left the three of them with one or two of their nurses, there was jealous vying for attention, but their teasing, pulling, and pushing of each other was welcomed short of hurt. Gradually they discovered that a dash up the hill brought an exciting flurry of "chase me." When Miss W. returned from vacation, John greeted her warmly, but on the first outing in the station wagon he sat jostling with Pat and Miss M. and ignored her. Today, if each of these boys has some time with his own nurse each day, they can sometimes go happily to school or to play as a group with any one of the three nurses.

LEARNING TO WORK WITH PSYCHOTIC CHILDREN

In the earlier description of Sarah I touched on the major problem of how to help a child-care staff group learn enough about psychopathology, psychotherapeutic principles, and the effect of their own personal reactions on children's responses that they are able to contribute effective and consistent work in the presence of the massively indirect, hostile, demanding, and self-hurtful behavior of psychotic children. For quite a few years we have known some things that helped. All ward-care staff is included in as many of our clinical discussion groups as their time will permit. The children are cared for one hour a week by psychiatry trainees so that the entire nursing staff is free to meet as a group with each other and with me as the Assistant Director. Each nurse has weekly opportunities to talk with a more senior nurse and with the psychiatrist of her assigned child. These things help, but not enough to sustain the level of achievement, particularly at critical periods. Major or minor crises were precipitated by various situations: when a child's behavior was exhaustingly aggressive and hurtful to himself or others; when there was disagreement about what would be helpful to a child; when key members of the senior staff were on vacation, attending meetings, or busy preparing papers or budgets; when there was an unusual shortage or rapid turnover of staff; when some administrative policies of the Institute changed seemingly undesirably; or when there was concern that someone had been treated unfairly. We began to know, for example, that from June through August of each year, there would be a period of explosive staff tension and reduced therapeutic efficacy. June is a month when nurses get married and husbands finish medical or dental school. July is our time for turnover of psychiatric trainees, and August is the month best suited for our University faculty vacations.

Several facts became apparent, however. Those persons who were best able to maintain effective focus on the clinical task in times of difficulty were most often the professionally trained nurses who had already had at least a year's experience, and who at some time had been able to meet regularly with a truly experienced and capable nurse or with one of the senior psychiatrists.

It was these observations that were vital in shaping the form of the three-year NIMH Community Services project that I mentioned earlier. We are pleased enough with its preliminary results that we have applied for a two-year extension.

In each year of this project we have selected two registered nurses who had B.A. degrees and who had no professional experience with children. Each committed herself to at least two years of clinical work, which was to include study, detailed recording, and intensive supervision. Each has had a clinical assignment similar to that of the ward nurses, but is relatively free from the ward's administrative demands, that is, free to attend more meetings than ward nurses and free of weekend and evening assignments. They have three supervisory sessions weekly with Miss Jane Paynter, the project's Nursing Education Director, who works directly under my supervision and coordinates the work with the Superintendent of Nurses and the charge nurse.

In every instance these project nurses have learned more rapidly and more consistently than have staff nurses with less supervision or graduate students with less emphasis on the clinical experience. They have had the same discouragements and difficulties that all other child-care persons have had, regardless of training or experience, but they have recognized them earlier than others, found more constructive ways to work on them, and have been more consistent in their clinical work despite them.

We feel convinced that at least in our hospital setting, with very disturbed children, professional nurses can learn to do the psychotherapeutically oriented work we desire of our child-care persons. I doubt if anyone can learn to do it without a skillful and available supervisor.

There are of course problems in the employment of professional nurses. They are usually women, and it is probably important to have some proportion of men. Most are young and will on the average not stay many years because of marriage or pregnancy. Their degree of professional training and their scarcity permits them to command a relatively prohibitive high salary. It is also difficult to implement a scaling of jobs so that those who do not leave are not promoted away.

I have come to believe that some of the solutions to the problem of providing adequate child care are: to have intelligent, educated persons with a professional identification such as nursing; to have enough of such persons; to pay them attractive salaries; to provide them with far more supervision than is regularly recognized as feasible; to be prepared for the constant job of providing the clinical-administrative help for crises; and to expect the job of training new workers to fill the vacancies to be unending.

SECTION FIVE

THE INTERDISCIPLINARY CREATION OF A
THERAPEUTIC MILIEU

INTRODUCTION

It has become almost commonplace to include in the staff of an inpatient treatment center, in addition to the psychiatric nurse, specialists
from other disciplines that are important in providing opportunities for
children to reach their maximal development. Among these latter disciplines are those of education and occupational and recreational therapy.
When possible, some of the specialists are experienced in physical education and music.

The following section gives attention to how these specialists and the
nurses work together and with the psychotherapists to provide elements
essential to a therapeutic environment on the ward for the child. Their
work together provides both opportunities and problems for program
planning, and integration of such disparate disciplines toward the overriding goal of the child's optimal development. Their efforts need to be
simultaneously directed toward therapeutic reduction of the child's
disorder so as to make it possible for him to attain this goal.

CHAPTER 14

THE TEACHING OF SCHIZOPHRENIC CHILDREN

Shirley E. Forbing

I am just completing my fourth year as a teacher on the Children's
Ward at the Langley Porter Neuropsychiatric Institute in San Francisco,
California. My job is an unusual one, since my pupils are all severely
emotionally disturbed children up to twelve years of age. Many are diag-
nosed as having childhood schizophrenia, a severe mental disorder. The
Langley Porter Neuropsychiatric Institute, supported by the State of
California Department of Mental Hygiene, is a teaching and research
center. This article relates my teaching experiences on the Children's
Ward, and is not intended to be a description of how all psychotic children should be taught.

The teaching position on the Children's Ward of the Institute is under
the jurisdiction of the San Francisco Unified School District and its
program for the physically handicapped. Since there is no special credential available in California for teaching emotionally disturbed children,
a California General Elementary Credential is all that is required for this
position. At present it seems that experience at the primary and kindergarten level is the best preparation for the job. This is true because many
of the children have never attended school, or have attended only minimally because of the severity of their emotional disorder.

The nursing staff regularly gives valuable aid in the classroom by
caring for special problems that arise. They sit by a child to see that he
performs his tasks, guide those children who otherwise would not attempt work, see that noses are wiped and shoes tied, curb destruction
of school materials, see that paint goes on the paper instead of in the
mouth, and remind children to pay attention. Without this assistance,
I could not begin to handle such a classroom except by doing individual
tutoring.

The school calendar and schedules are the same as for the rest of the schools in the district. In addition to the regular school year, there are two five-week summer sessions. During the summer, the school day is cut to four hours, and these hours are arranged by agreement of the teacher and the ward staff.

I have often been asked why I decided to go into this field of teaching, as if I had special reasons for doing so. The matter was simple enough— I needed a teaching job, and this position was the only one available at the time! Until this time, like many other teachers I was not aware that any attempt was being made to educate emotionally disturbed children. My acquaintances seemed to think I was making a drastic mistake even to consider teaching psychotic children. I felt that it would be a learning experience and that if I did not enjoy it, I could transfer back to a regular classroom. By the end of the first year, I had just begun to understand and enjoy my special pupils, and so I decided to stay on to explore my new frontier.

Another question that is often asked of me is whether or not the work is depressing and whether I might not be so sorry for these children that I would be unable to work with them. The answer is that I am so busy trying to find new ways to help the children learn that I never think of being depressed. Of course there are times when I am discouraged, as I would be in any other position. While I am working, I do whatever I can as a teacher to help the children. After I leave work, I am quite occupied with my own family, and I do not think of my job until the next day. I am informed by the psychiatric staff that a person who is able to find satisfaction in his personal life and who enjoys helping children learn is better able to succeed in this type of work than one who channels all of his efforts day and night into his job in an effort to achieve all his satisfactions from his work.

One of the things that was most helpful to me when I came to work with emotionally disturbed children was the formulation of a certain attitude about what I hoped to accomplish in my work. I learned that only about 10 percent of the children would ever be "cured." And what of the others? I felt that whatever learning they could accomplish, even though minimal, might help them to be a little more self-sufficient and less frightened of the learning process.

Our experience is that a teacher, even though she may not have had psychiatric training, may be successful if she is versatile and can vary her approach to meet individual needs. While a psychiatrist's primary job is to try to understand a child's fears and to help him solve his emotional problems, a teacher must try to help a child learn; and although learning has a therapeutic effect on the child, the teacher's aim is not to do therapy. Some of my friends who are teachers have said that they would be afraid to attempt working with a disturbed child for fear of doing or saying the wrong thing. I have found that these children, while in school, can be treated as normally as possible and can be expected to conform within their individual limits.

There are fifteen inpatients on the Children's Ward, with one bed for a study case. With one exception, the children stay on the ward throughout the week and go home if possible on weekends. One child stays during the days only and goes home with his mother at night, this being a satisfactory arrangement for her.

Besides his school program, each child participates in occupational therapy activities, where he has an opportunity to learn arts and crafts. He also spends three hours a week in play therapy with his psychiatrist, and he goes on special outings with the nurses. Some of these outings may include such activities as picnics or a trip to the zoo, the aquarium, the dimestore, the beach, or a movie.

I regularly attend various staff meetings on the ward such as treatment reviews (presentation of case studies and treatment), rounds (where current work with individual children is discussed by psychiatrists, nurses, occupational therapists, social worker, psychologist, and teacher) and another meeting where the ward staff discusses ward activities. These meetings are beneficial to the teacher as well as to the other staff because they provide an opportunity to exchange ideas, to air problems, and to know what is happening to the child in other areas. The teacher's observations about what the child is doing in school contribute materially to the overall picture of the child, and sometimes may offer clues about the child's readiness to move ahead in other areas.

The classroom schedule changes with the needs of the ward, but generally it is as follows: During the first session in the morning, one group of children will be in occupational therapy, and the remaining group usually has some type of musical activity. This is one activity in which the children participate as a group. Next, the class meets as a whole for the flag salute, the daily news (the children love to see their names in print), a discussion of the daily activities, and a story. If, for some reason, we are not able to have these opening exercises, the children seem to feel that the day has not started right. In fact, some of the children may get the flag and have their own private salute. Routine seems important to these children, even more than it is for normal children. We break up into groups after that, and while I am working with one group, the nurses take care of the others. I have one group that is doing first grade reading and simple arithmetic. Another group has just finished some pre-reading material and is enthusiastically starting on the first pre-primer. In a group of four, I have a nurse to assist in keeping the children's attention on the book. Some of the children are unable to do any kind of work in a group, and these I take individually.

Some of the other activities consist of simple art projects, planting gardens, learning to use simple rhythm instruments, and writing group stories. Music is the one area in which almost all the children respond. They are especially attentive to classical music. Even such simple activities as learning to color and cutting on a line require a great deal of individual attention, and many children will not even try to do these things unless a member of the staff is right beside them, either giving verbal encouragement or actually guiding their hands.

Our school, like other schools in the district, is on a budget. Since the children are quite destructive, the materials do not last very long and are supplemented from other funds. Attempts are made to help the children be less destructive, and many of them have responded to our insistence that they take better care of their things. For some, this is the first step in learning. Once in a while, the ward receives donations of toys and records. Among the materials we have acquired for school room use are a piano, an autoharp, records and a record player (one of our most popular items), a blackboard, and a bulletin board.

When working with normal children, a teacher expects her class to go through a testing period at the beginning of each new year. This means that the child tries to see how far he can go; he wants to know where the limits will be set for him and what is expected of him. I have found that the emotionally disturbed child reacts in much the same manner as the normal child, except that the testing is more rigorous and re-occurs frequently. His methods of testing are seemingly bizarre at times. They may take the form of dripping saliva in odd places, eating crayons, depositing feces, pulling and tugging, screeching, destroying completed lessons, or tantalizing by doing a tiny bit of the assigned task perfectly and then refusing to complete it.

In dealing with these problems, consistent firmness pays off. Anticipating a child's behavior and being attentive to the first clues he gives of his moods helps to prevent a lot of difficulty. If the child is successful in provoking me, he will continue his testing. In the early months of working together there seems to be a great deal of this kind of behavior, but as a good relationship is established as a result of consistent and kindly firmness, the testing diminishes and sometimes subsides altogether. Some children, however, seem to need to do at least a slight bit of testing each time they are asked to do a task. The more quickly this is handled, the faster the child settles down to work. Establishing rapport seems to take less time as my experience increases, and the period of testing seems to get shorter for each new child that enters the group.

The attitude toward learning varies with each child, but for the most part, an emotionally disturbed child approaches it with varying degrees of resistance. For instance, a child may try to convince you that he is totally unaware of what is being taught by not hearing, not seeing, not comprehending. This attitude can be handled in various ways, according to the child. One can learn by trial and error which method to use with a child. The child who is openly negative is much easier to handle than the one who is quietly negative. For example, when a child flings her pencil across the room and throws her paper away, I quietly pick up the paper and pencil and assure the child that she has to do the work, even if I have to help her for a while by guiding her hand. It is more difficult to help another child who, given the same lesson as the first one described, will pretend not to hear. If I try to guide his hand, he will let his hand go limp. It is difficult not to ignore a child of the second type when the child of the first type demands attention in such a way that disastrous things will occur if the situation is not immediately handled.

When teaching these children to read, I employ many of the techniques used with normal children. The main difference is that I must simplify much of the material to adjust to their short attention spans. I may read to the mute children while they follow with their eyes. I must use a lot of repetition in the lessons, since the children seem to learn more easily by rote than by the reasoning process. Many children have difficulty in applying what they have learned in one situation to another situation. The ability to use reasoning in problem-solving seems to increase when a child is more relaxed and less concerned about his personal problems.

With disturbed, as with normal children, learning seems to follow a pattern. For instance, in learning to write, a child may insist that he cannot use his hand unless I place mine over his to guide him. After guiding him in this manner for several months, I may loosen my grip on his hand so that he is doing the guiding. If I stop using the pressure of my hand before I feel his hands are ready to take over, the child may stop entirely, or if he is ready to go ahead, he may trace over letters that I have made. After this he may try to make letters by himself. The writing may be large, shaky, and done with very light pressure. As the child's confidence increases, the writing improves until it is farily normal.

Once a child experiences success in learning, he seems to learn more things at a faster rate; if he is being helped in other areas, then everything moves smoothly. As an example of this, I recall one bright boy who was mute for psychological reasons; when invited to school, he would throw a big temper tantrum. I told him that he would come to school even if he could only stay ten minutes a day at first. So, when I wanted him, I had to pry him loose from his bed and carry him (while he screamed and kicked) to school. At first the tantrums were violent, but gradually they changed quality, so that finally they seemed to be a device for "saving face." If he thought I was not going to notice that he was under his covers on his bed, he would let out a little screech to attract my attention. Once he started accomplishing his tasks in school and experiencing success in them, he moved ahead rapidly. In fact, I found it difficult to keep up with him. Instead of my having to come and get him for school, I found him waiting for me, and the moment I opened the door in the morning, he would rush me down to the cloakroom and pull my coat off and then take me to the classroom. A short while after he became interested in learning to read, he preferred to read out of encyclopedias and medical and scientific books.

Psychological muteness is common among severely emotionally disturbed children. However, although I found this a handicap at first, I soon discovered that there are many ways of communicating with these children. One day when I was completely mute from laryngitis, I was surprised to find that I could communicate almost better than usual with the children. There are ways in which I am able to know whether or not a child is learning anything, even if he will not speak or write. The boy I mentioned in the above paragraph developed his own sign language. Once the nurse assigned to him brought him into the classroom and very excitedly wanted to show me that he could comprehend the meaning of pictures in a magazine. She then drew a picture of a bar of soap on the blackboard and stood back, waiting for him to make the motions of washing his hands. It was a surprise to both of us when he picked up the chalk and wrote "Ivory" inside the picture of the soap. It was doubly amazing since he had never before written anything!

Quite often a child, while pretending extreme indifference, will absorb the lessons, and then reveal his knowledge at a much later time outside the school setting. I am working with a child at present who refuses to write at all unless I guide her hand. The lessons I present to her appear afterwards on the chalk board, on scraps of paper, and occasionally on the walls. Still another child who will not read from her pre-primer will use the words that are presented as new vocabulary in her social patter. For instance, if I present the word "run" and ask her to identify it, she will be quite negative, but a moment later may say, "Mike is running past my chair," which actually is not true.

Another example of belated response is that of a girl who had difficulty referring to herself in the first person. If she wanted a piece of candy she would say, "You want a piece of candy." After correcting her many times with, "Not *you,* but *I* want a piece of candy," we realized that she had learned the right way to say it. One day she went riding in the park. One of the nurses pointed to a tree and said, "Jane, see that tree over there? That's a eucalyptus tree." She countered with, "No not *eu*calyptus—*I*-calyptus."

There are some subjects such as music and rhythmic activities in which the whole class can participate effectively. The flag salute and sharing of the daily news are others. Play activities using clay, tinker toys, puzzles, and blocks can be done as a group. In these experiences, children learn to share and take turns. Their playing is, for the most part, parallel rather than interpersonal. Games such as enacting "Jack-Be-Nimble," in which a child or the group recites the rhyme while the children take turns jumping over the candlestick, is more successful than "Drop the Handkerchief." In the first instance, the action and result are completed without the interaction of the other children. If the child who is running with the handkerchief decides to use it as a scarf instead, then the game is lost.

Subjects such as reading, writing, and arithmetic are best taught either individually or in small groups of not more than four. Children who cannot tolerate being taught in a group are first tutored individually and, when ready, are transferred to the group. These subjects require great effort and concentration on the part of the child. I have found that it does not work out to have other children present in the room when these children are being taught, since almost none of the children are able to work alone, and they end up vying for my attention. When one child is being settled, the others start acting up, and vice-versa. There is a tremendous difference in the quality of work that is supervised and work that is given to the child to complete by himself. If someone sits quietly but attentively by, a child may put forth a certain amount of effort, while if left alone he may destroy the paper, write on the desks, or simply daydream. Because these children require so much individual attention, each of them ends up receiving only a little bit of schooling. Some of them could tolerate no more than this meager amount, but others definitely could use more school time. The only solution to this would be to have more teachers in such a classroom.

Sometimes a child moves so slowly that his progress is not discernible except over a period of time. Some children make very little progress in school work. Grade placement as such is impossible. A teacher's knowledge of the norm in scholastic attainment is beneficial when a comparison is to be made between the level of a disturbed child and what he should accomplish at his age. By the time a child approaches what should be his normal achievement, he is usually ready to be discharged.

A child may be making steady progress and then, because of emotional disturbances, he may hit a plateau or regress. Such was the case with one boy who was promised by his parents that he would go home if he improved. The child worked diligently and was making progress in practically every area. The parents, who were in therapy, did not improve as fast as the boy did, and by the time he was ready, they decided they were not. The boy's regression was immediate, especially in his reading and writing. His writing reverted to a shaky, illegible scrawl, and finally he made very little attempt to do any school work. Another boy, once he became interested in school, began to make rapid progress in reading. When the doctor praised the boy for his efforts, the child was all smiles and full of enthusiasm about reading. I made the mistake of asking the boy if he would like to read for his mother that afternoon, to which he responded willingly. Upon hearing her son read, the mother froze and stared disbelievingly. Shortly after this episode, the boy's therapist completed his training and left the Institute. The child's interest in reading suddenly waned, and it has taken me two years to get him back to the level at which he originally read.

During the four years I have worked with emotionally disturbed children, four have gone on to public school. One of these had been in school before coming to the clinic, and one had had a certain amount of schooling at Sonoma State Hospital. Another was dropped from school a short time after she entered. The fourth child had never been to school before and from our clinic went to the third grade in a regular public school. He entered at the mid-term and was promoted to the fourth grade the next year. This is a child who had just begun to talk at about the age of eight years and was barely intelligible when I first started teaching on the ward. He now speaks very well when he wishes and has quite a sense of humor.

When a child is ready to go on to public school, conferences may be arranged between the school (teacher, principal, school psychologist) and our staff (which usually includes the teacher, the child's therapist, our psychologist, the social worker, and the child's nurse). Evaluation is made of the child's scholastic ability and how he would adjust emotionally to the new school. In some cases a summary letter to the interested school is all that is required. In any case, our staff is willing to meet with the school if necessary or when special problems arise. The child generally continues his therapy with the outpatient department.

There are several ways a child may fit into the public school program. Several of our patients were accepted into the regular classroom. Others have home teachers or may attend school for just an hour a day and gradually increase this until they are going to school full-time. Another possibility is for the child to enroll in an adjustment class in the public schools. These classes usually emphasize remedial work.

Some schools, especially in the larger cities, have what are called Point I and Point II programs. The Point II program is for mentally retarded children who are trainable but not teachable, and whose IQs are under fifty. The Point I program is for children with IQs from fifty to seventy-five, and it is usually set up so that half of the time is spent in learning crafts and the other part in learning academic subjects. In this program, children are at different levels within the same class, and it is set up so that children who make good progress may be placed back in the normal classroom. One of our patients may be enrolled shortly in the Point II program, even though it is felt that her IQ is average. There are, as far as I know, few special classes for emotionally disturbed children in the public schools. However, there are some school districts that are cognizant of the problem and are exploring the possibilities of adding such classrooms to their schools.

I have thoroughly enjoyed my work with emotionally disturbed children. They have both provoked and elated me, but no moment was ever a dull one. Once I was asked which child was my favorite, and to my utter surprise I could not single out one!

CHAPTER 15

THE OCCUPATIONAL THERAPY PROGRAM*

Marietta C. Eng, O.T.R., Maleta J. Boatman, M.D.,
Joanna Gewertz Harris, B.S., M.A.

EDITORS' NOTE, 1970

The material in this chapter was written originally with the hope that other clinicians, particularly rehabilitation therapists, would find it detailed enough to have practical application. We hoped it was also theoretical enough to clarify the kind of multidisciplinary psychotherapeutic milieu in which it had evolved and in which it might be useful. It was written between 1959 and 1960, at the point when the ward's official capacity was being decreased from fifteen to fourteen, and when children, although always admitted under age twelve, still sometimes stayed until age fourteen or fifteen.

---

*The material in this chapter was originally presented as two separate papers. They are combined here for the sake of completeness with minimal repetition. Parts One, Two, Four, and Five are reprinted from *American Journal of Occupational Therapy*, Proceedings of the 1960 Annual Conference of the American Occupational Therapy Association, 33-36, where they appeared as: "The Occupational Therapy Program on a Ward for Psychotic Children," Eng, Marietta C., O.T.R., and Maleta J. Boatman, M.D. As originally published, it contained a very short description, now omitted, of the use of Creative Rhythmic Movement, and made reference to an unpublished paper that had been read at the 1959 Annual Meeting of the American Orthopsychiatric Association: Eng, Marietta C., Joanna Gewertz, and Maleta J. Boatman, "A Creative Rhythmic Movement Group for Psychotic Children in a Psychotherapeutic Program." Part Three of this chapter substitutes the unpublished paper for the omitted brief description [1-6].

PART ONE: DEVELOPMENT OF OCCUPATIONAL
THERAPY ACTIVITIES

Each activity for the twelve to fourteen psychotic boys and girls hospitalized on the Children's Ward at the Langley Porter Neuropsychiatric Institute is considered to be an integral part of the psychotherapeutic program. Occupational therapy activities became a carefully planned part of this program four and a half years ago when, early in 1956, the Rehabilitation Services Department assigned one occupational therapist to work at least ten hours a week on the Children's Ward. Since that time, this therapist and the child psychiatrist administratively responsible for the ward (Dr. Boatman) have met regularly together. The therapist has also participated in all ward conferences and has conducted at least one forty-five-minute activity session daily. Three sessions in crafts, one in singing motion games, and one in creative rhythmic movement have been included. At times it has also been possible to include tumbling and folk dancing.[1]

Prior to four and a half years ago (1956), the rehabilitation therapy staff of three to five persons provided daily sessions in the occupational therapy department for some or all of the children. Activities planned were those suited to children in general, and a good deal of free play was allowed. This staff group received general background information about each child and consulted with the psychiatrists regarding critical problems. However, except for brief, informal exchanges with whichever nurses accompanied the children to the sessions, there was no time for regular two-way communication with the ward staff. Under this arrangement, the child psychiatrists and the rehabilitation department mutually recognized an increasingly urgent need for an occupational therapy program planned and carried out by someone who could work as an integral part of the ward staff.

The present occupational therapist started on the Children's Ward with more than average preparation for the work. There were, however, aspects of it which she found unusual or difficult, and it was some time before the program attained its present effectiveness. Since these factors helped to shape the program, and since some of them may be encountered by others in similar settings, it may be useful to describe them briefly.

---

[1] Three paragraphs describing the ward setting and patient population are omitted to avoid repetition in this volume. See Chapter 4 for this background material.

Problems of Staff Interaction

Being as experienced as she was, it was difficult to feel and to be
treated as the "novice" within an established staff group that already
had so much experience with these impulsive children. It was difficult
for her to exercise the prompt firmness needed to meet an occasional
aggressive outburst from a youngster, particularly when the attack came
in response to encouragement or praise. Working with so few patients,
with the opportunity to work more intensively and effectively if an
adequate staff-patient ratio could be set up, was a new experience for
the therapist. This, however, required having nurses present at all sessions,
which at first seemed strange and sometimes difficult. They brought with
them their knowledge and familiarity with individual children, but were
relatively unfamiliar with craft skills. They tended to concentrate on
their individual relationships with the children and sometimes doubted
that the occupational therapist's expectations for the children were
realistic. The occupational therapist, on the other hand, felt uneasy
about how much direction to offer the nurses when she felt they were
disinterested in an activity or were doing too much for a child. As she
became aware that these problems were largely the result of the nurses'
uncertainty about the craft materials and goals, she began to recognize
their need to learn. She and the senior ward staff developed ways for
her to orient new nurses, to discuss differences in approach after an occurrence, and to talk to the whole staff more often about her plans and
goals. Although the problems have not been entirely resolved, they are
greatly reduced. Perhaps the necessity for such definition and clarification
helped the therapist in her own formulation of goals and methods. It certainly influenced the procedure that evolved for the conduct of the various
sessions.

PART TWO: CRAFT ACTIVITIES

Background

At the time the occupational therapist began to develop the current
program, the children were accustomed to having considerable choice
as to free play or participation in the planned craft. As few as two nurses
would bring six or seven of the children to the occupational therapy department, where several occupational therapists and a student would be
preparing materials for their arrival. When the group of children entered
the department, it immediately became as disorganized as though a big
wind had blown in and scattered a stack of papers. Alice would head

directly for the corner cabinet where the nylon stockings were kept and pull them out to slip on her legs. Billy would go to the window to look out. Robin would find a magazine from the rack and frantically leaf through it. Frances would be at the sink pulling paper cups from the dispenser, one after the other, filling each with water and drinking it.

Out of this chaos it was practically impossible to marshal all the children to one table to settle on one activity. So much time and energy were spent urging and helping them to put away what was pulled out that there was little time left for the proposed craft. The rehabilitation staff was also uninformed about the children's current moods, and the nurses were unprepared for the activity.

Procedure

As the occupational therapist became more familiar with the youngsters, she divided them into two groups, according to ability and interest rather than age. Each group came twice a week after breakfast for a forty-five-minute craft period. For various reasons it was gradually possible for more nurses to come with the children. The occupational therapist's daily participation in ward conferences made it possible for her and the nurses to keep abreast of plans and problems.

Also under the new plan, the occupational therapist swiftly moved in with the sample of a planned project, demonstrating it as a salesman would do, to attract the children's attention and to distract them from going their separate ways. The materials for the first step would be ready on the table so that the children's automatic handling of them would be entirely appropriate. A staff member would help each child get started. She was there to guide him step by step, giving explicit instructions such as "Saw on the red line." Sometimes the adult actually did a step with the child to help him overcome some initial resistance to trying it. For example, the nurse might hold the child's hand on the saw handle as she helped him actually experience how it felt to push and pull with long strokes. Materials for succeeding steps would be close at hand to make it easy to direct the child to them. The child was prepared for the approaching end of the session by being asked, or helped, to mark his name on his project and to assist in the cleanup. If the child had completed the project, and if he had reached the point of being able to enjoy what he had made, he would take it with him as the group returned to the ward.

Goals and Methods

It was in the setting described above that the following goals and methods were developed for the craft program.

1. Crafts are used to offer each child the opportunity to experience and explore a large variety of materials. There can be therapeutically needed sensory gratification in *feeling* sand trickle through the fingers, *seeing* the color and shape of crayon strokes on paper, *hearing* the whirring sound of machinery when the electric switch is turned on, *smelling* peppermint-scented paste, and *tasting* the flavor of gummed stars when licked with the tongue.
2. The motions involved in crafts provide a physical outlet whereby the energy behind aggressive and destructive emotions may be channeled into constructive uses. Examples are: pounding with a hammer on the resistive surface of wood or metal, and using the whole body to push and pull a hand saw.
3. It is hoped that the sessions will help the child learn the fun of working with another human being. Having an adult with each child provides someone attentive and interested to help hurdle a task that is new and strange, to cushion failure and help make repairs, to be a witness to achievement, and to help the child accept success.
4. The variety of craft materials and tools is used to help the children learn the names of objects and their purposes and proper use.
5. The regularly scheduled sessions and their planned pattern offer the children the security of meaningful routine and help them develop a sense of the use of time.
6. It is hoped that the child will gain some sense of self through creating an object of his own making, labeling it with his own name, and having it to hold on to or to do with as he wishes.
7. Crafts are chosen with an eye to stimulating interest and providing pleasure.
8. It is hoped that the satisfaction of constructing things time and time again may build up happy memories so that such endeavors in the future may be met with eager or willing acceptance rather than with inhibiting fear.

Planning

In order to achieve the foregoing goals it is essential that the planning for each session be adequate and precise. In addition to the time allowed prior to each session for organizing and arranging materials in the work areas, at least half an hour weekly is set aside for advance planning of the whole week's craft sessions. This planning is often done with occupational therapy students and, recently, with a few of the nurses. The following considerations are included in regard to each project suggested:

1. If there is to be a sample to show the children, will it have eye appeal in appearance, color, texture, and movement? If there is no sample, does the verbal description stir up interest through some previous association or remembered performance?
2. If there is a design involved, is it meaningful to the child?
3. Is there enough variation in the working processes to avoid boredom for those unable to retain long interest in one activity?
4. What physical motions are involved, and what degree of coordination and manual dexterity is required? Are they familiar or new ones?
5. How much previous learning of craft skills is required?
6. What kind and what volume of sound would be created? Is it soothing and rhythmical or loud, unexpected, and irritating?
7. What other types of sensory stimulation are offered by the processes or project—olfactory, kinesthetic, or what?
8. Are the dimensions of the pieces of workable size?
9. What is the approximate time necessary for completion of the project? If too long for one session, what procedures can be eliminated or what materials can be substituted to hasten the completion? If too short, what can be done for the remainder of the session? If it is to be a two-day project, can the children maintain interest the second day?
10. What would be the staff ratio needed to supervise the children in this activity?
11. How much briefing must be given to the nurses; what, when, and how should it be said; what should not be said in front of the children; and will time other than that during the session be necessary to communicate the information?
12. What are plans for the finished product? What should the staff response be if the child refuses or ignores it; if he wishes to take it home, to leave it on the ward or for occupational therapy display; or if he wants to give it as a gift? Should the decision be on his own initiative or from staff suggestion?
13. Is the finished article safe for handling by children? Is it free of jagged edges and loose or sharp parts? Is it toxic if taken internally? Will it stain clothing?
14. Would the cost of any needed material for the project be too great, and if so, can something be substituted for it?

An example of this type of project is the making of a wooden marionette. This attractive toy, familiar to the children, is simple to construct, and bounces with a springy motion and an interesting clatter.

Other Activities

Although crafts have continued to make up the major portion of the occupational therapy program, two other activities have also been included as part of the regular program. Each is an activity that can be held on the ward, requires slightly less staff, and can include all the children who are present and interested.

PART THREE: CREATIVE RHYTHMIC MOVEMENT

Rhythm music and movement activities have been held on the ward frequently since its inception in 1944. A rhythm instrument group has been a regular part of the occupational therapist's program since 1956. Creative rhythmic movement as described in this paper has been utilized since 1958. Some of the methods derive from established dance skills but are used in a less formal, less structured approach to the movement idiom that is flexibly adaptable to the needs of each child.

Described here will be the history of and the procedures, clinical observations, and conclusions derived from the first five months' experience with weekly creative rhythmic movement sessions in 1958.

Background

The three authors involved in the work described here were the occupational therapist assigned part-time to the ward, a volunteer dance teacher, and the child psychiatrist directly in charge of the ward. The psychiatrist felt, from her ten years on the ward, that planned rhythmic activity had potentialities of being very therapeutic for many psychotic children. If skillfully and sensitively carried out by the staff, it seemed likely to provide opportunities for: (a) needed "regressive" sensual gratification; (b) discrimination of this from the glee of sadomasochistic fear and hostility; and (c) the more integrated but basic satisfactions of learning bodily skills.

Rhythm activities of some type had usually been part of the program. For two years prior to the inception of the creative rhythmic movement group, the occupational therapist conducted a weekly rhythm group with the help of the nurses. She had seen how frequently inhibition of coordinated motor activity was part of the children's symptomatic expression of their emotional difficulties. This included such varied signs as rigid posture, limp passivity, ungainly or airy random movements, rhythmic rocking, and explosive pounding. She had also seen indications that total involvement of the body in planned rhythmic motion offered opportunity for rechanneling such behavior in a way that contributed to relaxation and satisfaction. However, she began to feel the need for assistance from someone who could offer a wider and more varied content to this activity, and who could better help the participating nursing staff gain a clearer understanding of and greater confidence in the use of movement skills.

Coincidentally, an experienced dance teacher was seeking opportunity to explore in what ways her skills could be of use in a psychotherapeutic program with psychiatric patients. In eight years' experience with normal children, she had noted that the dance medium offered them a vehicle for becoming kinesthetically aware of themselves and for improvement in body tone and coordination. She hoped it might benefit psychotic children similarly.

It was felt that with her skill, her personality, and her genuine interest in working closely with the staff, she could contribute to the ongoing program. In January 1958, she joined the occupational therapist in planning the weekly creative rhythmic movement sessions. For the next five months she led the group.

Procedures

In developing the procedure for the Creative Rhythmic Movement Group, the occupational therapist and the dance teacher pooled their own and others' [7-19] past experience and combined and modified techniques as they proceeded. Although adaptation of method to individual needs was a major part of the procedure, it will be described later as part of the clinical observations.

The ward group consisted of ten girls and five boys, aged four to twelve. Many were mute. Most tended to be preoccupied and isolated. A few could not tolerate even such physical closeness as a friendly hand on the shoulder. During physical activity, there were frequent impulsive or aggressive acts such as wild hugs or purposeful body collisions. There was frequent symptomatic behavior such as rocking, saliva play, masturbation, and tense shrieks of excitement or unhappiness.

Each Wednesday morning at 8:45 A.M. the dance leader and the occupational therapist with her two students would enter the large ward playroom to begin the thirty-minute activity. The children and four or so of the nursing staff were waiting. Some would help move chairs and toys against the wall. The phonograph was set up, and all would be ready.

Most sessions fell into five sections: (a) Lead-in; (b) Exercise and Body Awareness; (c) Introduction of New Material; (d) Individual Performance; and (e) Group Skills. These were sometimes presented in a different order or combined, but always proceeded without interruption since movement, rhythmic or music transitions were used. After the initial greeting of each child by the leader, the adults joined hands with the children in a circle. This was facilitated by familiar marches or other four-four time music of a simple folk dance nature.

The Lead-in activity usually consisted of a march in circle formation with the leader expressively offering such instruction as: "Now go the other way," "Walk with your body as tall as it can be," or "Walk with your body bending low." "Slow and Fast" walks were geared to suitable recorded music, or the leader's drum provided stimulus for the rhythmic change. All verbal direction was accompanied by simultaneous demonstration and, as needed, by an encouraging hand.

If the second section was the Introduction to New Material, such as a new record, a new pattern, or a new motor skill, the music that accompanied it was introduced during the Lead-in period, or some previous experience was drawn on as a springboard. The material offered consisted of basic locomotion organized in simple patterns, using folk dance music. Some sliding, marching, and hopping dances were adaptable for use. Examples are: "Seven Steps," "Carousel," and "Crested Hen." Their simple melodic lines had the useful qualities of strong beats, little syncopation, and consistent repetition. They had to be rechoreographed, however, to use simpler spatial patterns and formation and less complex skills.

Sometimes the second section was an Exercise and Body Awareness period. The group would then remain in the circle, either standing or sitting on the floor. Simple bends and stretches utilizing torso, head, feet, and arms would be directed. For example, the words "Yes" and "No"—and the corresponding head and torso movement that accompany them—formed the basis for one exercise.

A sitting period was included in each session, and was often used to initiate the fourth or Individual Performance section. Each child was encouraged to perform a skill (such as a jump, bend, or hop) in the center of the circle. The leader assisted the child with this unless he started it without too much hesitation.

The whole group resumed activity for the fifth section, that of Group Skills. Transition was often made by trying a movement initiated by an individual in the preceding section. Group participation at this point seldom took the form of full unison performance, but rather that of active locomotor patterns (hops, skips, runs) in groups of two or three. The small groups might work face to face, hands joined, or in a side-by-side position in threes, the leader or other adult holding each of two children around the waist. It was possible to follow more complex activity in these small, close formations.

Depending on the skills used in the other parts of the session, the concluding group participation would be either quiet movement or an active structured activity. Thus swings and sways in various directions or a simplified "Virginia Reel" might be used. A single line marching around the room might become a train making a journey up and down a mountain. Essentially the conclusion was aimed at being unified, pleasant, and leading to a feeling of achievement.

Modifications of Method

The foregoing method varied from that used with normal children primarily in timing and emphasis. The Lead-in period was made more stimulating, and the pace of presentation was much slower. Constant simplification and repetition were needed. Imaginative play in response to verbally presented images such as "Move like an elephant," so immediate to normal children, brought little response in these sessions. Movement skills were presented very objectively, therefore. Demonstration, music stimulation, and verbal and physical direction were the methods employed.

After each session the rhythm staff group met to exchange ideas and observations. The occupational therapist answered questions about the children's behavior in terms of probable reasons for it. The dance volunteer explained her presentation of material. An evaluation was made of what had been successful, what should be improved or deleted, and what needed a follow-up to test its true value. Clinical observations of individual children were later reported and discussed with the rest of the staff at ward conferences.

Observations and Impressions

The authors concurred that the experience of these five months confirmed their prior impressions of the value of planned rhythm activity for these children. Although no child showed major generalized improvement from this activity alone, a few gave evidence of its contribution to their progressively more integrated behavior. In addition, each child showed that most of the sessions afforded him some of the kinds of experience that this staff considers therapeutic. That is, within the sessions, each child repetitively experienced reduction in fearfulness, resolution of specific moments of conflict, and periods of increasing pleasure in his own activity and in relating to others. The clinical observations that follow illustrate and elaborate these points more fully.

Pleasure in use of body. Vera, age eleven, was a petite, pretty child who showed little expression and was practically mute. Isolated play, such as smearing saliva on her favorite toy, was frequent. Although initially she would allow herself to be led into the circle, she would soon leave. When, with apparent indifference, she began to stand with the group during stretching exercises, the adult at her side would lift her arms and guide her through the motions. Giggles of pleasure, rarely heard in other situations, became frequent. Gradually she began to follow the verbal instructions and to sustain attention on the movements for longer periods. At the end of the five months she still awaited a personal invitation to join the group, but often came without being led, and stayed throughout the sessions. Her reduced inhibition and increasing pleasure showed in her more alert facial expression, quickly hidden smiles, and more prolonged and skillful participation.

Vera was one of the many children for whom the rhythm group provided opportunity to experience a pleasurable rather than anxiety-provoking activity requiring some sustained attention and following of directions. This example also gives some indication that the rhythm sessions did result in tension release and improvement in body tone and coordination. This was often quite apparent as tight grasps relaxed, range of joint motion increased, and ability to follow the movement patterns appeared. Smiles and giggles were frequent signs of pleasure.

Social interaction. Increased social interaction was also apparent in the responsiveness of each child to particular adults. The activity also provided an unusually effective means of achieving parallel action and some degree of mutuality among the youngsters:

Alice was an obese, ungainly twelve-year-old whose frightened, distorted yearning for affection was apparent in her jealous and demanding behavior. Her parents, themselves emotionally deprived and unusually "helpless," constantly compared her unfavorably with her younger siblings. On the ward, she had frequent anguished temper tantrums and resisted most activity by stubbornly refusing to move or by gleefully disrupting an activity by precise clumsiness. Her assigned nurse attended the rhythm sessions, offering her gentle but firm encouragement. Alice found that her lack of willing participation in this activity did not lead either to her exclusion or to her forced participation. When, in the moving circle, she sat down unbudging on the floor, staff hands closed the gap and the group calmly moved on. If she did not respond to invitations to rejoin the group, she soon found herself again in place as the sitting period was initiated. Although, in the five months she did not reach the point where she felt it safe to show her interest or ability very openly, she did come with her nurse more readily and began to follow the group more closely. She less often leaned her weight gleefully on others, and would surreptitiously make the appropriate movements for the exercises.

Conflict reduction. The rhythm group did offer many children the kinds of experience that could be most precisely helpful to them in their resolution of internalized conflict. Its multi-faceted and flexibly adaptable form made it possible for the staff to offer each child opportunity for that kind, or combination of kinds, of experience that he most needed. The rhythmic nature of the action utilized as a starting point the twirling, swaying movements already familiar to them as a frequent form of expression of distorted sensual feelings, of conflict tensions and their compromise solutions. Even the child who rocked on the sidelines gained some sense of beginning participation. He could later join the group with less fear, and his subsequent experience tended actually to reduce fear and lead to pleasure:

Because of Lennie's persistent violent thumb-sucking in the first year of life, his anxious parents had, for eighteen months, followed a pediatrician's advice to splint his arms. In the period that followed, he had remained mute and expressionless except for resistance of others' expectations through violent tantrums. When admitted to the ward at age four he had been fearful of all physical contact and reluctant to use his hands except in autistic play with saliva-wet string.

At the time the creative rhythmic movement group was started, Lennie, then nine, was still learning to discriminate between trying something for his own pleasure and being made to do something *for* someone else. When asked to join hands in a circle, he would now willingly hold those of other children. But, with frightened defiance, he still often refused the hand of an adult unless he himself had extended his own first. The staff utilized the frequent opportunities the circle formation provided to allow him to make his decision according to his readiness. If he did not initiate the contact, an encouraging hand was proferred. If he refused it, the circle was allowed to move with a temporary gap, or positions were shifted so that he stood next to a child whose hand he might take. As the weeks passed, and as his fear that he was giving in to adult force or expectation slowly gave way to spontaneous pleasure in the activity, he participated more.

Closeness facilitated. The following example shows even more clearly the ways in which inhibited and distorted forms of expression of frightened yearning for emotional and bodily closeness could be appropriately incorporated into this activity. It also illustrates the way in which the rhythm group facilitated prompt, nonretaliative adult behavior that could help a child discriminate between anxiously hostile or sexually aggressive action and that which could actually lead to sensual gratification and learning:

George was a handsome, slender, nine-year-old Negro boy, who showed his tension and despair through taunting, sly, seductive gestures toward adults' breasts, and through harsh, unhappy laughter that sometimes gave way to asthmatic wheezing with spitting and smearing of saliva. These symptoms were most severe when his parents visited irregularly during periods of exacerbation in the mother's sexually tinged paranoid delusions. George seemed to seek and need much physical contact and personal warmth, but his conflictful distortions about closeness were clearly conveyed in the frequence of the anxious sensual and hostile behavior. The rhythm group offered opportunities for the bodily contact that both the staff and he felt at ease with, because the focus was on the activity and the position was impersonal. If his pleasure shifted to anxious sexual excitement or hostile glee, this contact could be promptly terminated by the adult without censuring or leaving him. It was seldom necessary, however, to make such behavioral discriminations for him. He also enjoyed the opportunity to demonstrate his considerable grace of movement and rhythmic ability in individual performance of newly learned motor skills or of original steps and shuffles. As the group supported him by praise and hand-clapping accompaniment, his smiles were those of genuine pleasure rather than of mixed fright and taunting glee.

Satisfactions of mastery. Similarly, with other children, it was found that the rhythm-group experience facilitated conflict-reduction and afforded effective opportunities for more integrated behavior. In simultaneously reducing fears and offering learning possibilities, the rhythm group resulted in the increased confidence that made greater socialization and mastery of skills possible. This was most strikingly apparent with Nancy, the slender but sturdy twelve-year-old who was the star pupil of the group. On admission to the ward two and one-half years before, she had been an extremely fearful child who shrank from people and activity. She had appeared deceptively frail and her parents were over-anxiously preoccupied with concern for her health. Although her major improvement was clearly related to progress made in psychotherapy, some of her most integrated behavior on the ward appeared first in the rhythm groups. She had gradually been able to master motor skills and had finally become eager and enthusiastic about rhythm activities. In the new creative rhythmic movement group she participated fully and with pleasure, showed confidence, learned rapidly, and soon developed ability to lead.

The foregoing observations are not meant to indicate that every session of the creative rhythmic movement group proceeded smoothly. At times the group seemed unusually disturbed from tensions arising

228

before the activity started. Interest and participation was then difficult
to elicit. At other times the staff was unable to anticipate or understand
a child's reaction in a given situation promptly enough to avert or resolve
his mounting anxiety before an outburst occurred or he became noisy
and violent enough to disturb the group. The authors hope, however,
that the foregoing brief observations have illustrated the clinical bases
for the following conclusions.

Conclusions

Creative rhythmic movement—with its integration of auditory, visual,
tactile, and kinesthetic experience—seems particularly suited to affording
psychotic children opportunity for experiencing an activity as pleasurable
rather than as anxiety-provoking. The child's previously isolated and iso-
lating behavior can be utilized as the starting point for interaction in
which the sensitively participating adult may help him rechannel his behavior in a way that contributes to reduction of his fearfulness. The
subsequent relaxation and pleasure contribute to the increased confidence
that makes socialization and learning possible. In other words, the flexibly
adaptable form of the rhythm group makes it possible for the child to
experience whatever combination he may need of sensual gratification,
of discrimination of this from sadomasochistic behavior, and of the satisfaction that comes with learning and mastery of skills.

It may be of interest to mention briefly some of the other aspects of
the form of the activity as described here which proved to be of particular
value. The fact that adult participation was that of "doing with" the
children rather than remaining peripheral to the group seemed to facilitate
the ease of absorption of new or shifting personnel. This is in contrast to
many activities where the lack of total staff continuity or the presence of
a stranger often proves disruptive.

All the staff gained increased skill and confidence in using the movement medium from their work with the dance teacher. The nursing staff
developed an even more positive attitude toward the potentialities of the
activity, and some drew upon the experience in their work with the children on other occasions.

The occupational therapist found of particular value the arrangement
by which, after joint planning, another person carried the leadership in
the sessions. This freed her to be even more observant of the individual
children, both in providing for their special needs in a given session and
in gaining understanding of their reactions.

The dance volunteer's close collaboration with the therapeutically
oriented staff who knew the children made it possible for her to understand

the needs of the situation more quickly and to draw more valid conclusions than would otherwise have been possible.

This activity seems to be one in which staff persons from different disciplines can easily participate together, share each other's knowledge for the benefit of the children, and make pertinent clinical observations. Discussion of such experiences can be of help to the whole staff in following the needs and progress of individual youngsters and in learning more about the dynamics of, and effective therapeutic methods with, psychotic children.

In summary, it may be said that the five months' experience with a creative rhythmic movement group led to the conclusion that this activity can offer valuable contributions to the total treatment program for psychotic children if it is well-organized, well-directed, and carefully integrated with other aspects of the work. Although the volunteer dance teacher is no longer part of this staff group, the activity has been continued in a similar form as part of the treatment program on this ward.

PART FOUR: SINGING-MOTION GAMES

The third activity, singing-motion games, was started in 1958 to substitute for one craft session. The nature of the activity will not be described in detail since everyone is familiar with the use of illustrative hand and arm motions to accompany the words of songs. The activity was selected for regular use in this program because, on trial attempts, the children responded to it with more than average interest. Most of them were willing to join the informal seating arrangement in a circle. Many of them showed pleasure at hearing and seeing the leader's expressive words and amusing actions to such songs as "Eensy Weensy Spider" and "Hickory Dickory Dock."

The activity is carried out on the ward, so that less staff is needed, and the children can move in and out of the group more freely. Spontaneous singing without accompaniment is used so that the leader can watch the children more carefully and respond quickly to any sound or motion from one of them that would indicate a wish for repetition or for choice of a song. The informality allows the children to participate as much or little as they are ready for without disrupting the activity. The motion phase allows silent children to take part without feeling coerced into singing. It offers pleasurable sensory stimulation, encouragement of recognition and appropriate use of parts of their bodies, and interesting practice in motor coordination. The following clinical vignette illustrates the value of this activity:

Bessie was invited to join the group, but usually stood about in the ward hallway. She was often led to sit in the circle, but when no one could give her undivided attention, she made tense, flying leaps in the air, knocking over her chair. Sessions later, when invited again, she seemed less hyperactive and more integrated, sitting very still, watching what the group was doing. Gradually she decided to join in, partially hiding what she was doing by turning her body sideways and appearing to make only inadvertently a motion the group was making. For instance, using the right hand to scratch the eczema on her left arm, she too casually slid that hand under the left elbow, closely approximating the "Hickory Dickory Dock" motion the group was doing. At subsequent sessions when she was ready to participate more openly, she watched the occupational therapist's motions intently. Very precisely she matched her fingers to the occupational therapist's to form a diamond shape, or, in standing games, would inch her feet together until they were evenly spaced, and satisfied with these adjustments, was ready to stamp her feet for a marching song. Preliminary to undertaking a new motion she seemed to measure off space with her hands as a test, carefully exploring a few cubic feet of air in front of her, then tentatively but bravely waving two hands in unison. Later she was able to make more definite and wider swoops in the air and try a wider range of motions. Finally, in addition to joining in on the motions, she began humming, softly at first, then louder, and gradually mouthing and making sounds close to the words of the song we were singing.

PART FIVE: CONCLUSION

In summary, all aspects of the program described above have been developed to offer each individual child an opportunity to learn to experience an activity as pleasurable rather than as anxiety-provoking. The sensory experiences that are so much a part of each activity seem specifically suited to the needs of these isolated and fearful children, particularly if sensitively carried out by a participating adult. When there is reduction in fearfulness, the child's subsequent relaxation and pleasure make it possible for him to begin to learn. Each activity is carefully planned but adaptable so that there are learning opportunities for each child at whatever level is timely for him.

The occupational therapist's overall impression is that the development of the program in the past four and a half years, as described here, has offered her the same kind of learning opportunities, meaningful relationships, and sense of accomplishment that she and the ward staff have attempted to offer the children.

Although it is hoped that it will be possible in the not-too-distant future to include more occupational therapy activities, the entire Children's Ward staff feels that the occupational therapy program is now an important and valuable part of the psychotherapeutic program for most children on the ward.

* * * * *

ADDENDUM, 1970

Shortly after the original papers in this chapter were written in 1960, the Rehabilitation Therapies Department was able to assign the occupational therapist's position to the Children's Ward four-fifths time instead of the ten hours per week described here. The occupational therapist was then able to take a greater part in planning and collaborating in carrying out the milieu program as a whole. In particular, she was able to expand the use of cooking activities for all the children (see Chapter 17).

REFERENCES

1. SZUREK, S. A. Dynamics of staff interaction in hospital psychiatric treatment of children. *Am. J. Orthopsychiat.,* **17**:652-664, 1947.
2. ———. The family and the staff in hospital psychiatric therapy of children. *Am. J. Orthopsychiat.,* **21**:597-611, 1951.
3. ———. Some lessons from efforts at psychotherapy with parents. *Am. J. Psychiat.,* **109**:(4), 296-301, 1952. Reprinted in S. A. Szurek & I. N. Berlin (Eds.), *Training in therapeutic work with children.* Vol. 2, the Langley Porter Child Psychiatry Series. Palo Alto, Calif.: Science and Behavior Books, 1967.
4. SZUREK, S. A., and BERLIN, I. N. Elements of psychotherapeutics with the schizophrenic child and his parents. *Psychiatry,* **19**:(1-9), 1956. Reprinted in S. A. Szurek & I. N. Berlin (Eds.), *Training in therapeutic work with children.* Vol. 2, the Langley Porter Child Psychiatry Series. Palo Alto, Calif.: Science and Behavior Books, 1967.
5. SZUREK, S. A. Childhood schizophrenia: psychotic episodes and psychotic maldevelopment. *Am. J. Orthopsychiat.,* **26**:519-543, 1956.
6. BOATMAN, MALETA J., and SZUREK, S. A. A clinical study of childhood schizophrenia. In Don D. Jackson (Ed.), *The etiology of schizophrenia.* New York: Basic Books, Inc., 1960, Chap. 14, pp. 389-440.

232

7. ANDREWS, GLADYS. *Creative rhythmic movement for children.* Englewood Cliffs, N. J.: Prentice-Hall, Inc., 1954.*

8. BENDER, LAURETTA, and BOAS, FRANZISKA. Creative dance in therapy. *Am. J. Orthopsychiat.,* 2:235-244, April, 1941.

9. BOAS, FRANZISKA. Psychological aspects in the practice and teaching of creative dance. *J. Aesthetics Art Crit.,* 2(7), 3-20, 1943.

10. CAMPBELL, DOUGLAS. Your actions speak so loudly. *Impulse,* 1954.

11. CHASE, MARIAN. Dance as an adjunctive therapy with hospitalized mental patients. *Bull. Menninger Clinic,* 17:219-225, Nov., 1953.

12. _____ . Dance therapy at St. Elizabeth's. *Psychiatric Aide,* Sept., 1951.

13. _____ . Opening doors thru dance. *J. Am. Assoc. for Health, Physical Education, and Recreation,* March, 1952.

14. GENTHER, SHIRLEY. A place to begin. *Impulse,* 1954.

15. LABAN, RUDOLF. The educational and therapeutic value of the dance. In Walter Sorrel (Ed.), *The dance has many faces.* New York: World, 1951.

16. MARTIN, DONALD W., and BEAVER, NOHMIE. A preliminary report on the use of the dance as an adjuvant in therapy of schizophrenia. *Psychiat. Quart. Supplement,* 25:176-190, Part 2, 1951.

17. MAY, ROWENA. Modern dance as therapy for the mentally ill. *Occupat. Therapy and Rehab.,* 10, April, 1941.

18. ROSEN, ELIZABETH. *Dance in psychotherapy.* New York: Bureau of Publications, Teachers College, Columbia University, 1957.

19. WATERMAN, ELIZABETH. *The rhythm book.* New York: A. S. Barnes and Co., 1936.

---

*References 7-19 did not appear in the original article but in the paper that now runs as Part Three of this chapter.

CHAPTER 16

THE INTEGRATION OF ACTIVITIES ON A CHILDREN'S WARD*

Maleta J. Boatman, M.D., Jane Paynter, R.N.,
Berta Mejia, R.N., Esther Milnes, M.A.

EDITORS' NOTE, 1970

This previously unpublished paper was prepared for and presented at a Workshop on Psychiatric Nursing at the Annual Meeting of the American Orthopsychiatric Association in March, 1962, with the title "The Nurse in an Integrated Activity Program for Hospitalized Psychotic Children." Despite the specific emphasis on nursing personnel, it is included here in Section Five rather than Section Four because its general theme is the interdisciplinary effort to create a psychotherapeutically oriented milieu.

The authors wish to acknowledge the contributions of the other staff members of the Children's Service to the work described, and to thank in particular for their help in preparing this report the following: Matha Black, R.N., formerly Senior Psychiatric Nurse; Marietta C. Eng. O.T.R.; and Mary Kelly Seymore, M.A., formerly Speech Correction Teacher.

Since 1946 one of the major efforts of the Children's Service of the Langley Porter Neuropsychiatric Institute in San Francisco, California, has been the development of a psychotherapeutic program for psychotic children and their families [1-8, 10-15]. A central part of this effort has

---
*This work was partially supported by the National Institute of Mental Health Project Grant No. 5-R11-MH-234-3, entitled, "Nursing in Hospital Psychiatric Therapy for Psychotic Children."

been to develop an inpatient program on the twelve-to-fifteen-bed Children's Ward[1] that would permit and if possible enhance the psychotherapists' work with even the most severely disturbed of such children and their families [2-6, 8, 13, 15].

The ward staff's early endeavor to do the best they could with what personnel had been provided by the State Department of Mental Hygiene eventually evolved into an effort to achieve and to test a particular method of using nursing personnel as an integral part of almost every aspect of each child's hospital program. The nurses thus became the persons whose constant presence and participation were major factors in integrating into a unified program the activities planned not only by themselves but also by the various professional disciplines. This method and five years' experience with its development since 1957 form the subject of this paper.

Even prior to the period described in this paper, one or more of the nurses had always accompanied the children to school and occupational therapy. They had in fact, in the first year of the ward, tried to provide school, craft, and other activities without any specialized help. Other important aspects of the current program had also already developed. Each child was assigned to one or more particular nurses for special attention and care. The children were frequently divided into groups according to age, ability, and interests, for special outings or activities and for specific parts of the school program. Some of the nurses and the teacher assigned full time by the city's school district participated with the psychiatrists, psychologist, and social worker in almost daily clinical staff meetings and weekly treatment reviews.

PARTICIPATION OF ALL DISCIPLINES

This participation in all clinical conferences by each staff member whose time permitted reflects a certain concept about inpatient therapy that may well be basic to the program that has gradually evolved. From the very beginning in 1946, the Director of the Children's Service, Dr. S. A. Szurek, had encouraged *each* staff member to view his clinical goal with child patients as two-faceted: to behave at all times in the precise manner that might, first, help the child to reduce his disorder (that is, his internalized conflict), however it manifested itself at a given moment or in a given activity; and that might, second, provide opportunities for the development of more integrated behavior at whatever level was timely for the child's own particular maturational and emotional capacities [9-11].

[1] For a description of the ward, its general program, and its staff, see Chapter 4. The details are omitted here to avoid repetition.

In other words, every moment of staff-child interaction was considered
to be potentially therapeutic; the specific skills of each discipline were
considered important in providing multiple learning opportunities for
the child; no staff member's observations and experiences were considered
more or less important than another's in gaining as full an understanding
of the child as possible; and, since the primary goal of each discipline was
the common therapeutic task, adequate achievement of the specific goals
of each was considered vital to the work of all the others. Within this
concept it becomes increasingly clear that each staff member contributes
most to the mutual therapeutic goal by maintaining a focus on developing
and performing the specific functions of his own discipline regardless of
the situation or activity in which he may find himself with the child or
with other staff members.

CONTRIBUTIONS OF NURSE TO ASPECTS OF PROGRAM[2]

It had always been clear that one of the nurses' particular contributions
with seriously disturbed children lay in helping them learn in the daily activities necessary to living, such as rising, bathing, dressing, toileting, playing, eating, going to bed, and sleeping. It had not seemed so clear that the
nursing concept of "total patient care" inevitably extended into activities
that were in the provinces of the teacher or the rehabilitation therapists.

However, as the proportion of psychotic children on the ward gradually increased until it was nearly 100 percent, the teacher and the occupational therapists found themselves less and less able to provide adequate programs for more than a few children at a time. They needed and
wanted assistance, but felt self-conscious and hampered by the presence
of more than one or two nurses. Conversely the nurses did not see their
job as one of "helper," and tended to question the time such assignments
took away from their "own" work. They felt that their own professional
identification was threatened. Had the staff been able to, they might well
have hired more activity specialists at that point. Since this was impossible,
several other things were tried instead.

One of the Institute's occupational therapists was assigned to work at
least ten hours a week with the Children's Ward and to plan and direct
all rehabilitation therapy activities for them. She joined the clinical conferences help on the ward, decided with the nurses which children would
come to any given activity in the occupational therapy shop, and planned

---

[2] For a more detailed account of each step by which the staff arrived at
the current program, see Chapter 11.

several recreational activities, such as a rhythm dance group, that could be carried out on the ward. She began to notice that the children whose participation and skill progressed most tended to be those whose assigned nurses most frequently accompanied the group to activities.

The psychiatric trainees began to care for the children one hour a week so that the whole ward staff could meet together. The psychiatrist with most immediate clinical responsibility for the inpatient program began to have regular individual conferences with the occupational therapist and with the teacher, in addition to her regular meetings with the charge nurse. A weekly administrative planning meeting for these four people was instituted.

The Nurse in the School Program

One of the first decisions made in this planning meeting was to see what would happen if two summer medical student externs came to school daily with the same three children for a reading class. Willing to give the medical students this experience but fearful of the consequences of their inexperience both with child psychiatry and with education, the teacher was amazed and gratified to find that the three children progressed more in these three summer months than they had in the whole preceding year.

Encouraged by these observations, the charge nurse began to send the nurses assigned to the most disturbed children with them to all activities as consistently as possible. One very self-hurtful and aggressive child who, during six years of hospitalization had been able to participate only minimally in those group activities that were held on the ward or on outings, began to tolerate some hour-long sessions in the school room and occupational therapy woodshop if her nurse were present. Her progress was very slow, but within a year her most satisfying hours were those spent in school, and she had begun to write and draw as well as to offer appropriate verbal responses to the lessons.

ACTIVITY PLANNING AND SUPERVISION

For a detailed account of the sequences by which the staff arrived at the current program, see Chapter 11. Two major steps need mention here, however. The advent of post-master's nursing students and project nurses made it possible for the first time to allow a few nurses to spend four to five hours daily with their own assigned children, Monday through Friday. Each of these was able to use her close relationship with her child and her intimate knowledge of him to facilitate his utilization of the learning opportunities and activities provided. She was also able to help him use what he was learning in O.T. and school in other situations throughout the day.

The major step in the program came through adversity. Major reconstruction was planned for the ward, and it proved impossible to arrange it to fit the ward's needs. In San Francisco's wettest, coldest season, the heat was turned off. The workmen arrived to do this the day the children returned from a week at home planned to accommodate it. It took longer than planned, and each step proved relatively unpredictable. Past experience with such construction had led the staff to discuss ahead of time how they would manage these weeks should they turn out adversely. Parents had been asked to take children home more consistently on weekends. Staff who had previously been reluctant, seen no need, or been given little opportunity to participate in activity planning began to be quite creative in thinking of things to do with a group of children contained in one room, and in finding places in the community where outings could be held. They planned carefully and closely with the teacher, occupational therapist, and project nurses. By the end of reconstruction, everyone was convinced that activity planning was desirable for the therapeutic work and that they were capable of participating in it. The psychiatrists had seen the results of utilizing more staff on the weekdays, and continued to explain its advantages to parents so that they could plan more carefully for children's weekend and overnight visits.

As a result of all these experiences, the current activity and staffing pattern was instituted. For activities, the children are divided into three groups according to age, interests, and capabilities. For each group the mornings are divided between school, recess, occupational therapy, and lunch. Each group has a weekly afternoon educational play period with the teacher and a cooking session with the occupational therapist. The groups take turns at the Wednesday outing when the ward has the use of the Institute's station wagon. Daily nap-time, weekly swimming, and rhythm dancing are total ward activities. As nearly as possible, there is one nursing staff person available to attend all activities with each child. For the most part, the psychiatrists have been able to schedule each child's playroom appointments (three to five per week) and the weekly meeting with the child's assigned nurse so that they fall in afternoon hours that do not disrupt the other schedules. Individual tutoring or speech therapy sessions are arranged for some children, also in afternoon time. Staff meetings are held between one and three p.m. so that both morning and afternoon nursing shifts may participate. Each nursing person has one weekly supervisory session with a more senior nurse, attends the small clinical staff meeting at which her child is discussed, participates in the ward care staff planning meeting for the group to which her child belongs, attends the total ward care staff meeting, and regularly meets with her child's psychiatrist. The nurses take turns attending the weekly treatment review and the staff meeting at which all ward psychiatrists and senior Children's Service staff are present.

EVALUATION OF PROGRAM

This complicated structure for intercommunication presents some of the greatest problems we have encountered. It is difficult to schedule staff time; it takes many hours of staff time away from the children; it is hard for everyone to speak freely and pertinently enough in groups to achieve the level of communication that is sought. These are not problems that appeared anew with this year's program, however; and the degree of staff participation and exchange of ideas, as well as the children's progress, would seem to indicate that it is well worth the effort.

The changing program has both necessitated and provided opportunity for closer involvement of the psychiatrists in these aspects of the work. It seems unlikely that the several disciplines involved could so easily have resolved some of their differences in integrating their work if the ward psychiatrist were not closely in touch with each and helping all to maintain the focus on the mutual clinical goal.

The charge nurse's central role in arranging staff time to meet the needs of the total program as well as of care, and in integrating the work of the three groups is a difficult and an arduous one. It has even raised new questions as to what the responsibilities of the charge nurse might ideally be, how many other supervisory persons are also needed, and how best to integrate the mutual clinical administrative responsibilities of the charge nurse and the ward psychiatrist.

The teacher, the speech therapist, and the occupational therapist are, on the whole, pleased with the current method of working. Their initial fear that as many nurses as children in the room would interfere with the task at hand has disappeared. With each child attended to, they have found themselves freer to present the work, to pick up minimal clues of trouble or interest on each child's part, and to turn their attention to the group or the individual as indicated. They can rely on the nurses to keep the faster children interested while the slower ones complete a task, and to reduce the latters' discouragement and jealousies. They can, in other words, have a group activity for children whose illness prevents them from being able actually to function as a member of any group.

INTEGRATION OF INTENSIVE CARE AND ACTIVITIES

This maintenance of the advantages of the one-to-one nurse-child relationship within activities best suited to and providing the advantages of groups is perhaps the greatest achievement of this method. The nurses who have come to understand this seldom feel that their psychiatric nursing is being interfered with. Problems do still arise for many of them at some times, however. Perhaps this is still a measure of lack of time for all of them to become familiar enough with the methods and purposes behind the suggestions of the activity specialists. Perhaps it indicates disadvantages not yet understood. That it occurs more frequently in recreational areas and in O.T. than in school or cooking would seem to indicate the former. Everyone seems to assume that learning to read and write is an integrative experience and that baking and eating one's own cookies is fun. All are not quite so sure that learning to hop or to paste or to saw is either fun or useful unless it is initiated spontaneously by the child. It is also harder for them to learn to feel competent in these areas.

In any event, when a child resists an activity there is sometimes a question of who should decide what response may be the most therapeutic one. This difficulty may be compounded when for other reasons either the nurse or specialist is currently having difficulties in her general relationship to the child. Already in temporary doubt about her current therapeutic efficacy and judgment, either person may interpret any suggestion made by the other as a critical demand. The specialist tends to offer too many anxious suggestions or to withdraw her technical support too soon. The nurse, on the other hand, may take the specialist's suggestions so literally that the task gets done by her instead of the child, or she may feel overwhelmed by the suggestions, and in a kind of passive paralysis allow the child to remove himself either literally or figuratively from the learning opportunity at hand.

Progress outweighs the vicissitudes often enough, however, that few if any of the staff would choose to stop trying to develop the method further.

The following example is illustrative of the contribution each discipline makes to an activity when the staff has achieved mutual understanding of the common therapeutical goal and has succeeded in coordinating their planning:

For a number of weeks, planned activities had a central theme of transportation. One highlight of this was to be a visit to a helicopter. The teacher arranged the trip through one of the psychiatrists. The helicopter was to land, and the group would tour the interior. Thus informed, the nurses used various opportunities to talk with their assigned children

240

about the coming outing. The speech therapist and teacher made murals of aerial scenes, emphasized whirring and buzzing sounds, and read stories about helicopters. The occupational therapist helped the children construct helicopters in the woodworking class.

On the trip, the nurses were attentive to each child's indications of pleasure, excitement, fear, or disappointment. Using the close individual knowledge they had of particular children, they were able to help the youngsters who became upset because of the loud noise and dust from the rotating blades, or who felt too confined sitting in the small compartment. One boy needed encouragement to take his turn at trying the seats when he found it was not going to take anyone for a ride. After the return to the ward there was more talk about the helicopter by the entire staff. During the rhythm dance session, the volunteer teacher encouraged the children to spread their arms out and fly across the room like the helicopter they had seen. One group of children made scrapbooks of airplane pictures to take home to their parents. One little boy's sister even became very envious of her hospitalized brother when she heard from him that he had had such an exciting outing.

Perhaps the following excerpts from the work of one project nurse with one boy will indicate the unified nature of the nurse's role in all areas of the child's life on the ward:

Pat is a slight, sandy haired, seven-year-old schizophrenic boy with an aloof manner and a handsome, wistful face. When admitted as a day patient at age four and a half, he was mute but constantly hummed or ground his teeth as he sat absorbed in repetitive skillful manipulation of small objects. His facial expression, for the most part bland, was sometimes a frozen empty smile or scowl. Small and chubby like a toddler, he was an appealing child. The staff's initial reaction of wanting to pick him up and cuddle him was short-lived, for he would stiffen, push away, and whine at any approach. Although he would casually saunter away from any greeting, if it was offered without physical contact he would return, perhaps circle the quietly waiting adult and, as he walked by, brush against him. He seldom looked at anyone and never made direct eye contact. He isolated himself from other children or activities, but the areas where he chose to sit were always strategic ones for keeping a furtive eye on everyone. This indirect watchfulness enabled him quickly but gracefully to saunter away from darting children no matter how rapidly they approached. From time to time he would excitedly run up and down the hall emitting a series of frenzied sounds. This child's elusive behavior, resistance to physical contact, and self-absorbed play gave him an air of self-sufficiency and of not wanting or needing anyone. The busy staff unintentionally withdrew any consistent effort to reach him.

Miss M., one of the nurses on the NIMH Project, has been able to spend four to six hours a day with him for the two years since she came. She has been able to attend all scheduled activities with him—school, O.T., educational play, cooking, swimming, dancing, as well as outdoor play and lunch. Miss M. has had daily contact with one or both parents, giving them the opportunity to exchange information concerning Pat's day at the clinic or evening at home. This has enabled her to gain more understanding of Pat's difficulties.

Initially Miss M. met with various of the activity specialists and gradually started to structure Pat's mornings so that he had a predictable routine. His reaction to these activities varied in degrees of fear, negativism, and anxiety. When exposed to unfamiliar places, sounds, sudden movement, or animals he would clutch her skirt, whine, grind his teeth, hum, or else run blindly ahead into greater hazards. When she succeeded in interesting him in a toy, he would seem to explore it, then subtly begin destroying it. On those rare occasions when he spontaneously looked at or fingered a toy, he did not seem to know what to do with it; if Miss M. tried to demonstrate its use, he would walk away without looking or shriek as she attempted to guide his hand. When it was time to pay attention to the teacher reading a story or to listen to a record, he would bury his head in Miss M.'s lap, look out the window and hum, or try to leave. If requested to dress himself after swimming, he stood motionless with an uncomprehending stare. His hold on tools—drills, hammers, saws—was putty-like. If he did grasp, he seemed unable to lift or to use them. He was unable to catch a ball. When one was placed in his hands he would let it roll away. All this was in marked contrast to his exceptional hand coordination in fine movements.

His refusal to look at what was shown him and his inhibition in using gross body movements were the two major problems Miss M. continually met in trying to help Pat utilize the various opportunities to obtain pleasure and to learn new skills. She finally tried insisting that he look at and pay attention to his surroundings. Verbally she emphasized the color, shape, and name of things. She often pointed to things while they were on outings or on the way to and from scheduled activities. At times she took his head in her hands and gently but firmly turned it in the direction she wanted him to look saying such things as: "Oh, look Pat, there's a yellow and black car just like your daddy's." "Look at the helicopter; it's like the one we made in O.T." "Look at the duck. It's like the one in the book. Listen to the duck quack. It sounds like the record in school." At the end of two months he began occasionally looking, but still turned quickly away with an irritated shrug. Sometimes a comment like, "Oh Pat, you're not looking, sweetheart," would bring a quick glance in Miss M.'s direction with either a sheepish smile or an angry whine.

She then tried getting down to his eye level to observe the shift of his eyes so that she could call his attention back to the task at hand more promptly. After many hours of attentive observation, she found that with her face beside his, he would look longer. If she could get in position to allow him to rest his cheek against the back of her hand, he would watch a demonstration. In trying to make full use of her observations, she sometimes found herself in awkward and grotesque body positions.

After another six months, Pat could frequently sit quietly watching the teacher while she read a story. He occasionally would try to imitate what was shown him. He learned to dress himself. As a jet passed over one day, he looked up, pointed, and said "plane." He began to make definite eye contact with Miss M., particularly when they roughhoused on the beds, for he now enjoyed being tickled and tossed about by her. If she leaned over him, he stared at her and, as if he hadn't seen her before, touched her eyelashes and nose and opened her mouth and examined her teeth. He started to babble more and to repeat an occasional word or phrase she had been saying, such as "ump again," "do it again," "no, no, no." If she playfully repeated his sounds correctly he would laugh and respond with a new sequence of sounds. They played making sounds into a tinker toy can, and she found that he would mimic her without hesitation. This method was later also utilized successfully by the speech therapist. In school, Pat would give no indication of having listened to a phonetic song, but on the ward he would practice all the sounds of the alphabet.

As his willingness to look directly increased, it became much easier for Miss M. to pick up cues indicating his readiness to enter an activity. In the initial period of working with Pat, she had once tried to introduce him to roller-skating. He had shrieked and kicked in a terrified manner. Three months later she observed him watching another child play with the wheels of the skate. When the child put it down, he picked it up and started playing with the wheels. She put his foot on the skate. He shrieked and ran off, but returned and sat in her lap as she sat on the floor playing with the skate. Later as she put the skate on *her* foot and moved, he screamed, took her foot off the skate, and kicked it across the room. When she picked it up, he grabbed and sat on it. He allowed her to pull him about the ward as he sat on the skate, and during the following two months he eventually allowed her to put the skates on his feet as long as they were not fastened. Two months later she noticed him watching other children skating. At that time he allowed her to put the skates on properly, and within the following two weeks he had learned to skate without assistance. It took a total of nine months from the initial introduction before he was able to skate for the fun of it. For several subsequent months, he demanded his skates as soon as he arrived and tried tenaciously to wear them everywhere, even at nap and outdoor play periods. The only time he took them off without a tantrum was when his doctor took him to the playroom or when he was going on an outing.

As Pat began using his body more skillfully and became freer to look at surroundings with interest, he became generally more animated and more open in his enjoyment of activities and accomplishments. He began to smile, laugh, and speak when happy or pleased. He also began to show his anger more openly and directly when he was disappointed, irritated, or frustrated. This he did by crying, stomping his feet, and occasionally trying to kick, pinch, or pound.

DISCUSSION

This paper has attempted to describe some of the advantages and problems a particular staff group has experienced through intensification of active participation of the nurses in every aspect of the children's activity program. Although it has increased opportunities for staff communication about each child's clinical progress, it has also created scheduling problems and has highlighted the potentialities that might lie in using a more adequate number of staff of all disciplines and at all levels of experience.

Plans are being made for earlier and more thorough orientation of new staff in all areas of the ward program. It also appears that more consistent attendance at given staff meetings may gradually reduce some of the existing barriers to full exchange of ideas and concerns between all persons working with the children. Repeated efforts are being made to enlarge the staff gradually and, in particular, to create some new positions for experienced nursing supervisors.[3]

The entire staff is encouraged by their recent experiences with the program. It has afforded each child more varied opportunities for activity and for learning. Most particularly, it has provided greater continuity of each child's relationship with his nurse, and through this has reduced the perhaps inevitable fragmentation of a child in an institutional setting, and has increased the frequency with which staff-patient interaction has facilitated each child's conflict reaction and therapeutic learning.

---

[3] For some of the developments that have occurred since this paper was written in 1962, see Chapter 4.

REFERENCES

1. BOATMAN, MALETA J. and SZUREK, S. A. A clinical study of childhood schizophrenia. In Don D. Jackson (Ed.), *The etiology of schizophrenia.* New York: Basic Books, Inc., 1960, pp. 389-440.

2. BOATMAN, MALETA J., PAYNTER, JANE, and PARSONS, CORINNE. Nursing in hospital psychiatric therapy for psychotic children. *Am. J. Orthopsychiat.,* **32**:808-817, 1962.

3. ENG, MARIETTA, and BOATMAN, MALETA J. The occupational therapy program on a ward for psychotic children. Proceedings of the 1960 Annual Conference, *Am. J. of Occupational Therapy,* 33-36.

4. ENG, MARIETTA, GERWERTZ, JOANNE, and BOATMAN, MALETA J. A creative rhythmic movement group for psychotic children in a psychotherapeutic program. Unpublished paper at Annual Meeting of American Orthopsychiatric Association, 1959.

5. REID, JOSEPH H., and HAGAN, HELEN R. A descriptive study of the program of the Langley Porter Clinic, Children's Inpatient Service. In *Residential treatment of emotionally disturbed children.* New York: The Child Welfare League of America, Inc., 1952, pp. 200-221.

6. SHEIMO, S. L., PAYNTER, JANE, and SZUREK, S. A. Problems of staff interaction with spontaneous group formations on a children's psychiatric ward, *Am. J. Orthopsychiat.,* **19**:599-611, 1949.

7. SZUREK, S. A. Childhood schizophrenia: psychotic episodes and psychotic maldevelopment, *Am. J. Orthopsychiat.,* **26**:519-543, 1956.

8. _____. The family and the staff in hospital psychiatric therapy of children. *Am. J. Orthopsychiat.,* **21**:597-611, 1951.

9. _____. Playfulness, creativity, and schisis. *Am. J. Orthopsychiat.,* **29**:667-682, 1959.

10. _____. Remarks on training for psychotherapy. *Am. J. Orthopsychiat.,* **19**:36-51, 1949. Reprinted in S. A. Szurek & I. N. Berlin (Eds.), *Training in therapeutic work with children.* Vol. 2, the Langley Porter Child Psychiatry Series. Palo Alto, Calif.: Science and Behavior Books, 1967.

11. _____. *The roots of psychoanalysis and psychotherapy, a search for principles of general psychotherapeutics.* Springfield, Ill.: Thomas, 1958.

12. _____. Some lessons from efforts at psychotherapy with parents. *Am. J. Psychiat.,* **109**:296-302, 1952. Reprinted in S. A. Szurek & I. N. Berlin (Eds.), *Training in therapeutic work with children.* Vol. 2, the Langley Porter Child Psychiatry Series. Palo Alto, Calif.: Science and Behavior Books, 1967.

13. _____. Some observations on the dynamics of staff interaction in hospital psychiatric treatment of children. *Am. J. Orthopsychiat.,* **17**: 652-664, 1947.

14. SZUREK, S. A., and BERLIN, I. N. Elements of psychotherapeutics with the schizophrenic child and his parents. *Psychiatry,* **19**:1-9, 1956. Reprinted in S. A. Szurek & I. N. Berlin (Eds.), *Training in therapeutic work with children.* Vol. 2, the Langley Porter Child Psychiatry Series. Palo Alto, Calif.: Science and Behavior Books, 1967.

15. SZUREK, S. A., SHEIMO, S. L., and PAYNTER, JANE. Problems encountered in dealing with handicapped and emotionally disturbed children. *Am. J. Occup. Ther.,* **3**:303-307, 1949.

CHAPTER 17

FOOD-CENTERED SITUATIONS*

Maleta J. Boatman, M.D.

PART ONE: INTRODUCTION

Food-centered situations are a prominent part of any type of residential program for children. In our psychotherapeutically oriented ward program for twelve (formerly fifteen) seriously disturbed youngsters on the Children's Service of the Langley Porter Neuropsychiatric Institute we have tried to ensure that such situations would enhance the therapeutic milieu for each child. We have noted that the degree to which we were successful in this often depended not only on how clear we were about the child's troubles and needs but also on how alert we were to our own difficulties with administrative realities, intrastaff communication, and personal attitudes about food.

Early Experiences

From the earliest days of the program over twenty years ago, the members of the nursing staff and the teachers have recognized opportunities for pleasurable learning that they might offer the children around food. A school-time outing to San Francisco's Farmer's Market provided experience with streetcar transportation, showed each child a myriad of garden-fresh food items, and allowed each to choose the potato he would scrub, bake, season, and eat later that day. Picnic outings have been times for learning about building and lighting fires over which to grill hamburgers and hot dogs. Learning about holidays has included making gingerbread houses at Christmas, heart-shaped red sugared cookies at Valentine's Day, and trick-or-treat bags for collecting goodies on Halloween.

---

*Unpublished paper, 1970.

Symptomatic Expressions of Conflict

As we increased the proportion of very severely disturbed psychotic children admitted to the ward, simply offering food-centered experiences that would have been pleasurable to most children was far from enough. These children experienced very little satisfaction in any activity, had great difficulty in learning, were reluctant to do things for themselves, and showed massive oppositional behavior to adults' expectations. Much symptomatic expression of conflict centered around what went into the mouth and how [1]. Many children made little effort to feed themselves, bit or chewed no solid foods even past age three years, had restrictive food preferences or phobias, or evidenced mealtime compulsions and rituals. Some had never explored the world with their mouths, not even their own thumbs, but others licked, sucked, or ate almost everything they could reach, including finger-paint, crayons, cigarette stubs from the street, toilet bowl water, sand, and tanbark. Playing with their own saliva and chewing on their tee-shirts until the fronts were wet and foul-smelling occurred frequently. Children who usually seemed to remain aloof from adults who tried to engage their interest would often run up eagerly and clingingly if their hands and faces were smeared with food or sticky with saliva. These were also the children whose proffered kisses sometimes turned into bites, and who frequently asked at meals for more food, only to dump or throw it.

It was in speaking of children such as these that a teacher expressed optimism about one newly admitted girl because she had stopped her isolated play to show eagerness and enjoyment in "scraping the bowl" to get the good-tasting remnants of a cake batter. It has been for such youngsters that our staff has tried to provide food-centered situations that would be as precisely therapeutic as possible for one or several at a given time. The following parts of this chapter are adapted from various staff members' descriptions of some of these specific undertakings.

PART TWO: A THERAPEUTICALLY DESIGNED LUNCHTIME ROUTINE[1]

In 1961, two psychiatric nurses who were participating for the second year in an NIMH-supported project each had as her assignment the total

[1] This part of this chapter is an expansion of a short article by Berta Mejia, R.N. and Rella B. Patterson, R.N., entitled "Lunchtime routine designed to help psychotic children." It appeared in *Food Talks,* a bulletin of Nutrition Services Section, Department of Mental Hygiene, State of California, April 1962, and is reprinted here by permission of the authors and publishers.

ward care of a young psychotic day-patient [2; see also Chapter 11].
Partly because of a shortage of staff nurses and partly because the project
staff wished to explore the application of principles of individual patient
care to group care, they also assumed partial responsibility for two other
young boys. The nurses recognized that each of these four boys had individual problems involving eating. Because there were many difficulties
in helping these children in the crowded dining room, their lunchtime
routine was changed in ways designed to meet their needs more closely.

Individual Problems

When the two nurses first worked with the boys, five-and-one-half-
year-old mute, aloof-appearing Sandy sat and stared at his lunch plate
most of the time. He made only tentative moves to eat food, and at the
slightest disturbance created by one of the other thirteen children would
run out of the dining room. His nurse gradually helped him stay longer
at the table by holding him on her lap, but he continued to be distracted
from eating by the behavior of the other children. His intake at home
each night was reported to be limited to a very narrow range of foods.

Six-year-old Timmy would make elaborate preparations with his
food. At any attempts to assist him or to shorten the time involved, or
at any interference by another child, Timmy would have a temper tantrum—screaming, dumping his food, and refusing to eat at all.

Eight-year-old Roy would eat only certain foods. Efforts to urge or
coax him to try others would often result in his darting from the table
and smearing handfuls of food in his hair and on any person or object
he passed.

Husky eight-year-old David greedily gulped any food he liked, yelled
for toast instead of bread, and insisted on separation of any mixed foods
before he would taste them. When his demands were denied, he objected
by loud shrieking or by leaving the dining room.

Group and Staff Problems

Just as each boy's problems were aggravated by other children's disturbances, so did his disruptive behavior interfere with others. The close
quarters of the dining room added other problems. When one of the
nurses responded to a particular child's behavior, either to calm him or
to try meeting his distress in a helpfully personalized way, other children
began to demand the same attentions. If, for example, toast was made
for David, more children demanded toast. It was understandable that a
nurse who was trying to be therapeutically helpful found herself sometimes willing to settle instead for merely avoiding a major scene.

Some of the children's individual requests could not be met because of the way the food was brought to the adjacent serving pantry from the Institute's main kitchen. Some could not be met because the relatively small size of the room made frequent moving from area to area on individual errands appear to be disorganized milling about. Some could not be met because of the small number of regular ward staff present. Furthermore, these staff persons sometimes suspected that the project nurses were pampering rather than helping the children.

The Experimental Changes

Having discussed the problems with each other and with the rest of the staff, the two project nurses decided to move the four boys to a quieter, less stimulating part of the ward at lunchtime. They hoped that if they could sit so that one of them was able to reach each child they could help all four sit at and stay at the table. The nurses believed that family-style serving would offer the children the opportunity to become acquainted with different foods. Service bowls provided by the dietary department were used so that the children could take as much food as they wanted or refuse it if they chose to do so. It was felt that if the children could see the food in open serving bowls and slowly become accustomed to it they might choose to eat it at a later date. Dessert was served along with the other food so that the children could eat this first if they desired. The idea was to eliminate any reward value connected with dessert and consider it as part of the meal. The main goal was to make mealtime as pleasant and relaxed as possible.

One of the things the nurses felt might have been extremely helpful to these children in trying new food and creating a more normal eating situation was to have the adults eat with the children. However, this was not possible under the existing conditions, which did not include facilities for preparing food for employees.[2]

Results

At first the problem was getting the children to sit at the eating area. A story was read to the children before mealtime to keep them together and relaxed. The storytelling dropped out as the children became interested in helping to set up the food cart and in assisting in food preparation and setting the table. The children soon became intrigued with

---

[2] A few years later it did become possible for the Institute to provide food for staff as well as children in the case of special outings and, occasionally, on special days.

the order of the routine, which included hand washing, going to the kitchen to make toast, setting up the food cart, and setting the table, as well as clearing the dishes and cleaning up after eating. The children gradually were able to sit for longer periods of time. They were able to accept new foods, even some they disliked, on their plates. Some of the four started tasting new foods.

Although for many more months these four boys were far from being good eaters, continued to have temper tantrums when their needs were not met, and reverted to old behavior patterns when there was a shortage of staff, they quickly improved in their ability to wait for mealtime. They accepted limits more readily and were able to eat in a more orderly fashion. Within several months they were able to pass food to each other as well as to take the initiative in obtaining their own food.

There were benefits for the whole ward also. Once this plan had been worked out for using a small serving cart to bring food to the table for one group of children, it was possible with the Dietician's help to obtain permission and equipment to expand it gradually to more meals than lunch and to the remaining children. Today the dining room serves only four or five children at any given meal. The others are served at group tables placed in other ward areas. This continues to facilitate individualizing facets of mealtime planning for diverse groups of children or for an individual child.

PART THREE: ANXIETY REDUCTION FOR ONE PSYCHOTIC CHILD[3]

Three-and-one-half-year-old Karen was one psychotic child who was completely unable to obatin any pleasure from eating. Her tremendous anxiety in food-centered situations was manifested as panic, rage, and rejection. Her nurse and the staff worked very hard to find methods to help her reduce the anxiety and thus modify her responses to the need to sustain life by eating.

On admission to our ward, Karen was completely nonverbal. Her mother stated that she had been a "problem eater" from birth and had suffered repeated, severe bronchial infections accompanied by anorexia. The child's thin, stunted body and unhealthy skin, nails, and hair supported this testimony. The clinic staff was confronted with a tremendous

---

[3] This part of this chapter is taken from a short article by B. Schuette, R.N., entitled "Anxiety reduction of a psychotic child in food-centered situations," which appeared in *Food Talks,* 1965; it is reprinted here by permission of the author and publisher.

challenge at Karen's first inpatient meal. It was described afterwards by one of the surprised, food-drenched nurses as "like a Roman gladiatorial contest."

Karen refused to feed herself or to chew food. She demanded a puréed diet administered without spilling any food on her and panicked if it touched even her lips externally. Only carrots, bananas, and ice cream were accepted with any willingness. A momentary inattentiveness or deviation by the nurse from the aforementioned procedure or diet unleashed a reservoir of rage. Screaming angrily, Karen hurled dishes and sent their contents cascading down staff and surroundings, tipped furniture, and ripped clothes. The apex of such a tantrum was punctuated with head-banging and attempts to hurt herself and staff in numerous other ways. Her profound need for individualized help was overwhelmingly apparent.

Therapeutic Objectives

The medical, nursing, educational, and dietary staffs conferred and agreed upon the obvious goal: reduction of mealtime anxiety. To achieve this, an approach was planned to attempt to make mealtime an interesting, enjoyable, socially pleasurable experience, while encouraging the development of eating skills. Improved nutrition with increased caloric intake was viewed as a desirable by-product concurrent with the primary objective of reducing anxiety.

To implement this goal, the dietary department was cooperative in providing Karen with a regular diet in addition to varied puréed foods. Her favorite between-meal nourishment, bananas and ice cream, was made available twenty-four hours a day.

For further implementation, a therapeutic mealtime setting was needed. The chaotically unsuccessful attempt to feed Karen in the limited staff group situation of the small dining room was immediately abandoned. Instead, a table and long sofa in a large playroom were used. A verbal, less ill peer was selected to occupy a table on the opposite side of the room. Each child was attended by a nurse well acquainted with both children and their problems. Thus a quiet, supportive atmosphere was provided that allowed much physical freedom while providing for prompt restraint when needed. It also afforded Karen the opportunity to hear her peer's verbalizations and to watch his more integrated behavior.

In this setting Karen's nurse made a concerted effort to be consistently attentive and meticulously neat while feeding her. Food accidentally spilled on the child or her surroundings was immediately removed with assurances of its harmlessness. The nurse talked of the texture, color, consistency, and origin of the various foods of the regular diet as she enthusiastically sampled them and demonstrated chewing and the use of the spoon. Gradually Karen was introduced to a more regular diet by the nurse's chopping or mashing it in her presence and adding it to the puréed foods. Eventually she was able to accept this modified regular diet exclusively. Variety was introduced gently by encouraging Karen to taste various foods, with the assurance that she need not eat them if she found them distasteful. This same persistent but not insistent encouragement was successfully applied to the use of the spoon. In the ensuing months Karen's lack of self control at mealtime diminished. When it did recur and resulted in destructiveness, she was consistently expected and aided to apply herself to cleaning up any disorder she had created. Violence directed at herself or others was responded to by prompt, nonpunitive physical restraint.

To expand Karen's experience with anxiety-free food situations, her teacher introduced food preparation and snack time into the nursery school session. This offered Karen the opportunity to watch and to participate in the preparation of simple foods such as instant puddings and fruit beverages. Frequent trips to grocery stores to examine products and to make purchases were also made a part of the school activities.

Result

Karen's reduced anxiety, as evidenced by her more integrated behavior at the end of one year, would seem to support the methods applied. By then she ate in the group dining room and would wash the table after eating. While the presence of a supportive adult was still required, destructive-aggressive acts became a rarity. She fed herself about half the time and consumed ample quantities of her modified regular diet, with its wide variety of foods. Chewing was not an established pattern, but was occasionally attempted in unstructured situations. Overt interest in food preparation was displayed, and limited participation was enjoyed. Spillage and handling of food no longer produced panic or rage reactions.

It is interesting to note that Karen's vocabulary of nearly three hundred words at that time began with the naming of foods and their related colors. She became most verbal, and frequently initiated word games at mealtimes.

There was physical evidence of her improved nutrition and increased caloric intake as by-products of the anxiety reduction goal. Her hair, skin, and nails appeared healthy, and there was a decrease in both the number and severity of bronchial infections. As already indicated, anorexia was no longer a problem. Weight increased by 8.4 percent, and she grew two and a half inches.

Karen's nurse felt that the support the girl obtained through persistent and unchanging affection from various members of the staff, who recognized and treated her as a desirable human being, was a major factor in the changes that occurred. She also gave equal recognition to the consistent cooperation of each discipline involved. Karen's anxiety reduction was gratifying to everyone, and the variety of activities and facilities available were recognized by all as major contributing factors. The senior staff members were most cognizant of the thoughtfulness and the complexity of the unstinting efforts of those members of the nursing and psychiatric staff who worked most closely with this child. They were convinced of the direct relationship between the staff's striving to be precisely therapeutic in their behaviors and the areas of steady achievement in the child's development of more capacity for experiencing and expressing satisfaction.

PART FOUR: INTRASTAFF COMMUNICATION

The preceding two examples of particular therapeutic efforts indicate only briefly the enormous importance and magnitude of the problems in maintaining adequate communication within a staff group when one major focus of a child's disturbed behavior is in food-centered situations. There are, of course, practical difficulties whenever a staff group is large enough to make the carrying out of individualized therapeutic planning feasible, and there are some emotional interferences whenever a patient's disturbed behavior is severe enough to be personally disturbing to most others who encounter it. We have come, however, to expect the latter to occur with great regularity when a child's symptomatic behaviors center around food.

Perhaps only when a child is even more overtly physically self-hurtful is there more likelihood of trouble in staff communication than around distressing eating patterns. To protect a child from physical hurt and to ensure that a child will be healthfully nourished are so synonymous with our concepts of ourselves as persons who "take care" that anything or anyone who threatens our achievement in these areas produces anxiety and anger. When the threatening person is the child himself, we seem to face an intolerable paradox. We may feel revengefully hurtful toward the child for not letting us keep him from hurting himself. Only when the threat is from other, usually respected, staff member's divergent ideas of "healthful nutrition" may we discover, with anxiety, how many and how absolute are the definitions of this concept—definitions held as unresolved remnants of earlier attitudes not yet modified by our clinical experience.

It takes frequent and thoughtful staff discussions in an atmosphere of concern for mutual clinical goals for each staff member to become interested and inquiring about his own judgmental attitudes concerning food and to become more tolerant of the time it takes others to perceive their own. As a group, a staff unquestioningly "knows" so many and such contradictory things: desserts should be eaten at the end of meals; snacks, however nutritious, are bad for children who do not eat at mealtime; forbidding snacks between meals is a cruel practice; children should not be allowed to play or dawdle with food; children should not be urged to eat food they don't like; a child should clean his plate (regardless of his weight); a child should not be offered "seconds"; vegetables are more nutritious than meat; protein should be eaten at every meal; meals should not be held for children to finish later; a child should be taught to share; children should not be expected to share their goodies; and so forth. The hallmark of all of these ideas is the accompanying feeling that the behavior is either "right" or "wrong." Inevitably there is difficulty in modifying the expression of that feeling. This is often so even after the person who experiences it can intellectually conceive that with particular children and for particular therapeutic reasons it might be helpful for the staff to behave in different ways for clinically relevant periods of time.

Thus Karen's nurse knew what a step forward it was when soft foods were accepted in chunks rather than having to be mashed. Nonetheless some of the staff could not help feeling guiltily critical of her for cutting Karen's ice cream. They were critical because they felt that she was overindulgent and prolonged the girl's helplessness. They felt guilty because they dreaded their own shorter periods of assigned work with this frighteningly difficult child. As is usually the case, the tension in such feelings diminished when they were expressed in staff discussions. As a result, some staff members began to be able to encourage Karen noncoercively to chew. Others were able to continue to help her feel accepted and pleased with her gains. Some were able to combine both attitudes flexibly in the way we consider most therapeutic.

PART FIVE: COOKING CLASSES[4]

In addition to continuing the staff's attentiveness to each child's needs at mealtimes, it became possible in 1961 to start the development of a cooking program with one group of children. Since that time, cooking classes have been held as a fairly regular part of the therapeutic program for all twelve children. They have most often been part of the program planned by the occupational therapist, but are sometimes carried out by the teachers or the nurses. The following is a description of the first four years of the development of this activity.

The Procedure for a Cooking Class

The setting was a comfortable recreation lounge, complete with a pantry equipped with a small, compact kitchen unit. Cooking done was usually one type of snack and a beverage. The occupational therapist did the major planning, which was tailored to the specific needs of each child or his group. Nurses and sometimes volunteers helped in the program. The procedure was to use a forty-five minute period to wash hands, don apron, prepare food, cook it, cool it, eat it, and clean up. One nurse helped each child with these tasks when possible. The routine was to help the children learn an organized pattern and to allow for some accomplishment and satisfaction in the limited time.

The menu was decided a week in advance to allow time for various arrangements. It usually fulfilled these six requirements:

1. What is to be eaten should be familiar, tasty, and tempting in appearance.
2. Tasks should require simple manipulation at the child's maturational and readiness level.
3. There should be enough tasks to keep each child engaged in the general theme, even during waiting times.
4. Some form of cooking with heat is preferable, as it releases usually aromatic odors. This step should not exceed fifteen minutes, and time must be allowed for cooling.
5. Ingredients should be inexpensive because of budget limits and inevitable waste during the learning process.

---

[4] This part of this chapter is an edited version of a paper by Marietta C. Eng, O.T.R., entitled "The use of foods and cooking in the treatment of autistic children," originally read at a workshop in 1965 at the Seventeenth Mental Hospital Institute of the American Psychiatric Association, September 26, 1965. It appears here with permission of the author.

6. Each session should add to some phase of the child's learning experience and give food a pleasurable image.

Some successful menus were: bread cutouts spread with softened butter, sprinkled with sugar and cinnamon and broiled; fresh orangeade or lemonade; ice cream made in a hand-cranked freezer, cookies or stiff dough shaped by hand; and fried donuts sugared by shaking in a paper bag. When a cooking class was started at a later date for a group of younger children, the menus were adapted to their need for immediate food gratification. Ready-to-eat products that required short preparation times were used to make such items as instant pudding, frosting, and candy.

Progress Made by Patrick

One child's experience will be described to illustrate how progress evolved. Six-year-old Patrick was one of a group of three boys, aged six and seven, who started cooking class early in 1962 with their nurses, who were on a National Institute of Mental Health supported project [2]. Pat resisted participating, running off instead to slam closet doors or to fidget with locks, thus increasing the tension in the group. Knowing his fascination for mechanical gadgets and his skillful manipulation of them, the staff tried to interest him in the cooking by inviting him to use the various utensils, such as the wire coil egg beater. Though he did not mind handling such clean metal or wood objects, he was repelled by messy, moist, or sticky substances. In paring a raw potato he used the parer well, but had to have his nurse hold the potato. When a peel fell to his lap he shrieked and grimaced in disgust. He was allowed to wash his hands frequently when handling such food, as proof to him that the messiness would wash off.

Pat usually ate only certain foods prepared in certain ways. At the start of the cooking classes, he did not eat foods he helped make even when they were among his few favorites. When his group sat at the table to eat what was prepared, Pat refused it adamantly. He suffered through the self-imposed ordeal silently by drinking glass after glass of milk. Over a period of several months, he gradually started and continued to eat with the others in the following sequence: he would watch his group of boys eat their food; he began to handle "messy" flour and wet dough while preparing food; he began to do some tasting; and he finally learned to make a decision about what to do with his finished product.

When Pat showed eagerness for a longer cooking time, and this became possible, he and another boy prepared their own lunches once weekly for three months. Pat's nurse and the occupational therapist worked closely on goals. Since the other child had problems mainly in *how* he ate, the menu planning centered around Pat's needs. Starting with what he already ate or the method of cooking, new foods and new textures were slowly added, always in his presence and with his involvement. The first cooking projects were dark browned and totally crispy foods. He nibbled the crumbs and scraps. Later French fries, a favorite food, were made partially soft. After Pat bit off all the crisp edges, he accepted his nurse's offering of the softer center portion. Eventually he learned to eat all parts of the French fry.

Catsup was a sauce Pat liked with all foods. Foods he had never eaten—shrimps, canned pineapple, and luncheon meat—were marinated in a barbecue sauce with a catsup-like flavor. After these were skewered and broiled, Pat first licked the sauce, then the sauce coating the foods, then the foods themselves. He was so involved during its preparation that when he was deveining the shrimp, he even spoke one of his infrequent words by complaining, "Dirty."

Three and one-half years after these classes started, Pat showed many signs of integration, including spontaneous participation and pleasure in what he was doing, the people he was with, and the guests invited for lunch. His accomplishments in cooking classes extended elsewhere. His nurse noticed that he ate about one new food on the ward each week and was also eating better at home.

All-Ward Luncheon

In the summer of 1965 it was possible for the first time, on a regular basis, for the staff to help the children by dining with them. The senior ward staff had long felt that this would be an important therapeutic step. Picnic lunches and parties had offered informal eating together, but these cooking sessions involved a complete mealtime in an actual dining setting. The staff decided that each week about ten of them would contribute toward the expenses. On the luncheon day they first helped the twelve children, divided into two groups, in the food preparations, and later all sat down to eat together.

Each of these meals became festive, like a party. It was the culmination of previous grocery shopping, menu studies in school, and that morning's sight, touch, smell, and sampling of the foods. There was the equality of self-service and second servings from the food-laden table and the mutuality of eating the same foods. There was the topic of food for table conversation and there were compliments to the chefs. There was the shared cleanup. Such a mealtime provided opportunity for staff to demonstrate their own healthier food attitudes to the children.

One meal that typified the successful luncheons featured a watermelon boat fruit salad, hot dog on bun, milk or coffee, and ice cream. This day everyone ate heartily, including some usually poor eaters who also happened to participate more than usual in the food preparations. It was fun for the groups to halve the large watermelon they had purchased the day before, use the melon ballers to scoop out the fruit and that of the cantaloupe, groove lines on the bananas before slicing them and the peaches, and pull seedless grapes from the bunch. The final product was tempting in color, moisture, and form; tasty with the combinations of flavors; and best of all, a result of everyone's contributions.

Difficulties for the Children

Frequently there was one child in a cooking group sitting at the table who, from some recurring fear of the consequences of human closeness in a temporarily pleasurable situation, would carry out a sudden taunting impulse to push over the pitcher of milk or someone else's cup of cocoa, then gleefully watch the staff reaction. His action usually created a moment of frozen silence, then a rush by the adults to rescue everything in the path of the milk flow and messy drip to the floor. Even new staff members soon learned that a nonretaliatory and calm attitude, aided by a large sponge on the table awaiting such an emergency, quickly ended the episode and soothed the atmosphere. A quick verbal reassurance to the other children in the group also averted a chain reaction. Often the nurses' attentiveness toward the child's positive behavior or an advance recognition of his possible desire toward destructiveness, stemming from some unresolved conflict, helped prevent such behavior from recurring.

Another situation that these acutely sensitive children were aware of was that supplies were limited. Eve was sometimes negativistic and hyperactive when reacting to any uncertainity or disagreement in staff about her. One day when she was about to measure flour, the occupational therapist hinted to the new nurse with her, "Have Eve measure accurately and not waste any." Ordinarily, a more open statement about material limits would have been made. In this case there was not an immediate serious shortage, and the therapist did not feel that Eve was able to handle such information because of her intense feelings of deprivation. The nurse, not knowing Eve well, asked sympathetically about the economy. The therapist was reluctant to say that the canister of flour was also for the use of the next group and that she was concerned there might not be enough for that day. In the meantime, Eve began spreading flour all over the table. Looking at both nurse and occupational therapist, she scooped handfuls of flour into her mouth, laughing mirthlessly, and spilling flour on the floor. The nurse moved in to stop her, and the therapist cleared the area and talked with Eve until she regained control. Later, in examining the sequence of events, it seemed that Eve had reacted in her typical self-destructive way because: (a) attentiveness was withdrawn from her during the staff conversation; (b) she could not tolerate sharing the flour with others; and (c) she heard and sensed staff anxiety as well as conflict about her.

A situation such as Eve's did not occur frequently after a cash donation by the San Francisco Mental Health Association made some food purchases possible. The Dietary Department continued to supply food ingredients in lieu of the children's between-meal nourishment for those days, and the small supplemental budget added extras. Important advantages included being able to plan menus creatively, purchase foods according to their timeliness in relationship to other activities, introduce more variety, and choose foods for their esthetic stimulus value. These improved choices also helped staff enthusiasm in carrying out the activity.

Difficulties for Staff

Two major difficulties that confronted the staff were meeting food handling standards while conducting a therapeutic activity and adapting or changing their own food attitudes to match the ability level of the children.

The dietetic staff prepared hospital foods under established public health standards. They had concern that the food ingredients they provided for the children's cooking classes be used with the same precautions. Since ward staff knew the importance of healthful use of foods and cooking with these children, they handled the responsibility by frequent consultations with the dietitian. Some of them completed a class in food handling and sanitation.

There were some adaptations of rules on a temporary basis. Like all children, these did not have dirt-free hands nor covered cough and sneeze habits. While the children were getting acquainted with the activity, staff did not insist that a child wear his apron if he was afraid to put the strap over his head, nor did they stop a child from eating his carefully baked cookies if they had accidentally dropped on the floor. With the vigilance of staff, the steady improvement of the children's health habits, the high heat of cooking destroying most bacteria, and the frequent physical checkups, no illness was ever reported as a result of food contamination.

The second area of staff difficulty was with their own established food attitudes when incompatible with treatment goals. When a child eagerly pressed the cookie cutter in the center of a slice of bread in his first try, it was automatic for a thrift-conscious adult to say, "You're wasting bread," instead of the therapeutic, "What a nice design you cut."

The occupational therapist found other staff attitudes that added problems for the activity. Some nurses felt that accurate measurements as she suggested them were a hinderance, since "Mother never measured." Most of the staff soon realized that beginners need some guide for accuracy and a successful outcome. Such common dinner table comments as, "I hate hash," were detrimental to a child's willingness to try the food or added to his already existent dislike of it. Adult criteria of how carefully a food item should be washed or prepared were sometimes over-applied. It could discourage the child if his task was redone for him. All the staff who worked with the cooking program over a period of time learned to offer a child recognition for his effort and not to be bothered by such harmless occurrences as having some green stem grated in with the orange carrot.

The nurses in turn found some difficulties in the occupational therapist's ways of presenting plans for the activity. As in the previously mentioned example of Eve and the flour, the therapist sometimes hoped they would follow her clues, although time had not been found for her to explain the goals and her methods or problems in advance. These difficulties diminished whenever it was possible for the therapist to offer some orientation sessions to persons new on the ward.

The foregoing description of the development of the cooking classes again highlights the importance of continuing alertness by the staff members to their own attitudes and to their openness with each other. It also offers further evidence of the need we find for dealing as effectively as possible with administrative realities such as space, institute policies, staff turnover, and budgets.

PART SIX: CONCLUSION

This chapter has presented three different descriptions of the development of specific therapeutic efforts in food-centered situations. It is also hoped that such sequential discussion of segments of one such important area of staff-patient activity (eating) will provide some feeling for the way in which programs evolve in relation to a steadfast effort to apply a stable concept concerning the nature of disordered behavior and of its reduction. Papers from the earlier periods on this ward reflect similar experiences with food-centered situations [1, 3]. Subsequent developments on the ward have had some of their roots in the situations described here [4].

The acquisition of a specially designed cart equipped with toaster, butter spreaders, and so forth has made it possible to include snack time in any part of the program, including that carried out in a schoolroom slightly separated from the ward. When our playground was remodeled, a raised fire-pit was included to facilitate weiner roasts and lunchtime cookouts.

Our summer program in 1966 was centered around weekly beach experiences. A major theme was menu planning, food purchasing, and the ultimate picnic that was part of each outing. The provision and preparation of food has been one highlight of overnight camping trips for most of the children in the past several years.

Food-centered situations are also utilized in helping parents and other Institute staff members feel more appropriately part of our ward program. Each child's birthday is celebrated with a party, and parents are invited to help plan it with the nurse so it will be most to the child's liking. Although cake with candles and ice cream are most common, potato chips and coca-cola have helped a child afraid of groups find enjoyment in his own party for the first time. Staff-provided food is the finale at an annual Christmas program and open house given for all children's parents, Institute staff, and volunteers, as well as children and staff who have recently left the ward program. An all-ward picnic usually introduces new trainee child-psychiatrists to the children and ward staff early in their two-year stay with us.

Nursing-care plans for individual children currently include eating as one of multiple areas of note. Special attention is given to: desirable seating arrangements; how much help is needed; presently suggested staff approach to particular problems about choosing, asking, or accepting; and degree of independence obtained, to be avoided, or being worked toward.

Thanksgiving of 1969 saw the most discrete example of the way in which all of the staff members of the several disciplines work together daily to bring their awareness of each child's needs to their contribution to all aspects of the program. All the children and all the ward staff members sat down together to a traditional meal that included cranberry salad, roast turkey, and warm pumpkin pies with homemade ice cream. Each child had taken part in its planning, decoration, and preparation in whatever ways fit his current capacities and needs as the staff understood them. The preparation for this event involved the efforts of the teachers, the nurses, the occupational therapist, and the speech therapist. It had occurred in the school room, on the outings, or in the evening activities. Areas of special achievement or anxiety had been shared with the psychotherapists, and the help of the dietician and the hospital administrator

had been sought. The staff's own questions about how to coordinate
their efforts and how to resolve any differences or doubts about a
given child's therapeutic needs were discussed in one or several of the
available staff meetings.

This year's budget includes the long-desired dishwasher for our ward
pantry as well as an increase in our cooking fund. The staff is already
considering which children may benefit from participating in this additional step in mealtime cleanup, heretofore forbidden for public health
reasons. They are also discussing the meaning that the now-possible
decorated dishes of our own choosing might have for particular children.
In these and other future developments of the use of food-centered activities, we anticipate the continuation of that kind of collaboration
among all staff members that we consider to be integration of the entire
staff in work toward a common therapeutic goal.

REFERENCES

1. BOATMAN, MALETA J. and SZUREK, S. A. A clinical study of
childhood schizophrenia. In Don D. Jackson (Ed.), *The etiology of
schizophrenia.* New York: Basic Books, Inc., 1960, Chap. 14, pp. 389-
440, especially pp. 397-398.
2. BOATMAN, MALETA J., PAYNTER, JANE, and PARSONS,
CORINNE. Nursing in hospital psychiatric therapy for psychotic children. *Am. J. Orthopsychiat.,* **32**:808-817, 1962.
3. BERLIN, I. N., BOATMAN, MALETA J., SHEIMO, S. L., and .
SZUREK, S. A. Adolescent alternation of anorexia and obesity. *Am. J.
Orthopsychiat.,* **21**:387-419, 1951. Also appears in Geo. Gardner (Ed.),
Case studies in childhood emotional disabilities. Volume 1. New York:
American Orthopsychiatric Assn., Inc., 1953, Chapter 3.
4. MORRISON, DELMONT, MEJIA, BERTA, and MILLER, DALE.
Staff conflicts in the use of operant techniques with autistic children.
Am. J. Orthopsychiat., **38**:647-652, 1968.

SECTION SIX

THE FAMILY AND THE INPATIENT WARD STAFF

INTRODUCTION

The efforts to work with parents, not only in therapy but through a variety of interactions with staff members involved with their child, has become an ever more important aspect of inpatient work. It increases the number of hopefully therapeutic contacts parents may have. These interactions not only influence their perceptions of how they interact with their child and other adults, but may also provide models with which to identify in terms of their mode of habitual interaction, expression of feelings, and awareness of the actual state of previously unperceived but present feelings, attitudes, and behavior. These aspects are dealt with in the following papers.

More recently, in addition to the above efforts with parents, a group therapy program with those parents willing to participate has begun. This is so recent that a report of it could not be included in this volume.

CHAPTER 18

THE FAMILY AND THE STAFF*

S. A. Szurek, M.D.

Discussions of practice and problems of a psychiatric inpatient service
for children in a hospital or a residential treatment center have emphasized many aspects of such a service. Cameron [1], for example, has
recently given a general description of an actual institution, with its
particular physical equipment and location, its personnel and organization,
its policies and program. Bradley [2] has discussed the advantages and disadvantages of residential treatment. Others have confined themselves to
a résumé of the experience gained with certain kinds of clinical problems
[3, 4]. Some with specialized interests have considered the advantages
of certain activities and programs under the guidance of specialists in
drama, music, dancing, or other physical activities [5], in addition to
those generally provided by a modern psychiatric hospital. Still others
have examined or reexamined the problems that a group of hospitalized
children poses to the nursing profession [6, 7] and to resident workers
[8, 9], or the particular contribution the nurses might make to the total
therapeutic program [10]. The effect of the group upon the individual
child has been described by Bettelheim and Sylvester [11]; and the general dynamic patterns of the group as a whole have been studied by
Redl [12, 13] and others.

Recently I have become more and more interested in two particular
problems. The first is the relation of the child's problems to the past
and current situation within his family; the second is the problem of
intrastaff relations. Both obviously are dynamic interpersonal situations
that may converge in their influence upon the child when he becomes a

---

*Reprinted by permission from *Am. J. Orthopsychiat.*, 21(3), July 1951,
pp. 597-611. (Copyright, Am. Orthopsychiatric Assn., Inc.)

patient on a psychiatric hospital ward: the family situation may contain not only those dynamic factors that have contributed to the genesis of his disorder, but also perhaps important assets or integrative potentialities for the amelioration of his emotional problems; and the staff may be considered the chief therapeutic agency available to promote or provide the atmosphere in which the child's conflict may be resolved.

THEORETICAL CONSIDERATIONS

There is essentially nothing very new about either of these aspects. For a long time many outpatient clinics for children have recognized the important part the parents or parental substitutes have in initiating and continuing the clinic's work. The part played by the conflicts within and between the parents in the genesis and maintenance of their child's disorder is being more widely recognized all the time [4, 14].

There remains, however, a considerable diversity of opinion as to whether those disorders of children so severe as to lead one to consider the advisability of separating the child from his home and the community are also similarly and genetically related to parental and intrafamilial tensions of conflict. To some, such disorders as may be classified as psychotic or severely psychopathic are either believed to be of unknown etiology, or are thought to be somehow transmitted through the genes. To others, even if the disorder of the parents is considered as having some etiological relation to the disorder of the child, it still remains important for various reasons to concentrate therapeutic attention upon the child.

Implied or stated in some of these attitudes and opinions are several conceptions: parents are as concerned about a child's mental disorder as they would be about any somatic disease; the offer of psychotherapeutic help accentuates their anxiety; parents who require assistance with their own internal conflicts should be referred to a psychotherapist interested in adults. At best, in order not to lose sight of the welfare of the child nor to be diverted in any way from the central therapeutic problem that his disorder presents, the therapist should see to it that parental participation in clinical work with the child is solely restricted to the usual parental duties; in this the parents may need some support, advice, guidance, or interpretation of the therapeutic efforts with the child, either from the child's psychotherapist or from some special collaborator who undertakes no therapy with the parents. At times it appears to some of those who hold such opinions that clinically scrutinizing the family may be an unrealistic effort to maintain the integrity of the family, when clearly the child's best interest may lie in a more permanent separation from it—especially from parents considered therapeutically more or less hopeless or more or less indifferent to the child.

Each of these opinions may contain some part of the truth, or at least point to potential errors in conception and practice that lead to relatively endless or futile efforts of the clinical staff with the family and child. Certainly there exists as yet no generally accepted and durably effective method to restore severely and chronically schizophrenic children to what is commonly regarded as "mental health." The psychopathic or the severe, impulsively hostile aggressive disturbances are still in the unsolved category of clinical problems; and the eclectic attitude that considers the possibility of hereditary transmission of some still obscure defect cannot be ignored. There is also the natural hope that a child offers a generally more favorable field for effective work than does the adult, who is often less responsive to modifying influences. Moreover, it is certainly always humanly possible to become over-identified with one's patient, if it be the parent, and perhaps lose some sense of the child's individual interest. It is, however, equally possible to over-identify with the child against his parents, in which case the child's interest may be poorly served, if not overlooked.

In short, the conception that all degrees of severity of mental disorder in childhood, however manifested symptomatologically, are reactions to living dependently with significant other persons who also suffer from some measure of mental disorder, is a hypothesis that probably requires much more documentation and testing. Perhaps before this validation can begin, a particularly pervasive and often insidiously disguised misconception may need to be removed or at least reduced. This may take many forms, but in essence it is the idea that to look for conflicts in the parents and to make an effort to help them resolve their conflicts is equated with "blaming" them for their child's disorder—blaming them for wanton cruelty to the child, whether this be identified as rejection, overprotection, deprivation of essential emotional warmth, interest, or some deficiency in that ideal complex of feelings called parental "love." It is extremely difficult for students of human behavior to achieve such complete "detachment" and "objectivity" of attitude as to be utterly free of some tendency to feel superior to and to derogate others, or to avoid arousing feelings of resentment in others whether or not they actually possess derogatory attitudes.

Here is difficult dilemma. On the one hand, restraint or censure of some sort is perhaps necessary in modifying the egocentricity of the human animal to permit some kind of organized group living; on the other hand, certain kinds or degrees of censure are conceived of as the source of mental disorder. Is it ever possible, then, to be free enough of mental disorder to conceive the problem dispassionately, let alone be fitted to treat it or discover it in others? The dilemma may, of course, not be actually as sharp or as insoluble as it sounds here. Differing intensities of conflict may still lead to sufficient qualitative differences between persons to allow for objectivity and dispassionate judgment. Does one nevertheless still face insoluble problems as to coercion against an individual's impulses—and while coercion is theoretically to be avoided, is it necessary for the protection of the patient himself as well as others?

INVOLVEMENT OF PARENTS IN THERAPY

Is it self-deception to consider it possible to offer parents therapy, when they complain chiefly of their child's lack of integration, without some subtle use of coercion against them? Is it not derogation and a form of censure to suggest to them that they are ill, that they need therapy, and that their child's chances for recovery may in part depend on the successful resolution of their presumed conflicts? Is not this attitude in itself potentially productive of conflict and illness in the parents, even if they are genuinely concerned about their child's illness and not at all ill themselves in any psychiatric sense of the word? What assurance is there that the psychiatrist is not exploiting the difficulties and problems of others for some unconscious motive of his own?

Nevertheless, even if the more favorable therapeutic results of concomitant work with both the child and his parents should be considered as no final proof of the hypothesis, the hypothesis itself needs to be no more destructive to anyone than any other working scientific hypothesis, provided the necessary self-critical attitude of its tester is present and always alive. Recently there has appeared a discussion in which the scientist's avoidance of errors of reasoning is likened to a disciplined steadfastness of moral integrity.[1] There is therefore perhaps no other

---

[1] "Axioms, that is, norms of thought, fully formulated and clearly understood, were accepted for methodological purposes as true, were consistently adhered to with utmost care in all deductive procedures. Yet the possibility was always left open for modifications of the initial premises when facts required them, and without undue concern over eternal verities the scientist frequently recast his axioms for greater conformity with the contingencies of direct experience. Nor did he see an inconsistency in this procedure.

"What he regards as inconsistent is failure to honor his tentative commitment to a formulated norm of thought during the process of deduction and empirical verification. He calls such inconsistencies errors of reasoning. Their avoidance is not always an easy matter; it often involves a degree of

bulwark against errors during the deductive reasoning from a tentative commitment to a hypothesis or during its empirical verification. Incidentally, this attitude of moral integrity, honesty, and critical self-scrutiny appears to me to be no different in any essential from that which is the only reliably effective one with the patient in psychotherapy as well.

Translated into other terms, all this might be expressed to the parents of the patient in some such words as the following: "I have a hunch that all or much of your child's difficulty is in some way connected with some difficulties you are experiencing. I may be wholly wrong in this. But I am willing to see you regularly and work with you, in addition to the effort we shall make with your child. My purpose is to see with you whether our work together to reduce any of your unhappiness will not also help reduce your child's difficulties. My hope is that any difference in your feelings that our work together may achieve will be of critical importance to your child as well as to you. I also feel that unless you agree with me and are yourself willing to see if such visits with me might be of some help to you, even if they may not be at all helpful to your child, there will be no great urge on your part even to begin all this. You cannot be at all sure beforehand that it will be useful to you alone. I cannot assure you that I can be useful to you. I can only say I am willing to try, always with the proviso that you may decide at any point to stop seeing me. If this should happen, we can then both discuss what alternatives to the present plan of keeping your child in this hospital there are, and which of these alternatives you may wish to select. I expect no promise now that either you or I will continue indefinitely in such work together, nor that either one of us may not get so discouraged as to wish to stop. I hope we can both be frank enough to express such feelings directly to each other if they should arise. Are you willing to try?"

---

tedium and of determination rivaling the disciplined steadfastness of moral integrity. Also, there are often personal advantages to be gained through scientific error which becomes a moral lapse when detected but not corrected. Indeed, there are places where the distinction between scientific and moral error becomes rather thin and where there is an overlapping of issues as in situations governed by a scientific code of ethics. At any rate, scientific sin is not commensurate with *doubt as to the axioms* of a given discipline; it is the *failure to honor a commitment* to a set of maxims, whether they are ultimately tenable or not.

"By axiom, or postulate, we mean here any basic (unproved) hypothesis which had deductive fertility." [15].

There is in this attitude no assumption that the child will necessarily be reunited more permanently with his parents. There is only the consideration of the possibility that if the mutual work of the parent and therapist is successful in releasing from stultifying and distorting conflict the parent's potentialities to feel more fully whatever his reactions actually are, then perhaps the parent will be enabled to free himself— and hence his child—from fantastic and guilty enslavement, whatever its particular form. To begin such therapeutic work with a child in a hospital on condition that the parents also undertake a therapeutic experiment themselves may be interpreted as a species of coercion of people who are particularly helpless, troubled, and hence unable to defend themselves against the imposition of harsh conditions dogmatically held. Although this may be a self-deceptive rationalization, it nevertheless seems possible that the function of a treatment hospital and the experimental attitude implied in the hypothesis can be honestly and firmly held with no insistence that the parents submit, but that their refusal even to begin the experiment, or a decision to stop it prematurely, involves and means a choice of an alternative institution. There is no implicit demand that they believe at the outset that the experiment will work, nor that they refrain from expressing to the therapist their doubts and difficulties as the work progresses; and it is made clear to them that the possibility of stopping the experiment at any point and thus ending hospitalization for the child is always present and available. This latter outcome hopefully will be accepted by the therapist without recrimination or rancor against the parents, but only with regret and with respect for the parents' right to terminate the therapeutic contract.

DISORDERED CHILD AND TROUBLED PARENTS

To state a hypothesis is relatively simple; to offer substantiating evidence quickly verifiable by other observers is a difficult matter. Statistically valid samples of psychological data are hard to accumulate, even over a professional lifetime. Clinicians' time-honored practice of offering a few, only partially describable samples may be useful for illustrative purposes, but it cannot contribute to a general validation of a thesis. An alternative to this method, perhaps no more satisfactory, is to make statements of one's increasing conviction, from long experience, that certain hypotheses are valid. In the absence of readily verifiable data, the following statements are presented in that spirit.

In all instances of mental disorder in childhood in which organic, impersonally caused disease is excluded from central etiological relevance, there is evidence of a less obvious disorder in at least one parent. Although direct, individual psychotherapy of the child is generally essential, psychotherapy of parental conflicts often offers an additional therapeutic lever that may prove of critical importance. Every detail of the child's symptomatology is finally related to particular experiences with both parents—chronologically and economically related to experiences with each of their conflicting attitudes. These statements have been borne out in all the instances I have thus far had the opportunity to study sufficiently, from the most transient and occasional nightmare or phobia, to the most severely schizophrenic autisms, including the overt, hostile-aggressive disturbances that in many ways are at the opposite end of the psychopathological spectrum.

Even when considerable therapeutic success with the child alone occurs, the likelihood of recrudescence of disorder upon his return to the parents is great if no essential change in their conflicts has taken place. In other words, the disorder of the child is an expression of crises within the family. His disorder can generally be understood at least retrospectively as the only adaptation possible for him alone, given the total psychological situation in the family. By the same token, parental attitudes are determined both by the remote past and the present situation, which includes the child's presence in the home with all his particular characteristics.

At the same time it is also true that the conflict of the parents that expresses itself toward and generates conflict in the child is only a part of the total attitudes of the parents and the child toward each other. There is generally an integrative emotional tie between them even if it is overshadowed by conflict in the severe disorders. But at a given point in their mutual lives, tolerance for each other may be strained to the breaking point by conflict, and it is at these periods that separation of the child from the parents is sought for the sake of all concerned.

HOSPITALIZATION AS AN INCIDENT IN THERAPY

If hospitalization of the child at these times is considered only an incident in the course of the total psychotherapeutic work of the staff with the members of the family, many practices and attitudes of the hospital staff follow naturally. Contact between parents and the child is not dictated by the staff as to its timing, frequency, or duration. Visits of parents to the hospital, or their taking the child home overnight, for weekends, or for short holiday periods, are matters toward which the staff maintains a therapeutic position in respect to both the child and his parents. In other words, conflict and anxiety about such contacts is examined and discussed like any other feeling and attitude that emerges in the process of psychotherapy. If the destructive factors in the relationship between the child and his parents are brought into the field of the transference with the therapist or therapists for working through, a progressive lessening of these factors will be observed. This does not mean that this process always moves in a straight line without retrogressions and reversals, especially in acute phases of the therapeutic work. Nevertheless, if transference attitudes are well established, the recrudescence of intense sadomasochistic episodes of child and parents toward one another becomes more and more obviously an acting out of the transferences, and can more and more often be analyzed with each of the patients in the therapeutic sessions.

THERAPEUTIC ATTITUDES

Every aspect of the child's and parents' behavior acquires dynamic significance in relation to the transferences and needs close attention from the entire staff, especially from the respective psychotherapists. The fees required and their regular payment, as well as their equitable adjustment to actual financial capacity to pay, may become the focus of the family's conflict. Similarly, the actual physical facilities of the hospital, whether as advantages or inadequacies, may evoke particularly characteristic tensions. The physical and medical care, the nursing procedures, the quality and amount of protection for the child from accidental or self-injury, or from the hostile aggression of other patients, the presence of other patients with particular traits on the ward, the food, the schooling, or the recreational opportunities may all at one time or another become the actuality toward which the child or the parents express ambivalent admiration or anxious derogation.

In all such situations, the attitudes of the whole staff, but particularly those of the psychotherapists, are of paramount importance as factors that can contribute toward the resolution of the conflict of each member of the family. The critical word in this last statement is *can*. There is no assurance that another person's conflicting feelings, attitudes, and behavior will be more or less durably modified as a result of the regular contacts with a psychotherapist or with the psychotherapeutic attitudes of a professional team. But whether the therapist remains quietly and firmly convinced of the *possibility* of resolution of the conflict during various types of crises is generally the final question. The extremely hateful, sadistic, and disruptive forces within each member of the family that were previously repressed, distorted, and expressed predominantly in the overt disorder of the child provide a crucial test of the psychotherapist's skill as they emerge, sometimes explosively, sometimes subtly.

The variety of attitudes and behavior of child and parents through which such self-destructive and revengeful feelings are expressed is inexhaustible. They may appear on the part of the parents as endless, insistent demands for proof of statements about the possibility of therapeutic resolution or for detailed advice as to behavior with respect to the child; or on the part of the child as insatiable insistence that the parents have no love for him, or as efforts to arouse the therapist's or staff's guilt, pity, or compensatory affection. Threats of separation, actual separation, and even moves toward divorce on the part of the parents are not at all infrequent. Transient episodes occur in which any two of the familial triangle form what has been called a mutually absorbing "two-world" excluding the third member, with appropriately violent reaction from the excluded one. This reaction, whether overtly or covertly hostile, is promptly used by one or both of the other two as further evidence of the bitter injustice they have endured.

Perhaps the most difficult burden for younger and less experienced therapists to bear is a persistent attitude of condescending indifference on the part of the patient; this often effectively reduces the therapist's precarious self-esteem. Again, a particularly seductive patient play is an extremely helpless, adulatory attitude toward the therapist, with subtle derogation of other therapists, members of the staff, and members of the patient's own family. Bitter resentment against the staff, over hospital facilities, fees, or some actual unfortunate incident, may also be loosed against the therapist, partly as a means of reducing the parents' own guilt and self-derogation, and partly as an effort to stir up uneasiness, uncertainty, and resentment in the therapist, at the same time reducing the parents feelings of inferiority. Episodes of intensified acute neurotic illness of one or the other parent, some of them severe enough to raise the question of necessity for hospitalization for the parent, or for treatment from nonpsychiatric physicians for somatic symptoms, are also seen.

COLLABORATIVE WORK

If collaborative therapeutic work by different therapists for the child and each of the parents is the mode of approach, any one of the patients may express more or less directly or indirectly some invidious comparison of his own therapist to one of the other therapists, or even make direct moves to get in touch with one of them without prior discussion with his own therapist. The child on the ward may for a time adamantly refuse to go to his own therapist and show greater interest in another staff member, whether a nurse, attendant, teacher, or the psychiatrist of one of his parents. Either parent may manifest similar tendencies by tardiness for his appointments, by sudden illnesses, by accidents on the way, and finally by actually forgetting appointments. A parent may discuss some of his feelings or some of his plans or wishes with respect to his child, often highly relevant to the whole treatment program, with other staff members such as nurses, attendants, schoolteachers, or others, and for a long time fail altogether to mention any of this in his therapeutic sessions. Or he may make plans with respect to the removal of the child from the hospital without mentioning these facts to anyone on the hospital staff. Parents have been known to express a desire to place the child, or to plan to place the child, in another institution where fees are demanded that they insist they cannot afford to pay to the present hospital; or they may repeatedly insist on knowing what the opinion of the supervisor or director of the staff is with respect to their child's progress or to the eventual outcome of therapy.

These and many other forms of derogation, simultaneously of self and of therapist and staff, constitute a barrage against their confidence and equanimity. It may be finally understood as a mixture of the two aspects of the conflict. On the one hand, there is revengeful hostility, contempt, extreme impatience, guilt, anxiety, and pervasively deep despair and pessimism about the satisfaction of certain distortions of basic impulses. On the other hand, there is an insatiable yearning for guiltless gratification of regressive needs and wishes, both active and passive (ontogenetically the earliest types), for exclusive, possessive, sensual contact. These, as one eventually comes to see, are evident in both child and parents. When they are directed toward the psychotherapists and others of the staff, it is little wonder, that severe staff problems arise.

THERAPIST'S DEVELOPMENT

Clearly the individual psychotherapist's clarity, precision of therapeutic behavior, capacity to persist in the work, and relative equanimity in the face of such untoward developments in the family are the result of many factors in his own personal experience. Training that has effected at least some loosening of any of his own defensive solutions about what is known as the primary narcissistic sensuality, and which has permitted some reintegration of it, is probably a general necessity. Experience of some success in therapeutic work with other persons, which gives him some sense of the time such work may require, is another very important factor. Another probably essential determinant is experience in direct therapeutic effort with parents and their children. This may provide him with evidence for the biologically given needs and tendencies of the child and the vicissitudes these undergo in subtle everyday interactions with the personal solutions to these needs that each of the parents has achieved in his own life. The psychotherapist's own current life satisfactions, both in his nonprofessional personal relations and in his professional relations, especially with the staff, are ever-present elements that variously affect his tolerance for the exercise of whatever skill he has acquired. These dynamically effective influences, as well as others, alter from time to time his work with the particular patient as well as the nature and quality of his collaboration with fellow staff members, which in turn may sometimes crucially affect the total work with the entire family.

THE ORGANIZATION, THE MILIEU, THE INDIVIDUAL

The interpersonal milieu in which each staff psychotherapist works is composed of others who not only in some measure participate in his work with the child and his family, but are also constantly aware of the results of the work at a given stage, both from direct contact with all members of the family and from staff discussions. For this reason, his and their mutual attitudes comprise a field of influence and interaction that has considerable effect on the outcome of therapy. Most hospital staffs, of course, are composed not only of different professions with differing backgrounds, traditions, and work concepts, but also of persons of varying degrees of competence, experience, and training—persons who differ from one another also in age, sex, sense of personal worth, security, achievement of life's satisfactions, and in aims for the future. These factors, plus the important fact that the medically trained psychiatrist has final clinical responsibility for many decisions as to the conduct of the service, require that the staff operate as an organized system or unity.

Any organization implies an orderly integration of a group for the performance of a task or function larger or more complex than any one member could easily accomplish. Hence, individual or more or less definable aspects of the total work require subdivision or differentiation of some members into particular subunits with particular functional responsibilities. Prompt and complete communication, not only between persons of the various subunits but also between the various subunits is as essential for the effective operation of the organization—the performance of its total task—as it is between the parts, systems, or organs of an individual organism for integrated living and adaptation within its environment. But individual human beings, however differentiated from one another in capacity by particular endowment, sex, age, training, and experience, are not structurally differentiated into separate cogs that fit into a total machine, to operate reliably until worn out by use and then to be easily replaced. Differentiation of functions in an organization almost inevitably carries with it anxieties about status, value, and the possibility that those in power will work to achieve and perpetuate personal prestige by derogatory subordination of others. Such tendencies in the persons fulfilling the responsibilities of integrating the whole organization intensify any readiness to rebel and to oppose that may exist in others. Since open nonperformance of function for which one is responsible in any organization is generally contrary to one's own self-esteem and is associated with the danger of censure, of loss of position, or of other penalty, conflict within the self is inevitable. Conflict, however, affects the promptness, thoroughness, and precision of one's functioning and the completeness of one's communications to one's colleagues in the organization in a deleterious direction, both from the point of view of the organization's work and of one's own subjective satisfaction.

Furthermore, time is necessary if one is to learn all the facets of one's job in an organization and to become acquainted with and acquire ease with the particular traits of one's colleagues—in short, to become integrated into the organization. It is in connection with this factor of time that difficulties in the organization's work arise from the presence of temporary or transient members whose term of duty or service may vary from occasional relief work to replace a regular staff member to a relatively short period of a few months or even a year. Depending on his degree of psychotherapeutic skill, a varying but usually a considerable period of time is necessary for the establishment of the transference bonds to the psychotherapist by both child and parents. The transference is probably the only means by which the conflict may be worked through to whatever degree of resolution all the factors in the situation permit; and this working through, which is the essence of the work, is time-consuming and requires continuity.

HIERARCHICAL PROBLEMS

It is a truism that the size of an organization affects not only the time necessary for it to become integrated toward the fulfillment of its function but also the quality of its integration and its work. The addition of each new person to an organization carries with it problems arising not only from his competence and the compatibility of his personality traits with those of the other staff members, but also from the degree of integration achieved by the rest of the staff prior to his arrival. The larger the number of persons composing the staff, the greater the difficulty for each staff member in achieving acquaintance and maintaining sufficiently direct personal contact and communication with all other members. This may be particularly important if the size of the staff precludes or reduces direct and sufficiently frequent contact of all members with those persons who have been previously called the "integrating persons"—leaders with final supervisory responsibility. This source of interference with contact and communicability serves unwittingly to increase what might be called the "psychological distance" between any one member and what Redl has called the central person or persons. Inevitably, even if the supervisory persons are not characterized by authoritarian tendencies, this psychological distance tends to be an obstacle to the integration of more peripheral members. In a hospital, even if the number of persons comprising the staff of a service is not too large for the possibility of fairly thorough integration, there remains the problem of integrating those staff members whose hours of duty are in the evening and at night.

A further problem for intrastaff communication and integration is the presence of more than one person of supervisory rank, each of whom may supervise different groups of individual members. Unless differences of attitude and opinion between the supervisors are openly expressed, discussed, and settled, subordinates are exposed to conflicts incompatible with the overall functioning of the staff, and are often tempted to utilize them for the expression of their own still unresolved conflicts. If supervisory persons differ as to rank, degree of responsibility for the entire service, experience, competence, and personality traits, and if unresolved and relatively unresolvable ambivalences exist between them, the disintegrating effects of such differences upon the other members of the staff may be of critical importance with regard to clinical behavior with particular problems.

DISCUSSION

The formation of subgroups with varying composition occurs within the staff even without divisive conflict between supervisory authorities. Such subgroups not only enable the individual members to express and discharge tensions of conflict with one or more other members of the staff against other members, but may affect all their attitudes toward particular patients and their families or toward the activities and behavior of all the patients in directions that are less than therapeutic. The deleterious effect of such intrastaff divisions upon the progress and behavior of a particular patient or groups of them has already been to some extent documented [16-20]. In effect, when parental surrogates or roughly equal authorities are in conflict, the patient, whether a child or not, experiences an increase of tension of his own conflict corresponding to the temptation to divide the authorities still further for more exclusive possession of each of them—always, however, with the danger of losing both.

These and probably many other factors within the staff composition contribute elements of experience, either integrative or disintegrative in their effect, to the individual psychotherapist, and through him to his patients. Any crisis, or what H. S. Sullivan [21] has termed a *disjunctive* tendency, manifested by the patients during the course of therapeutic work tends to influence both therapist and staff. The effect of this influence will depend on the therapist's own integration and the degree of integration already achieved by the staff, as well as in the integrative potentialities. It may evoke in the therapist a new attentiveness to the transference distortions expressed in the patients' tension and behavior, and with this may come a more thorough collaborative communication with colleagues working with the family; or it may arouse and intensify some conflict within the therapist himself, and promote divisive tensions of conflict within the staff as well; or finally, it may (and commonly does) result in some combination of both tendencies. How the integrative potentiality within the staff may be called forth so that each member may contribute at his point of contact with the child and family toward the resolution of the crisis constitutes a subject for separate treatment. However, it may be mentioned that smaller conferences between all the psychotherapists involved, together with the relevant other members of the staff with the supervisor, and more frequent individual supervisory sessions initiated either by the psychotherapist or the supervisor are probably the methods of choice. In these, all relevant facts and the chronology of events may clarify the meaning underlying the crisis, or its genesis. Any disagreement or tension within the staff may be ventilated and reduced. Especially in the individual sessions of psychotherapist with supervisor, what is known as the countertransference tension of the psychotherapist may be released and resolved, freeing him for more realistic appraisal of his patients and for more therapeutic behavior. Facing the possibility of failure in his therapeutic aims and sharing the responsibility with the supervisor for the possible outcome, he frequently realizes how he may have unconsciously participated in escalating the critical tension. These efforts, of course, do not always result in success as far as the crisis in the therapeutic work with the particular family is concerned, but they may at least decrease the tension of conflict within the psychotherapist and the staff, as well as adding to their clinical experience.

In these diverse ways the hospital psychiatric therapy of the severe disorders of children may be a constant experimentation with new ways

278

of living, not only for the child patient with other children with similar problems but also for the significant adults around him. It is an experiment in which tensions of conflict may find less destructive outlets as their resolution is achieved through newly acquired discriminations for the satisfaction of basic needs and through increasing self-awareness, lessening self-derogation, and dissolution of repressive self-stultification.

REFERENCES

1. CAMERON, KENNETH. A psychiatric inpatient department for children. *J. Ment. Sci.,* **95**:560-566, 1949.
2. BRADLEY, Charles. Indications for residential treatment of children with severe neuropsychiatric problems. *Am. J. Orthopsychiat.,* **19**:427-431, 1949.
3. BENDER, LAURETTA. Childhood schizophrenia. *Am. J. Orthopsychiat.,* **17**:40-56, 1947.
4. KANNER, LEO. Problems of nosology and psychodynamics of early infantile autism. *Am. J. Orthopsychiat.,* **19**:416-426, 1949.
5. VAN VLEET, PHYLLIS. Rhythmic activity—a project in group therapy with children. *Am. J. Orthopsychiat.,* **19**:79-86, 1949.
6. SUTTON, HELEN A. Some nursing aspects of a children's psychiatric ward. *Am. J. Orthopsychiat.,* **17**:675-683, 1947.
7. HART, RUTH GILBERTSON. Relationship therapy in a children's psychiatric ward. *Am. J. Psychiatry,* **104**:132-134, 1947.
8. ROBINSON, J. FRANKLIN. The use of residence in psychiatric treatment with children. *Am. J. Psychiatry,* **103**:814-817, 1947.
9. _____ . MAXWELL, ANABEL, and DOMINGUEZ, KATHRYN. Resident psychiatric treatment with children. *Am. J. Orthopsychiatry.,* **17**:458-467, 1947.
10. SZUREK, S. A. Dynamics of staff interaction in hospital psychiatric treatment of children. *Am. J. Orthopsychiat.,* **17**:652-664, 1947.
11. BETTELHEIM, B., and SYLVESTER, E. Therapeutic influence of the group on the individual. *Am. J. Orthopsychiat.,* **17**:684-692, 1947.
12. REDL, FRITZ. Group psychological elements in discipline problems. *Am. J. Orthophsychiat.,* **13**:77-81, 1943.
13. _____ . Group emotions and leadership. *Psychiatry,* **5**:573-596, 1942.
14. KANNER, LEO. Feeblemindedness: absolute, relative and apparent. *Nervous Child,* **7**:365-397, 1948, esp. p. 391.
15. MORGENAU, HENRY. Ethical science. *Scientific Monthly,* **69**:290-296, 1949, esp. p. 292.

279

16. STANTON, ALFRED H., and SCHWARTZ, MORRIS S. The management of a type of institutional participation in mental illness. *Psychiatry,* **12**:13-26, 1949.

17. _____ . Medical opinion and the social context in a mental health hospital. *Psychiatry,* **12**:243-249, 1949.

18. _____ . Observations on dissociation as social participation. *Psychiatry,* **12**:339-354, 1949.

19. SHEIMO, S. L., PAYNTER, J., and SZUREK, S. A. Dynamics of staff interaction with spontaneous group formations on a children's psychiatric ward. *Am. J. Orthopsychiatry,* **19**:599-611, 1949.

20. BOATMAN, MALETA J., et al. Can some efforts at collaborative therapy make a psychotic of a neurotic? Paper read at the 1949 Annual Meeting of the American Orthopsychiatric Association.

21. SULLIVAN, HARRY STACK. The theory of anxiety and the nature of psychotherapy. *Psychiatry,* **12**:3-12, 1949, esp. p. 11.

CHAPTER 19

NURSES WITH PARENTS AS AN
ASPECT OF THERAPY

Maleta J. Boatman, M.D.

EDITORS' NOTE, 1970

This previously unpublished paper was written for and read at the Annual Meeting of the American Psychiatric Association in 1958. In the light of recent developments in psychiatry it is somewhat difficult to recall that just twelve years ago, the amount of family involvement and the degree of overlapping of therapeutic roles between disciplines that is described here seemed unusual. Others have written on this subject since then, including one child psychiatrist who was a career trainee with us in 1960-1962 [12, 13].

After our staff reached the points of view represented in this paper, our concept of the ward nurses' therapeutic contributions to the total effort with the family changed very little, although there were continuing developments in its application. Facilitating factors in subsequent extensions included: the temporary increase in nursing staff because of our three-year National Institute of Mental Health-funded Project No. 5-R11-MH-234-3, "Nursing in Hospital Psychiatric Therapy for Psychotic Children"; the decrease in the official census of the ward from fifteen to twelve children in 1964; and particularly, the approval by the Institute's administration of having some of the twelve children as day-patients. All these innovations increased the time and energy available to the nursing staff for trying new things. Parents coming and going more regularly with day-patient children increased the opportunities for and the necessity for nurses talking with them.

In a number of instances weekly scheduled meetings of a parent or parents with their child's assigned nurse have been added to their regular interviews with their psychotherapist. These have focused on exchange of information about the child's care, behavior, and experiences. These meetings have sometimes provided a useful means of helping a parent become more aware of some of his own helpful or confusing responses to his child. With careful collaboration between nurse, psychotherapist, and a senior child psychiatrist, these meetings have occasionally been used to explore with parents the consequences of attitudes they continue to handle with denial in their therapy. This has included such approaches as a nurse's firmly stated expectation that if their child were to benefit from the program, age-appropriate or activity-appropriate clothing must be furnished by a family that had insisted their six- or seven-year-old boy was not ready for trousers that zipped or for sneakers instead of hard-soled shoes to climb in.

The problems and the advantages brought by this approach to the work of nurses with parents as well as children remain essentially the same as when this paper was written.

Experience on one psychiatric ward for children under twelve has led its staff to the conclusion that interaction between nursing personnel and parents can, if carefully reviewed and collated with other aspects of the total program, prove to be a valuable adjunct to psychotherapeutic work with families.

The particular clinical observations and conclusions on which this paper is based have been drawn from the author's 10 years' experience on this 15-bed ward, during which time approximately 135 children have been hospitalized for study or therapy for periods of a few weeks to 5 or more years. The material presented has been gained from individual psychotherapy with children and parents and from individual conferences of the ward staff.

Like any other aspect of the work of a given center, the nature of the integration of the nursing staff can be understood only in the context of the realities and philosophies particular to it [1, 2, 3]. The following facts about this center's setting and treatment attitudes are those that have most directly influenced the role of its nursing staff as discussed in this paper.

THE CLINICAL SETTING[1]

The ward for fifteen seriously disturbed girls and boys under twelve is physically small, with only limited areas where parents and children

---

[1] For further description of the ward and staff see Chapter 4.

may visit in semi-privacy and comfort. The twenty-four hour child-care staff includes six to nine psychiatric nurses and five psychiatric technicians. There is one school teacher and a part-time occupational therapist. The psychologist, social worker, and eight or more psychiatrists participate in outpatient as well as inpatient work. Although the Children's Service psychiatrists may be called at any time, medical coverage within the hospital during evening, night, and weekend hours is provided by a resident O.D. (On Duty) who is usually not familiar with this ward. Thus, it is the nursing personnel who provide staff continuity to children and parents around the clock. Perhaps this is sufficient detail to indicate that elimination of exchanges between nurses and parents would be difficult in this setting even if it were desired.

THEORETICAL BASIS

The philosophy of the staff has influenced the matter more profoundly than have the foregoing realities. For the past twelve years the primary research interest has been the clinical exploration of the possible psychogenic etiology of even the psychotic disorders of childhood [4]. Closely integrated with this has been the study of the therapeutic process [5] and methods of training [6]. The approach to these explorations has been primarily through concomitant psychotherapy with the child and, usually, with both parents. The preeminent psychotherapeutic goal has been the reduction of the internal conflicts of each family member [7]. Integration of the staff toward the common goal has been sought through supervision, collaboration, and frequent staff conferences for mutual review, examination, and collation of *all* experiences on the ward and with each child and family [8; see also Chapter 9]. As much encouragement and help as possible has been provided each staff member in his development of professional skill and personal maturity.

Among the therapeutic attitudes developed in this context [9; see also Chapter 18], several are most pertinent to this discussion. Hospitalization of the child is considered an incident in the total therapeutic work with the family. Parents' participation in decisions regarding the child and contact with him is assumed in the staff's methodology of psychotherapeutic work with the family. Since the staff's clinical method is presented to the parents in the initial stages of mutual planning, the subsequent participation of each available parent in all aspects of continuing work is assumed from his willingness to begin, however ambivalent it may be. Every contact of the parent and the child with any staff member in any situation in the hospital is viewed as potentially consistent with the psychotherapeutic goal.

In the clinical work derived from these attitudes, the therapists have no wish to proscribe the parents' contacts with a hospitalized child or with other staff members. Rather, any aspects of such contacts, including frequency or infrequency, that appear to be expressions of conflict are explored in the psychotherapeutic interviews.

NURSE-PARENT CONTACTS

Many parents choose to visit their child frequently on the ward and to take him home most weekends. With the agreement of the therapists, the nurses and parents usually make any necessary arrangements about these brief visits and about such matters as the child's clothing, laundry, and spending-money needs. Although there is no question but that the nurses' primary job is to look after the needs of the children, they are encouraged to consider how their discussions about these matters may be helpful to the parents as well.

The intensity of parental conflict and its anxious expression in the course of therapeutic work may shake the confidence of even relatively experienced psychotherapists [9, 10]. The staff recognizes, therefore, the additional difficulties potentially inherent in attempting to maintain psychotherapeutically consistent interaction of staff with parents in the day-to-day ward situation. In an effort to minimize these problems, the senior staff in the past sometimes encouraged the nurses to maintain minimal or limited contact with parents. At times of tension, a nurse was supported in any wish to refer parents' questions or complaints to the senior nurse. Clearly cognizant that her role was not that of psychotherapist, and hoping to encourage the discussion of obviously conflictful material in therapy, the senior nurse in turn often promptly referred the parent to the therapist. This practice seldom produced the hoped-for result of avoiding circular, anxious interaction: it seemed rather to increase the frequency and intensity of such interaction, often contributing to difficulties for child and nurse as well as parent.

Problems in Nurse-Parent Contacts

Already self-critical and fearful that the staff's willingness to hospitalize his child implied derogation of him, the parent often perceived the nurses' brevity as critical exclusion of him from his child's life. As a result, there was often intensification or prolongation of such anxious expression of conflict as avoidance of the nursing staff and hence also the child, persistent questioning, unrealistic demands, unfounded accusations of nursing negligence in care of the child, hostile flattery or emulation of the nurses, or increased helplessness with the child in the nurses' presence. The nurse herself, feeling inadequate in the situation, fearing that more extensive efforts on her part might fail or be criticized by the senior staff, and resenting any major deflection of her time from the children, did sometimes begin to feel angry at a parent, identify with a child against a parent, avoid or be abrupt with a parent, or "blame" a parent's visit for any particularly troublesome behavior of a child.

The occurrence of such feelings in the parents and nurses was, of course, not simply the result of the limitation of interchange between them [11]. Such anxieties are part of the transference and counter-transference phenomena that are probably an inevitable part of the work. Likewise, their eruption into behavior and their circular perpetuation rather than resolution is probably always influenced by multiple factors.

Nurses' Use of Problem Situations with Parents

The frequency, however, with which limitation of a nurse's response to a parent seemed to contribute to conflict, and the reduction of conflict when more spontaneous interchange was established led to the conclusion that the nursing staff should be encouraged and helped in more consistent interaction with parents about every matter pertinent to the ward situation. As in the following example, an effort was made to help them understand the parent's behavior and to discriminate what part of it could be met in the context of each current instance.

Eight-year-old Adrienne was mute, negativistic, obese, and disorderly. Her pretty but plump and often disheveled mother visited seldom and briefly, criticized the frequency of weekend home visits as arranged by father, and provided an inadequate amount of unattractive, ill-fitting, handed-down clothes. To the nurses' dismay, she consistently deflected the discussions about clothing and laundry to complaints of her own need for clothes and help. The evidence of need for a therapeutic resolution before such discussions could be more effective, as well as less difficult for the nurses, led to the decision that her therapist would accept full responsibility for trying to clarify the situation. The nurses, presumably still ready to talk with mother, stopped initiating any interchange with her. Finally, bringing some new clothes of the wrong size, she complained to the nurse of the trouble it would be to exchange them. The suggestion that she should have taken Adrienne along for fitting brought an angry tirade about the burden and embarrassment the girl was to her. Her subsequent accusations that Adrienne looked sloppy because the nurses let her get too dirty increased the already mounting frustration and anger of the staff. Many of the nurses began to avoid mother when possible, whereupon she began phoning the ward more frequently, complaining for long periods about Adrienne, the hospital, and her life in general. Requests that she talk to her therapist about these things only brought increasing helplessness to her complaints. She once called on a weekend, demanding that the nurse tell her how to stop Adrienne from flooding the bathroom at home. Adrienne herself began to gain weight and look even less attractive.

In frequent staff conferences, the therapists and nurses shared and discussed their frustrating experiences with this family. The senior nurses and psychiatrists acknowledged how difficult it was to maintain a therapeutic attitude toward this mother's behavior, but encouraged exploration of the longings, distortions, and fears that could have caused it and of the sequences of interaction that might be prolonging it. This mutual scrutiny and discussion of all the staff's knowledge of this child and family led the nurses as well as the rest of the staff to a better understanding of the dynamic significance of the mother's difficult behavior, and to the awareness that the nurses' avoidance of her had really been indirect and anxious interaction rather than decreased interaction with her.

The problems diminished, even though they did not disappear, when the nurses decided to try responding directly but considerately to all her demands. Lengthy phone calls were usually terminated when the nurse stated firmly that she was needed on the ward. Shoes that fit were brought when a nurse discussed the availability, relative costs, advantages and disadvantages of various types of shoes, and provided mother with tracings of Adrienne's feet to take with her to the store. Her complaints became more often focused in therapy hours after criticisms of her psychiatrist were met with the nurses' sincere conviction that talking these feelings over with him directly would really be of help to her. The nurses experienced satisfaction in their increasing ability to understand her behavior and to respond appropriately within the context of the ward situation. No longer so angry at mother, Adrienne's nurse also found that she really could do more to help the girl eat less ravenously, take some part in the care of her own clothes, and look nicer in whatever she had to wear.

INTEGRATION OF NURSE-PARENT CONTACT WITH TOTAL STAFF EFFORT

In the foregoing instance it was clear that the various frequent staff conferences played a part in the eventual establishment of less anxious and more effective interaction. Repeated experiences such as this have convinced the staff that failure to achieve this careful integration of nurse-parent contacts with all other aspects of the therapeutic program is often a factor contributing to interaction, which leads to increased difficulties. These experiences have also convinced the staff that mutual scrutiny, discussion, and collation by nurses, psychotherapists, and senior staff of all their experiences with a family can reduce the difficulties potentially inherent in nurse-parent interaction. Such staff discussions, between individuals and in groups, seem essential to achieving exchanges between nurse and parent that are, for the most part, consistent with the psychotherapeutic goal.

The staff has further been impressed with the multiple actual contributions made to the total work when the nursing staff achieves interaction with a parent that is based on understanding of the needs of parent as well as child, and which, although unhesitating, remains within the context of the current situation on the ward. In other words, such interaction is not merely consistent with the psychotherapeutic work with families—it is a positive addition to it, in that it provides valuable information to the therapists of child and parents, aids in the understanding of each child's individual needs, and affords an increased number of therapeutically oriented experiences for each family.

The following excerpts may indicate more fully some of the kinds of dynamically important information that may thus be provided to the therapists:

Robin, a mute, five-year-old Negro boy, was reluctant to use his hands except in saliva play. His alert watchfulness of the staff belied his apparent indifference to them. His well-educated, attractive mother and unassuming craftsman father both seemed genuinely warm toward him and uncritical of the ward program, to a degree that was unusual. Both, however, found therapeutic engagement with their psychiatrists exceptionally difficult. Their somewhat less guarded relationship with the nurses afforded the first precise confirmation to the clinical impression that their smiling cooperativeness actually covered considerable fear of discrimination and of retaliation for any negative impulses. Just as they had previously unprotestingly followed, and later blamed, a pediatrician's suggestion for many months of massive restraint of Robin's hands in thumb-sucking, they tended to emulate the nurses' care of the boy and report its failure to them as though they were responsible for it. For example, mother accusingly reported to the nurses that Robin had cut himself quite badly on the shampoo bottle she broke while trying to wash his hair the way she had seen it done on the ward. On one occasion she refused to believe the nurses when, informing her about a small scratch on his face, they said he made it himself when in a tantrum. She implied, rather, that the nurses deliberately allowed or encouraged the other children to abuse him. She always surveyed the ward displays of school and activity projects carefully. Although the nurses kept her informed of their relative lack of success in encouraging him to hold still for silhouettes or to draw pictures in school, she always said chidingly that they hadn't put *his* pictures up.

Shared with the therapists, such nurse-parent contacts as these aid in dynamic understanding, both through the nature of the interactions themselves and through the opportunities they provide for nurses to make meaningful observations.

The nurses' discussions with parents and observations of a child and a parent together may also contribute to a better understanding of how to help a particular youngster. This was illustrated by seven-year-old June who, on admission, talked incessantly about her dog and often acted out a phantasy where she was alternately the petted or scolded animal and the petting or scolding person. She talked with the nurses in varied pretended voices. She often greeted her mother with demands to go home to see the dog, and mother would agree. Although much therapeutic work was needed before this was understood more fully, the nurses were less hesitant about interrupting some of the girl's fantasies after they heard from mother that the family had had no dog since a short, pleasant period in their lives three years previously. With this knowledge, and sensing the girl's reaction to her mother's preoccupations and weary participation in her pretense, they were able fairly quickly to establish a more direct relationship with June by acknowledging her longing and disappointment in specific situations while being careful not to evade the facts of the matter.

In addition to the kind of understanding gained in the foregoing example, the nurses' discussions with the parents also give them useful information about such things as events on visits home, a child's special likes and dislikes, or the significance of some treasure a child brings to the ward. These discussions often contribute to reduction of parental anxiety about leaving the child on the ward and afford the parents and nurses opportunity for mutual planning of such events as birthday parties.

THERAPEUTIC CONTRIBUTION OF NURSE

The nurses' attentive interest and lack of anxiety around each of these matters can increase the number of therapeutically oriented experiences each family has with the staff. The following clinical examples indicate the even more precise nature of the contributions that nurse-parent interaction can make to the psychotherapeutic goal of conflict reduction:

The parents of nine-year-old Tim were constantly distressed and often angry with each other when the boy was home. It was clear to the staff from the parents' reports and from ward observations that each was unaware that *both* of them felt simultaneously helpless and jealous in Tim's presence. His constant clinging, seductive behavior with one or the other of them, accompanied by angry slapping of himself upon the other's approach, left the chosen parent feeling flattered but abandoned to a burdened isolation, and left the excluded parent feeling rejected and unwanted by anyone. The mother, who had attempted exploration of this problem many times in therapy, reported some greater emotional understanding of it after a nurse's resolution of a similar incident on the ward. When Tim had tried to cling and reject mother's visit, the nurse's easy statement, "Look what Tim is doing to us, playing us off against each other," had been followed by his smiling relaxation and fairly prompt turning to visit with his mother.

Perhaps even more difficult but equally helpful are the instances in which a nurse finds a way to help the parent himself interrupt a distressing sequence of interaction with a child:

Eight-year-old Jack had for many months needed frequent restraint from parents or staff to prevent self-destructive behavior of nearly suicidal intensity. During one visit father became so obviously discouraged and angry that he stood immobilized even when the boy resumed banging his head on the wall in the old vicious way. The nurse joined them and asked father if he would find it easier to help Jack control himself if they moved to a more comfortable and private place in the ward. Throughout the remainder of father's visit, he responded more quickly and directly to everything Jack said and did.

SUMMARY

The clinical observations and conclusions presented in this paper are not meant to indicate that this staff now achieves consistent success in the resolution of the difficulties inherent in interaction between nurses and parents on a children's psychiatric ward. It is hoped, however, that the material has illustrated some of the factors in their experience that have led them to the conclusion that such interaction can provide a valuable aspect of the psychotherapeutic work with families if it is carefully reviewed with other staff experiences and integrated into the total program.

These experiences have at least encouraged the staff to continue their exploration of the therapeutic potentials in nurse-parent interaction. They are hopeful of being able in the future to study this subject more intensively as part of an overall inquiry into psychiatric nursing skills and training.

REFERENCES

1. ROBINSON, J. FRANKLIN, ET AL, EDS. *Psychiatric inpatient treatment of children.* Washington: American Psychiatric Association, 1957.
2. REID, JOSEPH H., and HAGAN, HELEN R. A descriptive study of the program of the Langley Porter Clinic Children's Inpatient Service. In *Residential treatment of emotionally disturbed children.* New York: The Child Welfare League of America, Inc., 1952, pp. 200-201.
3. BOATMAN, MALETA J., BYRON, HELEN, GALLAGHER, URSULA, and DEVRIES, ROBERT. *Residential treatment for emotionally disturbed children.* San Francisco: Community Chest of San Francisco, 1954, Section II.
4. SZUREK, S. A. Childhood schizophrenia: psychotic episodes and psychotic maldevelopment. *Am. J. Orthopsychiat.,* **26**:519-543, 1956.
5. SZUREK, S. A. and BERLIN, I. N. Elements of psychotherapeutics with the schizophrenic child and his parents. *Psychiatry,* **19**:1-9, 1956. Reprinted in S. A. Szurek & I. N. Berlin (Eds.), *Training in therapeutic work with children.* Vol. 2, the Langley Porter Child Psychiatry Series. Palo Alto, Calif.: Science and Behavior Books, 1967.
6. SZUREK, S. A. Remarks on training for psychotherapy. *Am. J. Orthopsychiat.,* **19**:36-51, 1949. Reprinted in S. A. Szurek & I. N. Berlin (Eds.), *Training in therapeutic work with children.* Vol. 2, the Langley Porter Child Psychiatry Series. Palo Alto, Calif.: Science and Behavior Books, 1967.
7. _____ . Some lessons from efforts at psychotherapy with parents. *Am. J. Psychiat.,* **109**:296-302, 1952. Reprinted in S. A. Szurek & I. N. Berlin (Eds.), *Training in therapeutic work with children.* Vol. 2, the Langley Porter Child Psychiatry Series. Palo Alto, Calif.: Science and Behavior Books, 1967.
8. _____ . Some observations on the dynamics of staff interaction in hospital psychiatric treatment of children. *Am. J. Orthopsychiat.,* **17**:652-664, 1947.
9. _____ . The family and the staff in hospital psychiatric therapy of children. *Am. J. Orthopsychiat.,* **21**:597-611, 1951.
10. BERLIN, I. N., BOATMAN, M. J., SHEIMO, S. L., and SZUREK, S. A. Adolescent alternation of anorexia and obesity. *Am. J. Orthopsychiat.,* **21**:387-419, April 1951. Also appeared in George Gardner (Ed.), *Case studies in childhood emotional disabilities,* Vol. 1. New York: American Orthopsychiatric Association, Inc., 1953.
11. HARTRICK, PAULETTE. *Nursing Outlook,* **4**:146, March 1956.
12. CHRIST, A. E., CRITCHLEY, D. L., LARSON, M. L., and BROWN, M. The role of the child psychiatric nurse. *Nursing Outlook,* **13**:30-2, 1963.

290

13. CHRIST, A. E. and GRIFFITHS, R. Parent-nurse therapeutic contact on a child psychiatry unit. *Am. J. Ortho.*, **35**:589-93, April 1965.

INDEX[*]

---

[*]Bold page number indicates bibliographic reference.

292